HUMAN PATHOLOGY

- BACTERIOLOGY
- PARASITOLOGY
- GENERAL PATHOLOGY
- SPOT LIGHT

With Sample Papers

HUMAN PATHOLOGY

INCLUDING MICROBIOLOGY & PARASITOLOGY IN QUESTION-ANSWER FORMAT FOR HOMOEOPATHY STUDENTS

Dr. BALARAM JANA

B. Jain Publishers (P) Ltd.
USA—EUROPE—INDIA

HUMAN PATHOLOGY

First Edition: 1985
8th Impression: 2012

Note From the Publishers

Any information given in this book is not intended to be taken as a replacement for medical advice. Any person with a condition requiring medical attention should consult a qualified practitioner or therapist.

Published by Kuldeep Jain for

B. JAIN PUBLISHERS (P) LTD.

1921/10, Chuna Mandi, Paharganj, New Delhi 110 055 (INDIA)
Tel.: +91-11-4567 1000   Fax: +91-11-4567 1010
Email: info@bjain.com   Website: **www.bjain.com**

Printed in India by

J.J. Offset Printers

ISBN: 978-81-319-0756-6

In the memory of my father

LATE BEHARI LAL JANA

To

Dr. Pareshchandra Paul

PREFACE

Since the discoveries of Louis Pasteur and Robert Koch the medical world has come to believe in the simple dogma **"kill the germs and cure the disease"**. But subsequent experience has revealed that there is an elusive factor call **susceptibility** of the patient which is behind infection and actual out break of disease. As homoeopathy is mainly concerned with reactions of the human organism to different morbid factors, microbial or otherwise. The role of bacteria or viruses in the production of disease is therefore in homoeopathy quite secondary.

But the knowledge of bacteriology is never the less important to become a complete homoeopathic physician as it is more important for the diagnosis, prognosis, prevention of disease and general management of a case. Similarly pathology gives us the knowledge for **disease determination, prognosis, for discrimination between symptoms of the patient and symptoms of the disease and for adjusting the dose and potency of indicated homoeopathic remedy.**

However only broad basic training in pathology, free from specialist bias, should be imparted to students. Teachers of pathology should never loose sight of the fact that they are training medical practitioners, especially homoeopathic practitioners, and not technicians and specialists in pathology. **The living patient, and not the corpse, should be the central theme in the teaching of the subject.**

Considering the above, I have humbly embarked myself on this arduous endeavour particularly to meet the requirements of the student to corelate the subjective symptoms with the objective ones, and to interpret clinical symptoms and their inter relationship on the basis of underlying pathology and also the practitioner for self guidance who have no laboratory near them in which pathological diagnosis is under taken.

As this book is written on a model of answers to questions of the important Universities, Boards and Councils the reader can be guided well about the important and practical aspects of this subject matter. As far as possible most of the subject matters have been covered and written in a concise and simplified form according to latest syllabus for degree, graded degree and diploma courses as prescribed by the Central Council of Homoeopathy, New Delhi (1983). To make it a **standard help as well as text book** in place of any standard text book the matter of this book has been derived from reference of different standard text books, research journals and papers on this subject, and are compiled in a compact and simplified form. The most important figures and latest concept of this subject have been incorporated whenever needed.

I am grateful to **Sri Birendra Nath Roy, Sri Sontosh Kr. Kar, Sri Tapas Kr. Roy, Sri Tarapada Mondal and Sri Bimal Kanti Malakar of Roy Book Stall** without whose efforts and active co-operation this treatise could not have been brought to light in time. It will be an act of great injustice on my part if I fail to mention the name of **Dr. Narendra Keshori Banerjee** and **Dr. B.N. Nandi,** of Bengal Homoeopathic Medical College and Hospital for extending his co-operative hand to complete the manuscripts.

Finally, I would like to state that it would be too much to hope the first edition should be entirely free of errors or omission and commission, and in conclusion, I shall consider my efforts fully recompensed if the book serves the purpose for which it is written and published.

BALARAM JANA

46/2, Narasingha Dutta Road,
Howrah-711101, W.B., INDIA.

CONTENTS

CHAPTER—1

STUDY OF PATHOLOGY

PART—I
BACTERIOLOGY

CHAPTER—2
GENERAL BACTERIOLOGY

[*Page 19 to 44*]

CHAPTER—3
IMPORTANT COCCI

[*Page 45 to 62*]

CHAPTER—4

IMPORTANT BACILLI

[*Page 63 to 110*]

CHAPTER—5

VIRUS

[*Page 111 to 120*]

PART—II
PARASITOLOGY

CHAPTER—1
PARASITES

CHAPTER—2

HELMINTHOLOGY

HELMINTHES

[Pages 157 to 212]

PART—III
GENERAL AND SPECIAL PATHOLOGY

1. INFLAMMATION

[Pages 213 to 336]

2. NECROSIS

3. GANGRENE

4. OEDEMA

5. THROMBOSIS

6. EMBOLISM

7. INFARCTION

8. DEGENERATION

9. TUMOUR

10. JAUNDICE

11. ANAEMA

12. IMMUNITY

** 13. AIDS

14. PEPTIC ULCER

15. CARCINOMA OF STOMACH

16. CARCINOMA OF LIVER

17. LOBAR PNEUMONIA

18. BRONCHOPNEUMONIA

19. PULMONARY TUBERCULOSIS

20. ADULT TYPE OF TUBERCULOSIS

21. BRONCHOGENIC CARCINOMA

22. GLOMERULUNEPHRITIS

23. NEPHROSIS

PART—IV

SPOT LIGHT

I. PRACTICAL EXAMINATION

N.B. – Any one should be done in Practical Examination.

II. FOR ORAL EXAMINATION

INSTRUMENTATION

CONTENTS
FOR QUICK REFERENCES

PART—II

PARASITOLOGY

CHAPTER—1

PROTOZOLOGY [*Page 121 to 156*]

CHAPTER—2

HELMINTHOLOGY [*Page 157 to 212*]

PART — III

GENERAL AND SPECIAL PATHOLOGY

[*Page 213 to 336*]

PART—IV

SPOT LIGHT [*Page 337 to 397*]

** FOR DETAILS FOLLOW CONTENTS.

PATHOLOGY

DISCUSSION FOR LEARNING

I *Pathology*–Definition.

II Mode of Teaching.

III Disease or pathology in Allopathy and Homoeopathy.

IV What are the benefits, we can get from the knowledge of Pathology.

V "Where the Homoeopathic Pathology ends, the Allopathic Pathology begins''–Explain.

VI Why we should study the Pathology ?

Q. 1.1. What is Pathology ?

Pathology is defined as that branch of biological science which deals with the subject–study of disease in a systemic way and considers disease from all aspects; e.g., the cause of the disease, the course of the diseases, its diagnostic signs and symptoms, biochemical and structural changes and the complications that may occur, with the disease.

It is also defined *as a branch of medicine concerned with the study of cause, nature and evolution of the diseases and the changes in Anatomy, Physiology, and Chemistry resulting from there in.*

In short it is a '*Science of disease*'.

Q. 1.2. What are its Province ?

Pathology is the study of disease and one of the basic medical Science. Its essential foundations are derived from the study of the normal that is *Anatomy* and *Physiology*. Its province is extremely broad, for it deals simultaneously with the structural changes found in the organs of the diseased persons both before and after death, with the functional disorders that these may bring about and the adaptations often made by other organs to compensate for such defects, and lastly with the causes which are responsible for these changes and disorders. *Pathology* is thus primarily concerned with disease states and processes, and their pathogenesis.

It also leads the clinician to the footsteps of the diseases and leaves to *Clinical Medicine* and *Surgery* the task of discovering how these may be detected and treated at the bed side.

Q. 1.3. What are the various branches of Pathology ?

DIVISIONS OF PATHOLOGY

General	**Clinical**	**Special**	**Experimental**
[Includes the principle, theories, explanation of disease]	[Includes signs and symptoms, stages, course and diagnosis of a disease of a patient]	[Study of a disease of specific type like T.B., Cancer, Syphilis etc. to find out its course and exact nature and to decide whether the diseases require Medical or Surgical treatment]	[Study the disease under artificial condition i.e., in the laboratory. This is related with new discovery.]

It is also sub-divided into: —

1. Pathological Anatomy i.e. the study of the structural changes in disease, including *Histo-pathology* i.e. Gross pathology.

2. Aetiology—the study of the causes of disease.

3. Pathological Physiology—the study of the alterations of functions and metabolism in disease, including Pathological Chemistry or Chemical Pathology (Bio-chemistry).

4. Laboratory Pathology—includes the study of the disease by examining the blood, urine, stool etc. in a laboratory for the purpose of diagnosis of the disease of a patient.

5. Post-mortem Pathology—the study of the disease of the patient after his death.

Q. 1.4. What are the main objects of studying Pathology ?

Before the era of pathology, medical treatment was based upon speculation and was not on scientific basis. But since the development of pathology, the achievement in the medical, surgical and other forms of treatment have been improved by leaps and bound, so much so that many diseases have been completely eradicated. Although the main objects of studying pathology is to help the medical man to :—

1. *Prevent and cure the diseases,* and
2. *To manage the treatment of the patient in a suitable way with proper diet and nursing.*
3. *To give the correct diagnosis and prognosis of the disease,* whether it is curable, incurable, medical or surgical.
4. *Above all it gives all the information* for the treatment of a patient.

Q. 1.5. What is Pathology (in Homoeopathic view) ?

Pathology is the scientific study of the abnormal and of the abnormalities in structure of tissues, which may or may not be attended by disease when a departure from normal takes place disease results. The disease first manifests itself by subjective symptoms. To start with these is almost always a disturbance of function. If the function remains disturbed for a long time, some changes in the tissues or organs are bound to take place and objective signs and symptoms appear. Thus pathology tries to find out and makes a scientific study of the abnormalities in structure, which underline and are the cause of symptoms and disturbances of function. Such changes may gross and visible to the naked eye or may be detectable only by the microscope. Sometimes, it is not possible to find any visible alternation. As a working principle the presence of structural changes are taken as a cause of disturbed function.

It is here that Homoeopathy differs. The structural changes are called *lesions.* There are cases in which the lesions is two minute to be discoverable yet. Even the alterations visible under the highest power of the microscope are relatively gross. The lesions may be capable of resolution and a cure may take place and the parts may return a normal. But some lesions are permanent and the pathology is not reversible. All disturbances of function in disease produce alteration in the life of cells which is evidenced partly by damage and partly by increased activity. Each particular change found represents a stage in a series of changes. Pathology strives to discover the cause which has started the particular pathological process and has led to the departure from the normal. In Homoeopathy we not only presume but believe that it is the *Life Principle* or *Vital Principle* governing the cell which is primarily affected and deviates from the normal. When the cells of the body are thus placed under abnormal conditions a series of changes take place. Whether such processes are new or peculiar to disease or are merely physiological processes in abnormal conditions, are covered under pathology.

Q. 1.6. What would be the mode of teaching Pathology and Bacteriology in Homoeopathy ?

1. The Study of *Pathology* and *Bacteriology* should be done very cautiously and judiciously, as the *Allopathy* associated with the pathology of tissues and micro-organism with disease conditions and considered bacteria as conditioned cause of disease, *Homoeopathy* regards diseases as purely a dynamic disturbance of the vital force expressed as altered sensation and functions which may or may not be ultimate in gross tissue changes. The tissue changes are not therefore, an essential part of the disease as seen in Allopathy and are not accordingly in Homoeopathy the object of treatment by medication.

2. Since the discoveries of *Louis Pasteur* and *Robert Koch* the medical world has come to believe in the simple dogma "*Kill the germs and cure the disease*". But subsequently experience has revealed that there is an elusive factor called '*susceptibility*' of the patient which is behind infection and actual out break of disease. As homoeopathy is mainly concerned with reactions of the human organism to different morbid factors, microbial or otherwise, the role of bacteria or viruses in the production of disease is therefore, in homoeopathy quite secondary.

3. Knowledge of *bacteriology* is nevertheless necessary for a complete homoeopathic physician; but it is for purposes other than therapeutics such as for diagnosis, prognosis, prevention of disease and general management. Similarly knowledge of *pathology* is necessary for disease determination, prognosis, for discrimination between symptoms of the patient and symptoms of the disease and for adjusting the dose and potency of indicated homoeopathic remedy.

4. Only broad basic training in pathology, free from specialist bias, should however, be imported to students. Teachers of pathology should never loose sight of the fact that they are giving training to medical practitioners, especially homoeopathic practitioners, and not technicians and specialists in pathology. The living patient, and not the cropse, should be the central theme for the teaching of the subject.

5. The purpose of the instruction in pathology is to enable the student to correlate subjective symptoms with the objective ones, to interpret clinical symptoms and their relationship of the basis of undering pathology.

Q. 1.7. What are the basic differences between Pathology (or diseases) in Allopathy and Homoeopathy ?

In Homoeopathy	In Allopathy
1. According to homoeopathy the mission of the physician is to cure the sick individual.	1. The object of allopathy is to discover the specific nature of diseases and to manage, treat and prevent the problems arising from diseases involving on individual or a community.
2. In homoeopatny, every sick individual is different with regard to his constitution, cause of his sickness and peculiar character of his disease.	2. In allopathy, all patients suffering from the same disease are treated alike with special regard to the complications.
3. In homoeopathy, sickness of the individual depends upon the vital nature of the patient, sickness is represented by altered sensations and functions produced by inimical influences of the morbific agents on the vital force.	3. Allopathy is guided by cellular pathology. Altered functions and organic changes produced in disease due to internal and external factors from typical and atypical morbid conditions called diseases of specific nature.

4. In homoeopathy, constitution of the individual is prior to causation of his illness. Idiosyncrasy, conceptuality, reactivity, latency, suppression and expression of peculiar symptoms constitute dynamic nature of the sick individual.

5. According to homoeopathy, spiritual nature of the organism is to be considered in the treatment of the sick individuals.

6. In homoeopathy, feelings of the patients are of greatest importance, so long they are there and distress the sick, he requires treatment; the feelings of being well is of utmost importance in a healthy and fit person.

4. Allopathy consider s that endogenous and exogenous causes operate in the production of a disease. Constitution of the patient has no significance. Causation are considered supreme, primary and worth while.

5. In allopathy, the material nature of the organism is to be considered in the treatment of patients.

6. From allopathic point of view feelings are of secondary importance, so long as the physical examination and laboratory tests and other investigations are found to be normal a person is declared fit and healthy. This attitude is found to change with the discovery of psycho-somatic medicine.

Q. 1.8. What are the benefits, we get from the knowledge of Pathology ?

From the knowledge of pathology we can get the following benefits:—

1. The knowledge of pathology enlightens a homoeopath about *causation of diseases*. Dr. Hahnemann says in para 4 of the Organon that a physician can not remove the disease unless he knows the causation of diseases. The causations may be:—

(a) *Maintaining causes*—i.e., unhygienic surroundings, ill ventilated houses, living in damp places and unhealthy, dirty habits etc.

(b) *Exciting causes*—i.e., emotional excitements, anger, grief, mortification, frustrations, loss of sleep, change of weather, irregular diet, etc.

(c) *Specific causes*—like infection due to viruses, bacteria, parasites, chemical, poisons, drugs, etc.

(d) *The predisposing causes*—e.g. diabetes, gout, etc. due to disturbances of circulation, hereditary diseases, etc.

2. The study of pathology gives us a *knowledge about the kind of disease*.

(a) The kind of disease may be Acute, Sub-Acute or Chronic.

(b) The disease may be Benign or Malignant.

(c) The disease may be Surgical or Medical.

(d) The disease may be a minor ailment or a Constitutional disorder.

3. The knowledge of pathology helps a homoeopath to *differentiate between the common and uncommon symptoms of the diseases and characteristic symptoms* of the patient. This knowledge is very useful for the *selection of the appropriate homoeopathic remedy*.

4. The knowledge of pathology gives us the information by which we can judge the *progress of the disease or recovery from the disease*; e.g. by urine examination, we can find out the condition of the diabetic patient, from stool examination we can find out the condition of worms of the intestinal tract of the patient, by X-ray we can find out the condition of lungs in pulmonary tuberculosis etc.

5. By the knowledge of pathology we can understand the *deficiencies to be replaced for the recovery and cure of the patient*; e.g., in cases of severe haemorrhagic anaemia transfusion of blood may be necessary. In case of cholera the loss of water shall have to be replaced by saline injections, and in case of vitamin deficiencies, the proper supply of vitamins may be essential for the cure of disease.

6. The knowledge of pathology also helps a homoeopath to recognise the serious conditions in which the *treatment is possible in hospital only*; e.g., in a case of contracted pelvis, the safe delivery is possible only in a hospital where the surgical operation can be performed; or in case of head injury a surgical operation may be required to save the life of the patient.

7. The knowledge of pathology guides a homoeopathic physician in *preventing the spread of the diseases* e.g., in case of tuberculosis and other infectious diseases, isolation of patient and notification of the disease have been advised. He is also able to advise the patient about proper food and nursing and forbids all those conditions which will aggravate the diseases.

8. From the knowledge of pathology we can easily understand and describe the pathological changes which are occuring during the proving of certain drugs.

9. In certain conditions, homoeopathic remedies may be dangerous; e.g., in case of tuberculosis of the lungs when there are cavitives and fibrosis, Silicea, Phosphorus or Sulphur should not be used particularly when the vitality is very low. This condition generally known by the help of the knowledge of pathology.

10. The study of pathology also gives the confidence to the physician as well as to the patient and his relatives.

Conclusion :

But the domain of homoeopathic pathology lies in the investigation of the pre-pathological stage where there is no other evidence available than the presence of symptoms, due to disturbed sensation and functions, because of the deviation from normal of the vital principle. Even the minutes of the minute detectable pathological change is a gross change, as it has already passed through miles of pre-pathological or functional changes. Here is a meeting point of allopathic-pathology and homoeopathic-pathology. Where the latter ends the former begins.

Q. 1.9. What would be the disadvantages, if we do not know the Pathology ?

1. The common symptoms of the disease cannot be distinguished from the peculiar, uncommon and characteristics symptoms of the patient.
2. Diagnosis of the disease cannot be reached at.

3. Course of the disease cannot be known.

4. One cannot have the prognosis of the disease, whether curable or fatal.

5. One cannot advise the patient as far as diet, nursing and prevention of the spread of the disease are concerned.

6. Surgical cases cannot be shorted out.

7. In certain conditions homoeopathic remedy may be dangerous e.g. Silicea, Phosphorus or Sulphur in case of tuberculosis of lungs where there are cavities and fibrosis. So till we know the full nature of the disease, we cannot have the confidence in treating the patient.

Q. 1.10. What are the pathological symptoms to be taken into consideration while treating acute and chronic cases homoeopathically ?

Cure means the anhilation of all the morbid symptoms—subjective and objective, functional and pathological. So, we shall have to know the pathology as well. Some of the pathological symptoms or date that must be taken into account in the successful treatment of the patient are :—

I. Laboratory Examinations :

1. Sputum examination as in tuberculosis of the lungs.

2. Urine examination for sugar, albumen, pus cells, casts, R.B.C. etc. in a number of conditions, e.g. diabetes, nephritis, etc.

3. Blood examination in anaemia, leukaemia, diabetes (blood sugar), uraemia (blood urea), widal test, khan, etc.

4. Stool examination for the persence of worms and occult blood.

5. Examination of cerebrospinal fluid in meningitis, sternal puncture fluid in kalazar, pleural fluid in pleurisy with effusion, etc.

II. Radiological exmination particularly in the diseases of the heart and lungs.

III. Blood pressure examination.

IV. Sometimes Electrocardiography (E.C.G.), Electroencephalography (E.E.G.), Microscopic examination of tissue (Histo-pathology) etc. are also helpful.

Q. 1.11. "Where the Homoeopathic pathology ends, the Allopathic pathology begins" — Explain.

Homoeopathy means *Homoeopathicity*. It is based on certain principles *similia, simplex, minimum* and *infrequent repetition of the medicine*. It takes into account all the symptoms and changes, functional as well as structural, dynamic as well as physical; and the physical or structural changes are nothing but pathological changes or objective symptoms.

It is true that homoeopathy does not give such importance and significance to the pathological symptoms, because they are seen on the physical and material plane and not on the dynamic plane and also they do not help in individualising the patient. Homoeopathy believes that before pathological changes take place, there is always a disturbance of function even though microscopic investigations may fail to reveal any change. (This is called *Pre-pathological stage or Dynamic pathology*). When an evidence of pathology is present, however, early it may be, it is gross pathological change i.e. post-pathological stage of the disease.

Hence the domain of the science of pathology (Allopathic) lies in the investigating the changes which have already ultimated in pathology or where they have not established, may be early or advanced, i.e. post-pathological stage of the disease.

But the domain of homoeopathic pathology lies in the investigation of the pre-pathological stage where there is no other evidence available than the presence of symptoms due to disturbed sensations and functions, because of the deviation from the normal of the vital principle. Even the minutes detectable pathological change—is a gross change, as it has already passed through pre-pathological or functional changes. Here is the meeting point of *Allopathic pathology and Homoeopathic pathology. Where the latter ends, the former begins.*

Q. 1.12. Why we should study Pathology ?

In homoeopathy, *we treat the patient but not his disease*. So it is aimed more on the subjective symptoms than on the pathological changes or the objective symptoms because they do not pertain to the individuality of the patient. Pathological changes occur in the physical body much later, but the vital force is effected primarily and much earlier. So pathological changes are only the late manifestations of the disturbed *vital force*. But even then the knowledge of pathology is essential for a homoeopath as well as allopath due to the following reasons :—

1. FOR DISEASE DIAGNOSIS

Diagnosis is the identification of the disease from symptoms and signs and from the result of special laboratory tests. Symptoms and signs, the former noticed by the patient himself and the later detected by the clinician, are the manifestations of altered structure and functions which constitute the pathology of the case. The symptoms and signs can be understood and properly interpretted only in the light of pathology. The common symptoms generally give us the diagnosis of the disease whereas the peculiar symptoms help the homoeopath in the selection of the right remedy.

Beside this the first question that a patient or his party asks a physician—about the name of the disease he has been suffering from. Although they know only few common names of diseases but still they want a diagnosis which they consider to be the only criterion to judge the merit of a physician or after knowing the name of the disease the person concerned can understand the nature of his illness and become alert.

Beside these, Nosological diagnosis is necessary for giving a leave and death certificate, witness in court etc. and in such cases, the person concerned cannot understand the nature of illness unless we mention the name of the disease after diagnosis.

2. FOR PROGNOSIS AND TREATMENT

The art of predicting the likely outcome of the disease in a particular patient, clearly depends on a sound knowledge of pathology, as it requires on the one hand to understand the natural history of that disease in general and on the other hand, assessment of its severity and extent of its lesions in the particular case, both of which are in the province of pathology.

In homoeopathy prognosis may also be presumed by observing the effect of the 1st prescription. But a correct first prescription depends partly on the knowledge of pathology. If the 1st prescription is wrong as we observe in 1st and 2nd observations of Dr. Kent, the whole process of treatment of the case may be misdirected and the patient may be loss. Because prognosis and treatment depends on the seat of the disease, depth of the disease, stage and nature of the disease, its cause and the structure of the tissue involved.

3. FOR MANAGEMENT AND PREVENTION

Next to treatment the general questions which are commonly occur is the general *management* of a case. To determine the period of isolation, quarantine, diet, rest, exercise and other measures which are involved in the general management of a case, pathological knowledge is unavoidable.

As for example, in a case of Bacillary dysentery, whether the patient requires carbohydrate or protein diet, depends mainly on the type of infection. Naturally unless we can diagnosis the case properly, the patient may not be cured inspite of our correct selection of the medicine. Similarly rest in herart diseases, exercise, massage and physiotherapy in paralytic conditions, etc. depend mostly on diagnosis of the case.

Similarly in order to prevent the spread of diseases like measles, diphtheria, pox, cholera, whooping cough, tuberculosis, etc. know ledge of pathology is a must. Because, unless we possess adequate knowledge about the nature of diseases and their mode of spread from the pathology, how we can prevent them ?

4. FOR CORRECT HOMOEOPATHIC PRESCRIPTION

Q. 1.13. How does the knowledge of Pathology help us directly to make a correct homoeopathic prescription ?

1. FOR INDIVIDUALISATION AND EVALUATION OF SYMPTOMS

The basis of homoeopathic prescription is "*Individualisation*" which again depends on correct evaluation of symptoms. In the process of evaluation, the exciting, maintaining and fundamental causes of diseases are of supreme importance and thereafter the rare, uncommon, peculiar and characteristic symptoms of the patient. In all cases, we get some common symptoms of the disease and a few characteristic symptoms of the patient. Homoeopathic prescription depends mostly on these characteristic symptoms. The knowledge of pathology helps us to differentiate between common and uncommon symptoms of the disease and peculiar characteristic symptoms of the patient.

Examples : In a case of *Pneumonia*—fever, cough, dyspnoea, hurried respiration, rusty sputum, consolidation of lungs etc. are all common symptoms of the disease, but we cannot prescribe on these common symptoms alone, so we should observe the patient for the individualising symptoms.

Suppose, a *Pneumonia* patient is very much thirsty specially for icy cold drinks, the patient vomits after eating or drinking, is unable to lie on left side and there is burning all over the body. With all these symptoms we can safely prescribe *Phosphorus* for that case.

But suppose the patient is absolutely thirstless even with 104° -105° F temperature his tongue is absolutely dry, there is aggravation of all the symptoms in the evening and the stool is loose—the character of which is constantly changing. All these symptoms undoubtedly indicate *Pulsatilla* for that case. Similarly, if the tongue of the patient is absolutely clean with constant nausea ratling sound in chest, we should think of *Ipecac*. Thus, we see five pneumonia patients may require five different medicines. If we prescribe for the common symptoms of pneumonia, we may rarely be able to cure a case for which homoeopathy is not to blame.

So, *to make a proper evaluation of symptoms as to which ones are common or characteristic, we are essentially in need of the knowledge of pathology.*

As a homoeopath, we all know that stitching pain relieved by hard pressure is a characteristic symptom of *Bryonia*. But we also know from the knowledge of disease that this is common symptom of a case of *Dry Pleurisy*. Now, if we get this symptom present a case of dry Pleurisy, we cannot prescribe *Bryonia* if patient is thirstless and restless. Because, here this particular pain symptom is diagnostic of pleurisy and not of Bryonia. But, if the same symptom is present in a case of rheumatism or abdominal colic it may stand as a characteristic of Bryonia in the absence of individualising feature. Thus we see the same symptom may be common in one case and individualistic in another case. So to determine this knowledge of pathology is must.

Prescribing *Apis mel.* for thirstlessness and other common symptoms of Anasarca or *Opium* for common symptoms of coma, cannot result in success in homoeopathy, excepting occasional temporary palliation.

2. FOR THE SELECTION OF REMEDY IN SECOND PRESCRIPTION

Similarly, knowledge of pathology also helps to follow up a case properly, after *First Prescription and to make judicious Second Prescription*. Very often it is seen that the first prescription of a younger physician is generally correct, but the second prescriptions are not at all reasonable because of lack of proper follow up of the case and a correct assessment of the effect of first prescription. We know that various changes may follow the application of a correctly selected homoeopathic medicine. This has been very nicely dealt with by Dr. Kent in his observations, but it requires a keen sense of observation and adequate knowledge of pathology to follow the effect of a medicine. This is specially true for a homoeopath. Now-a-days, very often it has been observed that a patient knowingly or unknowingly gives the wrong report to his physician, the reason probably is the wrong idea of being cured quickly by exaggerating the complaints. Naturally, we are to depend more on our own observation. This observation includes a proper analysis and interpretation of the changed symptoms including physical and laboratory findings.

Explanation : Suppose, a patient comes after fifteen days or a month after the first prescription and reports that his or her condition is unchanged. But on examination it is found that the extent of enlargement of the liver is much less than what it was one month back or his blood pressure is less than before or his blood count has improved and so on. Naturally, we can easily understand that the patient is improving though he himself may not be able to understand or does not like to admit the same. Here, we are not to interfere with the action of the medicine already given, because if we change the medicine here the case may be spoiled. But it must be remembered here that the patient's general feeling as a whole must be better simultaneously with such improvement of physical and laboratory findings. Otherwise, the patient may symptomatically be palliated misguiding the physician in his second prescription and finally the patient may turn to be incurable. Here, the knowledge of pathology and the physician's own analysis following Kent's observations are complementary to each other.

3. ABOUT ESSENTIAL CAUSES OF DISEASE

Sometimes, *the patient forgets to mention many important points in connection with his past or family history. In such cases knowledge of pathology may help to arrive at the essential cause of the disease.*

Examples: From a patient of bronchial asthma, it was seen that his apparent symptom-totality was indicative of *Silicea*. But on routine examination, it was found that his chest was pigeon shaped. Then on further enquiry, it was seen that the patient in his childhood suffered seriously from whooping cough after one month of which he developed bronchial asthma. But at the time of case taking, he forgot to mention that important history. However prescription was "*Pertussin*" instead of "*Silicea*" for that patient and he was cured with "*Pertussin*" alone.

Similarly, *scar mark* on the neck of a patient may be suggestive of tubercular gland in the past, *Hutchinson's teeth* or cleft *palate* may be suggestive of hereditary syphilis and so on.

4. FOR MIASMATIC DIAGNOSIS

The knowledge of pathology also helps us in arriving at the miasmatic diagnosis or miasmatic dyscrasia of a case which is the main basis of our prescription in chronic diseases.

Examples: Congenital Hydrocephalus, Microcephale, Idiocy, Congenital ulcers, etc. are generally suggestive of syphilitic dyscrasia and Congenital overgrowth, Telipes, Haemangioma etc. are suggestive of sycotic dyscrasia. These are generally known as hereditary. In cases of acquired dyscrasia where the basic pathology of the disease is suggestive of ulceration from the beginning, the condition indicates syphilitic dyscrasia but if the pathology is suggestive of overgrowth, malformations and/or loss of co-ordination from the very beginning, it is suggestive of sycosis. Thus the pathological changes are very helpful in arriving at the miasmatic dyscrasia either hereditary or acquired.

Dr. Bogar also stresses the value of pathological generals as opposed to the diagnostic pathology. He feels that tnese are the pathological conditions which become characteristic of the patients and effect him in many parts. For example, warts, naevi, keloids, polypi, fibroid, tumours, corns, etc. tend to show the constitutional tendency of the person and are therefore, valuable generals for the constitutional treatment.

5. FOR THE SELECTION OF POTENCY

Next comes to the questions of potency selection of the indicated medicine and to avoid the danger of potency, knowledge of pathology is unavoidable.

Examples: We know that selection of potency depends on the susceptibility of the patient. It is still a difficult problem for us to select the correct potency necessary for a particular patient. Because the susceptibility cannot accurately be measured from outside. But from the knowledge of pathology, we may be able to assess the degree of susceptibility almost correctly in most of the cases, but with few exceptions. The more the structural changes are there, the more the susceptibility of the patient becomes lowered. In cases where the disease is still in the dynamic plane with preponderance of function symptoms, we may presume that the susceptibility of the patient is still high and the patient requires higher potencies. That is why we should not prescribe higher potencies in advanced stages of tuberculosis, cancer, diabetes mellitus, rheumatiod arthritis, Heart diseases, etc. whereas in acute diseases like Influenza, first week of typhoid, whooping cough, mumps etc. and in the begining of chronic diseases, we generally prescrible high potencies. Indiscriminate use of high potencies in repeated doses may even lead to death of the patient. For this reason, Dr. Kent has strongly warned us about the indiscriminate use of high potencies. So to avoid the danger of potency selection knowledge of pathology is must.

6. FOR REPETITION OF DOSES

After the selection of proper medicine and potency the next question comes about repetition of doses. Generally pathology helps greatly in this respect.

Explanation: We know the nature of acute diseases being very rapid and violent, they require frequent repetition of doses; as because, here the action of the medicine is very quickly exhausted from the system. But in chronic diseases the onset and progress of the disease is such that a single dose takes long time to completely exhaust its action and naturally they require less frequent repetition.

7. FOR THE STUDIES OF MATERIA MEDICA, REPERTORY AND THERAPEUTICS

Next comes to the use of the knowledge of Materia Medica, Therapeutics and Repertory.

Most of the Materia Medica and Repertories contain the names of diseases and pathological conditions in which they have been found useful. Unless we know the pathology it is not possible to follow Materia Medica and Repertory fully. Moreover, we may not be able to make necessary inference from the portraits of the dynamic pathology of drugs as stated in the Materia Medica. The same difficulty arises in studing the therapeutics. So the pathology is an indispensible auxillary branch to the study of the therapeutics. It is helpful in enabling the physician to group the symptoms of a case in a more rational way. Pathology acts not only as a guide in therapeutics but also acts as an instrument which he uses in studying the phenomenon which are the subject and agents of his therapeutic operation. When we take the symptomatology as a picture of totality of the symptoms, external and internal causes, and course of the disease, the pathology is indispensiable to therapeutics.

Conclusions

Dr. B.K. Sircar describes in his book that the knowledge of *Physiology* and *Pathology* is must for every homoeopath as the homoeopathic approach is based on the idea that similar beginning lead to similar endings. We are not able to match our remedies to the endings of the disease e.g. pathology of diseases through characteristic symptoms and on the hypothesis that thereby the ending must also match. But we must appreciate that this may not always be so and we must able to match the disease and the drug pictures both in their beginnings and endings e.g. both symptomatically and at the end (pathologically). Otherwise in this age when pathology has so developed and many disease processes present themselves only through their pathological symptoms, we shall be left behind with our imperfect methods and instrument of cure.

Summary

In summary, it is only through the knowledge of the pathology that the physician can diagnose, predict *the course and progress of the disease*, manage the case including dietary regime and prognosis of a case as well as prevention of a disease. But only by means of it, we can know the symptoms that are common to disease and those that are peculiar in the patient i.e. *individualise a case*. The pathological data has great importance in the homoeopathic *selection of remedy; 1st prescription and 2nd prescription, selection of potency, repetition of doses, miasmatic dyscrasia and use of Materia Medica, Therapeutics and Repertory*.

PART—I

BACTERIOLOGY

(Study of Bacteria)

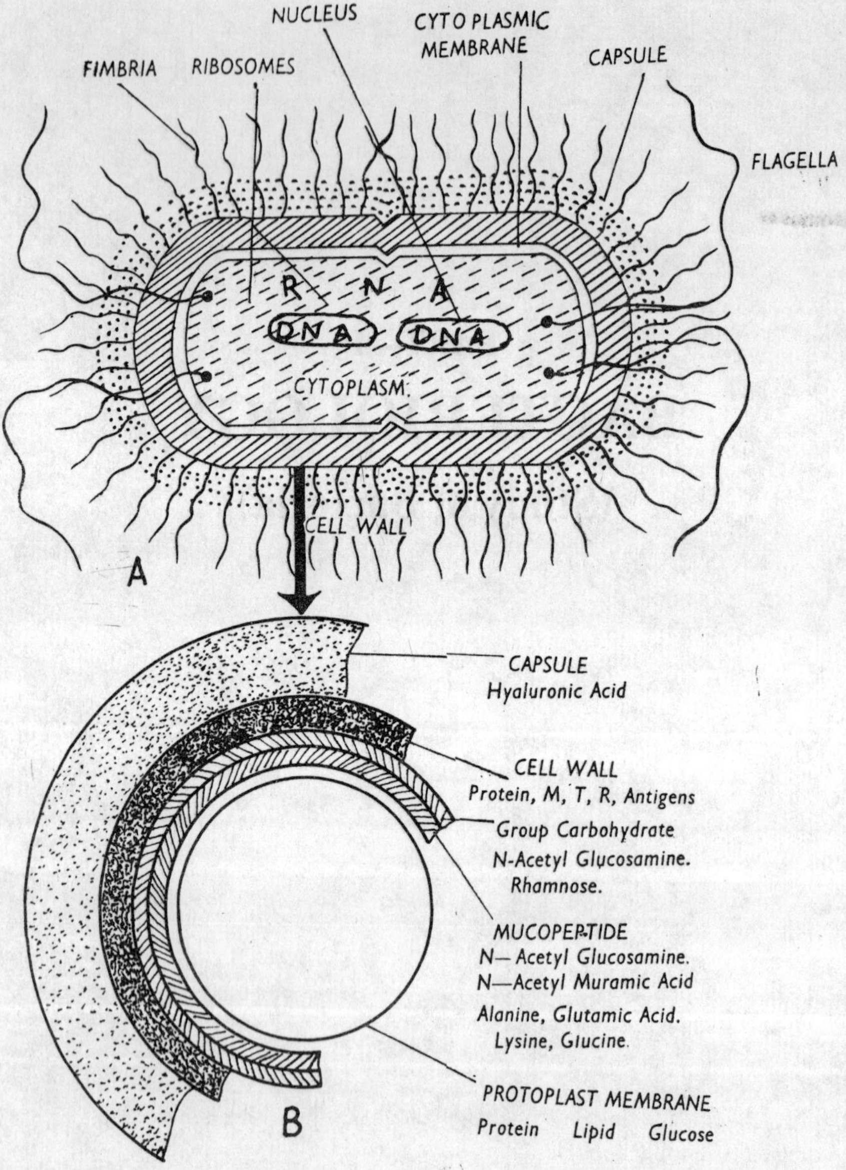

Fig. 1. Structure of a Bacterial cell and its cell wall compositions.

LIVING WORLD

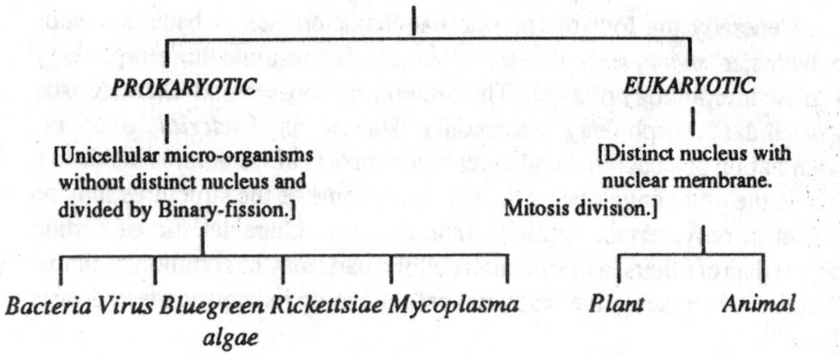

Latest system of classification by *Stanier and Van Niel* 1962, *Round* 1965.

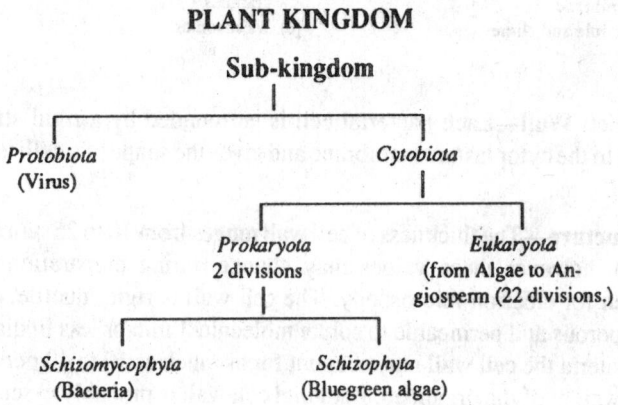

PLANT KINGDOM

Sub-kingdom

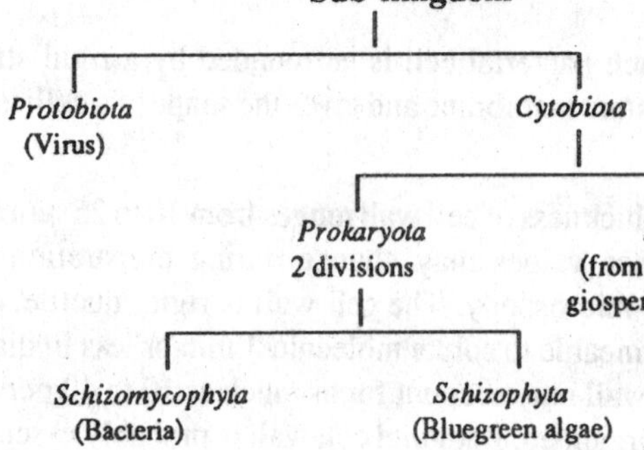

Q. 2.5. Name the various parts of a bacterial cell with special reference to the structure and composition of a cell wall.

Generally the four major external characteristics of bacterial cells i.e. their *size, shape, structure and arrangement* constitute the morphology or gross morphology of a cell. The bacterial cell possesses a characteristic intracellular morphology commonly known as *bacterial anatomy.* Examination of a bacterial cell reveals certain definite structures inside and outside the other envelope or the cell wall. Some of the structures may be present in only certain species; some are more characteristic of certain species than of others; and still other cellular parts may be common to almost all cells. A representative bacterial cell including its appandages consists of:—

BACTERIAL CELL

Covering	Nucleus	Cytoplasm	Protoplasmic appendages
(a) Cell Wall		(a) Ribosomes	(a) Fimbria
(b) Cytoplasmic membrane		(b) Inclusions granules	(b) Flagella
(c) Capsule and slime		(c) Mesosomes	

1. Cell Wall—Each bacterial cell is surrounded by a rigid structure external to the cytoplasmic membrane and gives the shape of a cell, is called *cell wall.*

Structure—The thickness of cell wall ranges from 10 to 25 µm (100—250 A^0), however these values may change during preparation of the specimen for electron microscopy. The cell wall is rigid, ductile, elastic, openly porous and permeable to solute molecules1 mm or less in diameter. In Eubacteria the cell wall may account for as much as 10 to 40 per cent of the dry weight of the organism. Bacterial cell wall is probably essential for bacterial growth and division as naked protoplasts are incapable of normal growth and division.

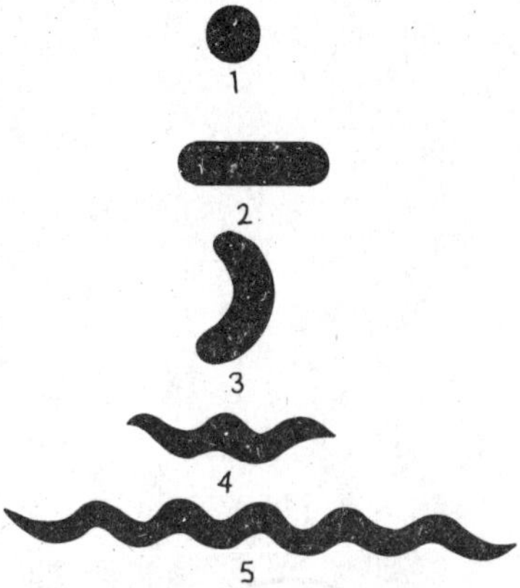

<u>Shapes of bacteria</u> : 1. coccus
2. bacillus 3. vibrio 4. spirillum
5. spirochaete

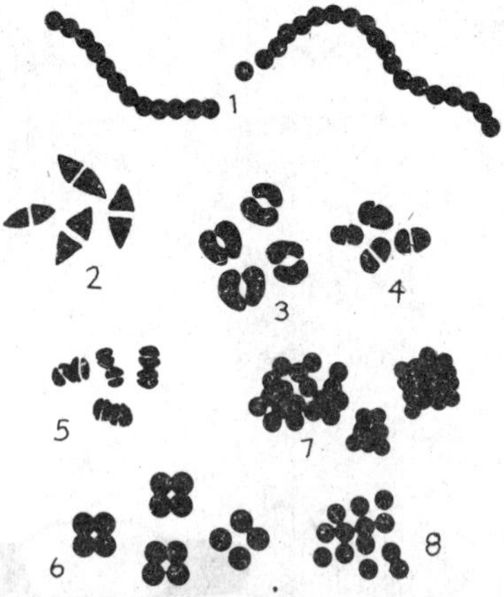

<u>Arrangement of cocci</u> : 1. streptococci
2. pneumococci 3. gonococci
4. meningococci 5. *Neisseria catarrhalis*
6. Gaffyka tetragena 7. sarcina
8. staphylococci

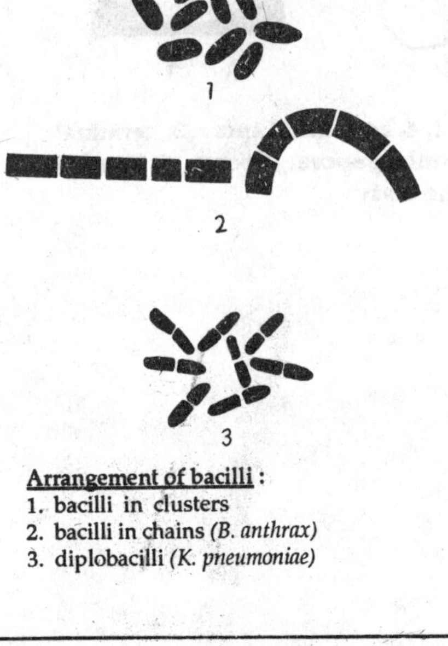

<u>Arrangement of bacilli</u> :
1. bacilli in clusters
2. bacilli in chains *(B. anthrax)*
3. diplobacilli *(K. pneumoniae)*

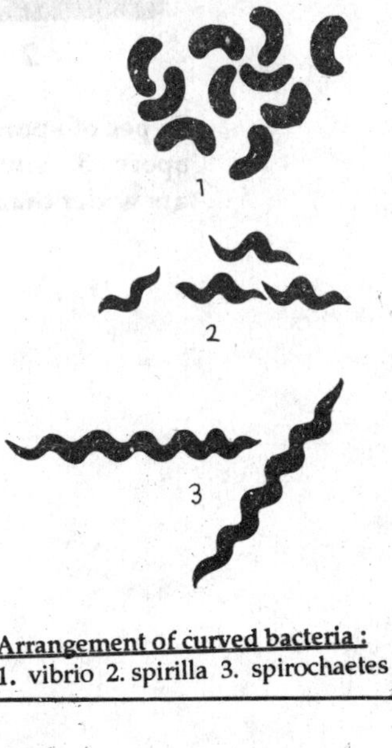

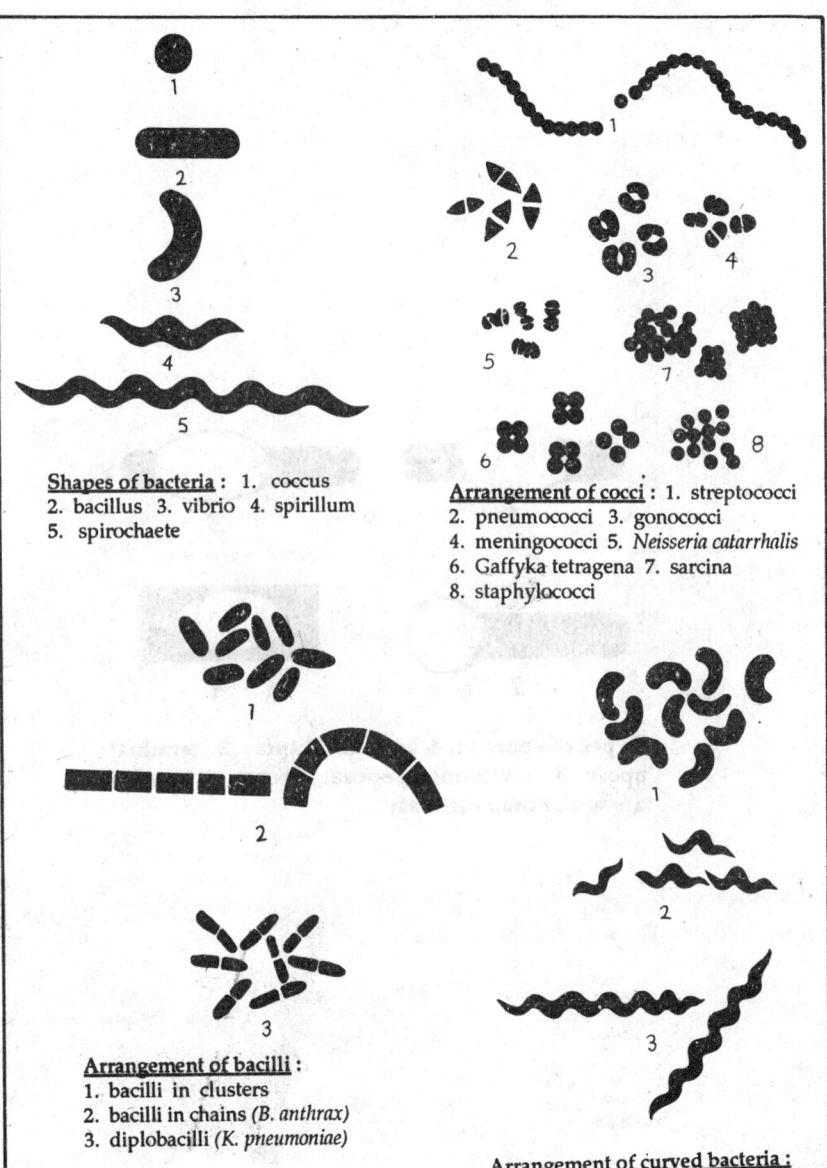

<u>Arrangement of curved bacteria</u> :
1. vibrio 2. spirilla 3. spirochaetes

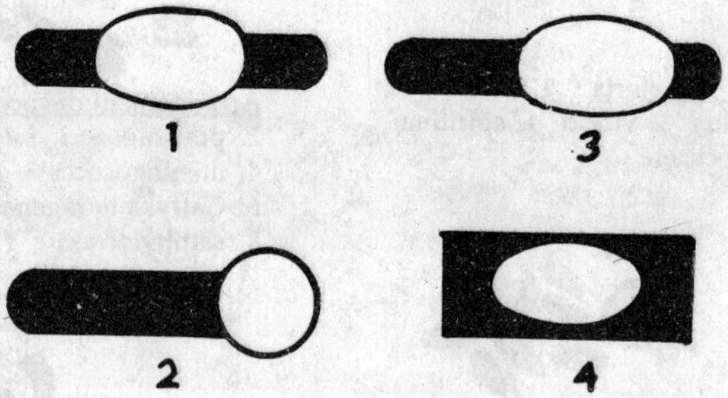

Types of spore : 1, 4. equatorial spore 2. terminal spore 3. subterminal spore. Spores 1, 2 and 3 are wider than the body

COMPOSITION OF A CELL WALL

Usual Components

(a) *Peptidoglycans or Mucopeptides* (Peptide amino sugar)

It forms the rigid component surrounding the cytoplasmic membrane and consists of Acetylglucosamine (AGA), Acetylmuramic acid (AMA) and a peptide consisting of four amino-acids of limited variety e.g. *D* and *L* alanine, Glutamic acid, L-Lysin, *Di-aminopimelic acid, Glycine*. These are attached as side chains to mucopeptides and linked among themselves by peptide chains. Mucopeptides constitute as much as 95% matrix substances of the cell wall in Gram + Ve bacteria and to as little as 5-10% in Gm-Ve bacteria.

(b) *Mucopolysaccharide* (Amino sugar)

(c) *Polyribitol-teichoic acid* (Containing Ribitol phosphate and Glycosophosphate)

(d) *Lipoprotein* (Lipid and Protein)

(e) *Lipo-Polysaccharide* (Lipid and Polysaccharide). In Gram-Ve bacteria Lipoprotein or Lipopolysaccharide are present at the outer layer, which form 80% of the cell wall.

Special Components
(Vary with species)

In Gm + Ve

(i) *Ribitolteichoic acid*

(ii) *Glycine*.

In Gm + Ve composed of 3 coats

(a) *Inner mucopeptide*.

(b) *Outer*—2 *Lipo-protein* and *Lipoplysaccharide*.

(c) The *matrix substances* (middle layer). In the walls of Gram Positive bacteria contain Mucopolysaccharides and Polyribitol teichoic acid. Teichoic acid molecules are covalently linked to Peptidoglycan.

Q. 2.6. Koch's Postulates.

The following are the four postulations of the Robert Koch in 1884.

1. The organism should be found in the lesion, in quantity adequate to account for its effect.

2. The organism from the lesion should be cultivated or grown in a pure state, in a suitable artificial medium, for several generations.

3. The organisms, from repeated subculture, should be able to produce similar lesions in members of the same species.

4. Circulating antibodies should be present against specific organisms, in (i) late stage of illness and (ii) during convalesence.

Q. 2.7. What are the significance of Koch's Postulation and their practical application ?

Significance

1. Diagnosis of infective diseases.
2. Criteria of pathogenicity of an organism.
3. Fundamental basis of experimental bacteriology.

Practical Application

Postulate—1 is for "*Direct smear and demonstration*".

Postulate—2 is for "*Culture*".

Postulate—3 is for "*Animal pathogenicity test*".

Postulate—4 is for "*Serology*" (This was added after Koch's time).

Q. 2.8. What are the falacies of Koch's postulations ?

FALACY OF THE KOCH'S POSTULATIONS:—

Postulate 1:

(a) In *Cl. welchi* and *C. diphtheriae* infections, the lesions are remote due to exotoxins. So there is no organism at the site of remote lesions. Only local lesions show presence of organisms.

(b) In Mycobacterium tuberculosis and Treponema pallidum, organisms act by hypersensitivity. So very scanty or no organism can be found at the site of lesion e.g. Gummata.

(c) Pathogenic-organisms may be present without lesions e.g. in carrier.

Postulate 2:

(a) M. leprae and T. pallidum, cannot be grown on culture media.

(b) Viruses require living cells for cultivation.

Postulate 3:

(a) In *M. leprae* no animal pathogenicity is possible.

(b) Human transference of disease is impracticable. So animal inoculation is used instead of this.

(c) In case of viruses the second and third postulates merge because viruses require living cells for growth.

[N.B.–Recently inoculation of M.leprae in mice foot pad and in golden hamsters have produced granulomatous lesions].

Q. 2.9. Notes on:

1. Nucleoid

Bacterial cells do not contain the nucleus characteristic of the cells of higher plants and animals i.e. a nucleus with nuclear membrane, nuclear reticulum, nucleolus etc. They do, however, contain DNA within the cytoplasm that is regarded as nuclear structure and variously designated as *nuclear material, chromatic body, nucleoid*, even *bacterial chromosome*. The portion of the cytoplasm occupied by the DNA is also known as nucleoplasm and is equivalent to a nucleus. The genetic material (DNA) due to the presence of gene is also termed as '*Genophore*'. The bacterial nucleus may assume various shapes, from a sphere to an elongated or dumb-bell or irregular specimen. The nucleoid consists of a single, 1100 and 1400 mm long, double-stranded, circular molecule of DNA which occupies one fifth ($^1/_5$ th) of the space of a cell. The DNA ring is highly folded (having 40 to 50 loops, the loops are held together by RNA) and attached to the plasma membrane at one point. In most bacilli two or more nucleoids may be seen, since nuclear division precedes cell division. In addition to the nucleoid DNA, subsidiary DNA is also present in bacteria in the form of *plasmids* or *episomes*. Plasmids are also circular DNA duplexes attached to the plasma membrane and are capable of autonomous replication.

2. Capsule or Slime Layer

It is a mucellagenous layer covering a bacterial body.

Structure : Some bacteria are surrounded by a mucoid envelop or slime layer forming a covering layer or envelop outside the cell wall and the organisms having it, is called capsulated. e.g. *Pneumococcus*, *Klebsiella*, *Bacillus anthracis*, *Clostridium welchi and some strains of Streptococcus.* Generally the capsule is secreted by the cell and due to its viscosity it is not readily diffused away and hence gives a coating to the cell wall. Its thickness is markedly influenced by the environment where the bacterium is cultivated. Thick capsules or macrocapsules are 0.2 mm thick and can be seen under the light microscope. Microcapsules are very thin and cannot be seen under the light microscope.

Chemistry: The capsule is usually composed of polysaccharides (dextrine, levan dextran, cellulose), but sometimes made up of polypeptides (D-glutamic acid).

Functions: (i) It is protective in functions. (ii) It resists phagocytosis. (iii) It forms partial antigens. (iv) It gives specificity to the organism, at least to different pneumococci types are distinguishable on the basis of slight differences in the chemical composition of the capsule. (v) It shows capsular phenomenon. It helps transformation of type characters from rough to smooth strains in some bacteria.

3. Flagella (Flagellum)

This is a thin hairlike contractile protoplasmic process present around the bacterial body.

Structure: These are filamentous, cytoplasmic appandages protruding through cell wall, found in all motile bacteria except spirochates. Generally they are originate from a granular structure or basal body just beneath the cell membrane in the cytoplasome. The length of the flagellum is usually several times that of the cell (may be up to 4—5 mm long), however, it is only 10—20 mm in diameter. The flagellum has three parts:

(a) *Basal structure or basal granules*—20-50 mm in diameter and consists of four ring arranged in two sets of two rings and anchored to the plasma membrane and peptidoglycan layer of the cell wall.

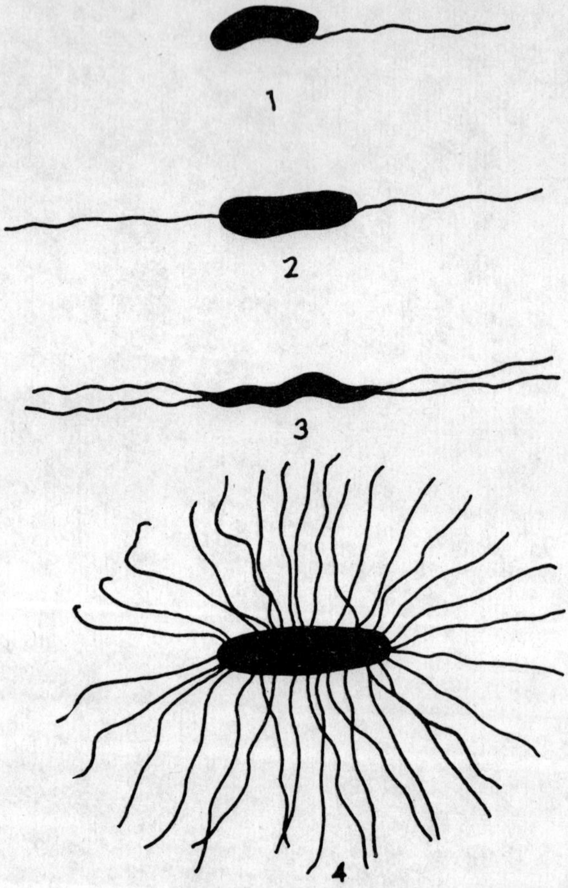

Types of flagellar arrangement : 1. monotrichate
2. amphitrichate 3. lophotrichate **4. peritrichate**

(b) *The hook structure*—is the middle portion, it connects the main filament with the basal structure.

(c) The main filament is 4-5 mm long and 10-20 mm in diameter and consists of a protein called *flagellin.*

Electromicroscopic examination, have shown these flagella to consist of a protein *sheath* and a hollow *core*.

Chemistry: Chemical analysis of flagella has established that they are composed of protein subunits called *flagellin* (similar to myosin). The amino acid composition of flagellin from different bacterial species differs to some extent.

Functions: *Flagella* are responsible for the mortality of bacteria. The movement of flagella may take place due to alternate contract and relax of the macromolecular protein chain producing a wave like motion which pulls or pushes the organism.

Flagella contains type specific antigens (e.g. 'H' antigens in salmonella), so that specific antisera can be prepared.

Arrangement of Flagalla

Depending upon number and disposition of flagella the following types of bacteria are recognised:

(i) *Atrichus*—Without any flagella e.g. all cocci, dysenteric group of bacilli, and P. pestis.

(ii) *Monotrichus*—Single terminal e.g. *Vibrio coma.*

(iii) *Amphitrichus*—Possessing a flagellum at either pole e.g. Spirillum *Volutans* (Non-pathogenic bacteria).

(iv) *Lophotrichates*—Possessing a tuff of flagella at one (*Pseudomonas sp.*) or both (spirillum serpens) poles.

(v) *Peritrichates*—With flagella arranged all round the bacterial cell e.g. *Salmonella typhosa, Escherichia coli, Clostridium tetani.*

4. Fimbriae or Pili

Some Gram negative bacilli (*shigella flexneri, salmonalla typhi*) possess small filamentous appendages different from the flagella are called fimbriae or *pili*. These are smaller, shorter and more numerous than flagella and they do not form regular waves as flagella. They can be seen only by electron microscopy. As the fimbriae are not related to mortality they occur in non-motile as well as in motile stains of bacteria. They are borne peritrichously by each cell. The function of these structures are not definitely known but they may probably (i) act as organs of adhesion for attachment of bacilli to surfaces of various kinds, (ii) during conjugation they form bridge, (iii) they help in the formation of pellicle on the surface of stagnant liquid media and (iv) causes adherence of RBC of pig or human being or sheep.

5. Cocci

The spherical or ellipsoidal bacteria are designated as cocci. The cocci are the second largest group of bacteria, the first being bacilli. Cocci are more drought resistant owing to their round form. In cocci various patterns of cell aggregation are found. Each of the pattern of cell arrangement is characteristic of a particular species of bacteria. On the basis of cell arrangement cocci are of the following types:

(a) *Micrococci*: In this the cells remain separate immediately after cell division e.g. Micrococcus flavus, M. nigra.

(b) *Diplocci*: In this type the cells divide in one plane and remain attached predominantly in pairs e.g. *Diplococcous pneumoniae*.

(c) *Streptococci*: In this type the cells divide in one plane and remain attached to form chains looking like beaded structure e.g. Streptococcus pyrogenes, S. mutans.

(d) *Tetra cocci*: In this type the cells divide in two planes at right angle to each other and the bacteria occur in groups of four cells. e.g. Gaffkya tetragena.

(e) *Sarcinae* : In this type cells divide in three planes in a regular pattern and at right angle to each other, producing a cuboidal arrangement of 8, 16 or more cells e.g. Sarcina maxima, S. lutea.

(f) *Staphylococci*: In this type the cells divide in three planes, in an irregular pattern producing bunches of cocci like grape bunches e.g. Staphylococcus aureus, S. epidermis.

6. Bacilli (Sing. Bacillus)

Rod shaped or cylindrical bacteria are termed bacilli. There are considerable variation in the size of the various bacilli species. Some are only slightly longer than they are wide (*Salmonella typhi*), others are several times as long as they are wide *clostridium sporogens*). Bacilli generally occur singly as unattached cells. Occasionally they occur in pairs (*Diplo bacilli e.g. Pseudomonas sp.*) or in chains (*Strepto bacillie e.g. Bacillus cereus*). Sometimes bacilli have a tendency to produce groupings of cells lined side by side like match sticks known as palisade arrangement e.g. Diphtheria disease producing bacillus *Corynebacterium diphtheria.* The tuberculosis disease (human) producing bacillus *Mycobacterium tuberculosis* may occur is an arrangement of three bacilli that give the impression of a branched structure.

7. Pleomorphism

It means variability in size and shape of some bacteria. So the existence of different forms in the same species of micro organisms is known as *pleomorphism.* Bacteria also show plemorphism, e.g. Azotobacter, *C. diphtheria*, Cl. tetani, P. petis, Haemophylus, Influenza, Mycobacterium, Rhizobium change their shape from rod to oval or irregular branched bodies.

8. Involution Form

These are degenerated out and destroyed form of a particular bacteria and is usually seen in old culture. The bacteria becomes swollen up and granular. This feature is commonly seen in diphther bacillus, meningococcus, gonococcus, P. pestis etc.

9. L-Form Bacteria

These are degenerate forms of bacteria due to defective cell wall synthesis, from bacteria of normal morphology. It was first described in Lister Institute, London. So named as L-form. It is seen in Cocci, Bacilli or is Vibrios. Their main features are (i) Non-rigid cell wall, so varying in shape and size, (ii) Repeated sub-culture is possible, and (iii) They can grow and multiply on ordinary artificial medium, e.g. *Stepto bacillus moniliformis.*

10. Bacterial Spores

Spores are highly resistant resting phase of a bacterium, formed in unfavourable environmental conditions like starvation and desiccation. They are of 2 types—(a) *Endospore* (true spore) and (b) *Exospores* (conidia).

(a) *Endospore* are formed within the parent vegetative cell and they become *central* (B. anthracis) or *subterminal* (Cl. welchi) or *terminal* (Cl. tetani) according to their site of formation.

(b) *Exospore* (conidia) are formed in higher (mycelial) bacteria like actinomyces and are extra-cellulary formed by abstriction from the ends of parent cells (conidiophores). Generally the spores are highly resistant due to:-

(i) Highly impermeable cortex and heat spore coat.
(ii) High content of Ca + + and dipicolinic acid.
(iii) Very low metaholic and enzymatic activities.
(iv) Low content of unbound water.

Under favourable condition i.e. in suitable temperature and moisture, germination of the spores takes place. By rupture of spore envelop or by absorption of spore coat, germ cells come out as out growth and gradually develop into mature vegetative form.

Or, How they form ?

1. At first in the vegetative form of bacterial cell condensation of nuclear chromatin (in a particular sport of the bacterial body) occurs which is well stained by ordinary stain.

2. Then there is a formation of a thick impervious wall around the condensed mass and at this stage ordinary stain cannot penetrate.

3. Finally, the rest of the bacterial body disappears leaving behind the spore only.

Q. 2.10. What is medium ? What are the various types of media used for bacterial culture ? What are the advantages and disadvantages of solid media and liquid media ? What is a carrying medium ?

Medium—It is an artificial environment with essential nutrients at optimum pH. suitable for growth of bacteria.

(A) TYPES OF MEDIA

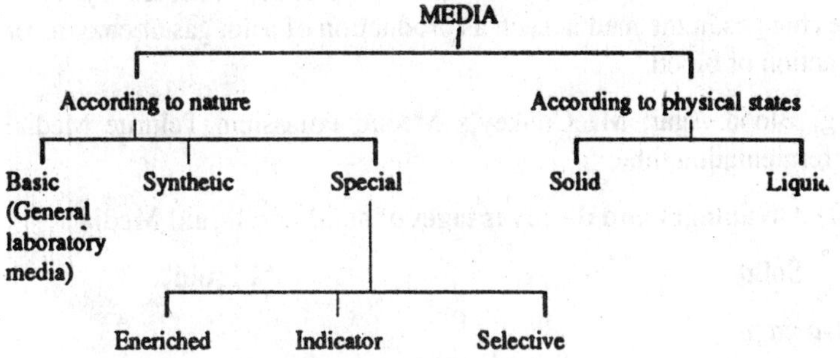

1. Basic media—must contain amino-acids, nucleic acids, carbon and energy sources, nitrogen sources, minerals.

Generally it contains hydrolysate of a cheap protein—>called peptone—>contains essential amino acids.

(i) *Meat extract or yeast extract*—>for growth factors and inorganic salts.

(ii) *Sodium chloride*—>to maintain osmotic tension of organism.

[*Advantages*:- Wide range of organisms can be cultured and easy to produce and it is very cheap.]

2. Synthetic media—In these specific nutrients (pure chemical substances) are added separately to produce a definite chemical product. They are only used for specialized bacteriological techniques, like microbiological assays and preparation of bacterial end products in pure form.

Example:-*Dubos medium*—>Twin (R) 80,—containing caesin hydrolysate, Bovine serum albumin, and Mineral salts.

3. Special media

(a) *Selective Media*: One which suppress growth of all bacteria except a single species or a particular strain. e.g. Lower Stain--Jensens' Media, MacConkey's Media and Loeffier's Media.

(b) *Enriched media*:- When some special nutrients are added to a media, for the purpose of growing a particular organism e.g. Robertson's Cooked Meat Media, Dorest's Egg Media, Blood Agar.

(c) *Indicator media*: One used to detect the colonies of particular bacterial species or strain by distinctive properties, indicated by some visible changes in the media, such as production of acid, gas or enzyme or by its action of blood.

e.g. Blood Agar, MacConkey's Media, Potassium Telurite Media, Sugar fermentation tube.

(B) Advantages and disadvantages of solid and liquid Media

Solid	**Liquid**
(a) *Advantages*:	
1. Colony pattern well marked.	1. Useful in promoting growth of organism when these are scanty.
2. Identification of organisms is very easy.	2. Exotoxin can be extracted.
	3. Motility can be studied.
(b) *Disadvantages:*	
1. Cannot promote growth at scanty organisms. e.g. Nutrient Agar, Agar Agar etc.	1. Isolation from a mixture of organisms is not possible.
	2. Indentification of individual organisms is different.
	3. Colony patterns not so well marked e.g. Nutrient Broth, Glucose etc.

(C) Carrying medium

A medium that is used for preservation and maintanance of a particular type of organism at a particular stage of growth, e.g. Stuart's media—used in *Gonococcus*, Bile salt—Gelatin Agar—used in *Vibrio cholera.*

(D) VARIOUS IMPORTANT MEDIA AND THEIR USES

Name of the Media	Uses
1. *Blood Agar*	For the growth *Streptococci* and *Pneumococci.*
2. Chacolate Agar	Cultivation of *Meningococci*, *Gonococci*, *Pneumococci* and *H. influenzae.*
3. *Loeffler's Inspissated serum media*	Cultivation of *C. diphtheriae* (6-8 hrs.)
4. *Dorset's Egg media*	For the growth of *C. diphtheriae* (in 1-2 days) and of *M. tuber culosis* (3-6 weeks).
5. *Potassium Telurite media*	*M. tuberculosis* (in 3-6 weeks). Selective media for *C. diphtheriae.*
6. *Lowenstain-Jensen media*	For the growth at *Myco-bacterium tuberculosis.*
7. *MacConkey's media*	For the culture of intestinal group of organisms E. Coli Salmonella, Shigella, Vibrios, Stepto fecales.
8. *Deoxycholate-citrate Agar* (DCA)	In bacteriologic examination of faeces, to exclude E. Coli and to isolate Salmonella and Shigella organisms.
9. *Tetrathonate broth and selenite-F-enriched media*	For the culture of Salmonella organisms.
10. *Nutrient Broth*	Growth of the organisms like Staphylococci and *E. Coli.*

Q. 2.11. What is meant by Gram Staining? How it is done?

Staining is essential for the study of the morphology and differentiation of bacteria under light microscopy. Gram staining is one such method to differentiate bacteria by their staining reactions. Gram stain was first introduced by *Christian Gram* (1884), a Danish physician.

1. Principle: In this process bacterial smears are first stained with *crystal violet* or *Gentian violet* or *Methyl violet*, then treated with *Grams* or *Lugol's iodine solution* and decolourised with a solvent like *Alcohol* or *Acetone*, washed and counter stained with *Saffranin* or *Neutral red* or *Ziehl's fuchsin*. Then it is seen whether:—

(a) The organism can resist decolorisation by retaining the dye-iodine complex being colored *Purple violet—Gram + ve*, or

(b) It is decolorised—*Gram*—ve.

(c) Which are decolorised and lose the vilot stain, take the counter stain only, hence appear red or pink in colour, and are called *Gram—ve.*

So all the bacteria are classified broadly into Gram—ve and Gram + ve groups according to whether they can retain or cannot retain the dye-iodine complex.

2. Procedure

(a) *Smear*

(b) *Fixation*—Passing the film twice or thrice through a flame.

(c) *Staining*—By methyl violet (0.5%) for 1 minute.

(d) *Mordanting*—Washed with water and added Gram's Iodine (Iodine in Potassium Iodite) for 2 minutes.

(e) *Decolorisation* — Washed with water and decolorised with Ethyl alcohol until the violet stain ceases to come out of preparation.

(f) *Counter staining* — Washed with water and treated with saffranin 0.25% for 2 minutes.

(g) *Examination* — Washed with water, dried and examined under oil immersion lens.

Q. 2.12. What are role of Iodine in Gram stain ?

Iodine—(i) Acts as a mordant.

(ii) Increases acidity of cytoplasm of Gram + ve organism.

(iii) Selectively decreases permeability of cell wall of Gram + ve organisms.

Q. 2.13. What is meant by Gram + ve and Gram – ve organism ? Name some organisms.

Those which resist decolorisation by alcohol or acetone; and can retain the dye-iodine complex, appearing purple-violet colour by Gram stain are known as Gram + ve organisms.

Those which are decolorised by alcohol and acetone; cannot retain the dye-iodine complex and take the colour of the counter stain (saffranin) that is pink are known as *Gram – ve organisms.*

Examples of Gram + ve and Gram – ve organisms

1. All pathogenic *Cocci* are Gram + ve, except *Neisseriae* and *Veillonela* which are Gram – ve.

2. All pathogenic *Bacilli* are Gram – ve, except acid fast organisms (*Mycobacteria*), spore forming bacilli (*B. anthacis, Clostridia*), *Corynebacteriae*—which are Gram positive.

3. *Actinomyces, Nocordia, Erysipelothrix, Listerie* and *Fungus* are Gram + ve.

Q. 2.14. What are difference between Gram + ve and Gram – ve organisms ?

Items	**Gram + ve**	**Gram – ve**
1. *Staining*	*Retain Gram stain to appear (Purple violet)*	*Do not retain Gram stain appear (Pink)*
2. *pH*	More acidic, 2-3	Less acidic, 4-5
3. *Permeability*	Less	More
4. *Cell wall*		
(a) (Mucopeptide)	Thick and stronger	Weaker
(b) Lipid	Low lipid content (1.4%)	High lipid content (11-22%)
(c) Magnesium Ribonucleate + Protein complex		
5. *Toxins*	Mainly produce exotoxins	Mainly produce endotoxins

Items	Gram + ve	Gram – ve
6. *Synthetic ability*	Less synthetic ability, Nutritional requirement relatively complex.	More synthetic ability, Nutritional requirement relatively simple.
7. *Susceptibility*	More susceptible to antibiotics.	Less susceptible to antibiotics.
8. *Lysis mainly by*	Penicillins, Acids, Basic dyes, Detergents	Antibodies, Complements, Alkalies, Enzymes
9. *Internal osmotic pressure*	High	Low
10. *Mechanical damages*	More resistant to physical disruption	Less resistant to physical disruption.

Q. 2.15. Whether or not we can make a Gram + ve organism to Gram – ve organism ?

By repeated sub-culture or in ageing culture and by the action of enzyme ribonuclease (which removes Mg-Ribonucleate protein complex), we can make a Gram + ve organism to Gram – ve organisms.

Q. 2.16. Why the bacteria are stained by Gram stain ?

Or, Describe the possible mechanism of Gram staining.

Mechanism of Gram staining is not clearly known till today. Possibly staining is due to fundamental differences in morphology of Gram + ve and Gram – ve organisms.

Although the possible theories are:

1. pH of organisms

(a) pH of Gram + ve organism's cytoplasm is more acidic (2-3), then pH of Gram – ve organisms (4-5).

(b) Iodine makes cytoplasm of Gram + ve organisms more acidic.

(c) So Gram + ve organisms have more affinity for basic dyes, can retain basic dyes like methyl violet.

2. Permeability of cell wall

Cell wall of Gram + ve organisms is less permeable than the wall of Gram + ve organisms, due to thicker and stronger muco-peptide coat. So dye-iodine complex on treatment with decolorises, easily diffuses out of Gram – ve one (as more permeable cell wall), and organism is stained pink, due to counter stain. On contrary, the dye-iodine complex does not pass out of Gram + ve organisms (less permeable); the dye is retained; there is no decolourisation and hence the organisms are stained purple violet.

3. Integrity of cellular structure

Gram + ve organism contains at their surface, ribonucleate magnesium-protein complex. This is mainly responsible for Gram positive. But if this ribonucleate complex is removed by enzyme ribonucleas the organism becomes Gram – ve.

Q. 2.17. What is meant by chromogenic bacteria?

Chromogenic bacteria means pigment producing bacteria. These are:

Staphylococcus aureus	—	Golden yellow pigment.
Pseudomonas pyocyanea	—	Bluish green pigment.
Chromogenic mycobacteria	—	Photochromogens and Scotochromogens.
Bacillus prodigiosus	—	Red pigment.

Q. 2.18. What is meant by exotoxins and endotoxins ?

Exotoxins: These are extracellular poisonous soluble toxic substances which diffuse radially from the body of the bacteria into surrounding media, in which these have been grown and the vitality of bacteria not been injured. They are formed by Gram-positive bacteria such as *C. diphtheriae, Cl. tetani, Cl. botulinum, Cl. welchii, Streptococcus haemolyticus and Staph. aureus*. Chemically they are unconjugated proteins. Heating destroys them readily. They are highly *antigenic* and so *antisera* are available against them. The latter are used to neutralise toxicity of exotoxins. *Exotoxins* differ widely in their effects.

Effects: *Diphtheria exotoxin* is lethal to cardiae muscle whereas toxins of clostridia are neurotoxins. *α-toxin of Staphpyogenes* causes shattering of the lysosomes of leucocytes. *Enterotoxin of Staphylococcal* origin gives rise to food poisoning. In most cases effects of exotoxin are irreversible and lead to death of the affected cell. In some cases, exotoxins appear to act as enzymes. For example, *α-toxin of Cl. welchii* is a lecithinase, and its other toxins are collagenase, protease, hyaluronidases etc.

Endotoxins:

Toxic substances which are heat stable lipopoly saccharides and associated principally with the cell wall are called endotoxins. Unlike exotoxins these produce similar effects irrespective of their origin. However, they differ in potency from species to species. In small doses they cause sharp rise in temperatures. The same is called endotoxic shock. This type of shock is a feature of severe infection with Gram-negative organisms in elderly persons. In comparison to exotoxins, they are less toxic. Endotoxin though stimulate production of specific antibodies in animals, are but not neutralised efficiently by them. That is why, antiserum therapy is ineffective with endotoxin produceing bacteria, such as a Gram-negative bacteria (M. meningitidis, Salm. typhi or V. cholerae). Endotoxins are liberated only after destruction or death of the bacteria.

Q. 2.19. Name some bacteria which produces exotoxins and endotoxins?

Exotoxins producing organisms	**Endotoxin producing organisms**
Mainly Gram positive organisms Corynebacterium diphtheriae, Cl. groups. Strepto, haemolyticus Pneumococcus, Shigella dysenteriae.	*Mainly Gram negative organisms E. Coli, Salmonella, Shigella, Brucellae, Neisseriae, Vibrio cholerae, Pseudomonas pyocyanae.*

Q. 2.20. What are the differences between exotoxins and endotoxins?

Items	Exotoxin	Endotoxin
1. Liberation	The toxins are produced as a result of cellular activity so being soluble come out of the body of bacteria.	It is intimately connected with the body of the bacteria and as it is insoluble it does not come out of the body of bacteria — only comes out during bacterial disintegration.
2. Action of heat.	Heat liable except-Botulinilum toxin. Loose its properties at 65 °c.	Thermostable. Retains properties after heating at 100 °c.
3. Lethal dose.	It is deadly even in small dose.	Large amount of it may be lethal.
4. Selective affinity.	Specific for particular tissues or organs.	No specific effect on particular tissue.
5. Toxicity.	Living organisms toxic highly toxic	Weakly toxic
6. Diffuse into media.	+ Hence present in bacterial free filtrate.	— Bounded in the bacterial cell.
7. Composition.	Simple protein.	Complex protein (Protein+Carbohydrate + Lipids).
8. Antigenicity.	It is antigenic and so when introduced in the system produce antibody.	Antigenic action poor, so when introduced, less formation of corresponding antibody.
9. Union with antibody.	Simple reaction— precipitation.	Complex reaction agglutination and complement fixation.
10. Role of antibody.	Protection.	Variable, some protective, some are not.
11. Convert-able into	It may be converted into toxiod by heating or by formalin, so that antigenic property retained.	Cannot converted into toxoid.

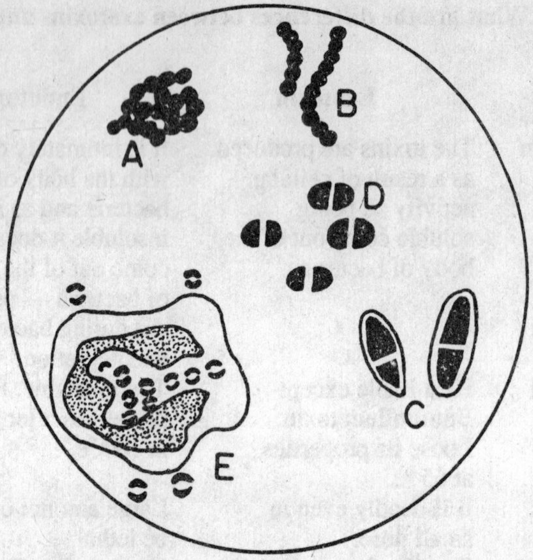

Fig. 2. Some Important Coccic

A. Staphylococcus.

B. Streptococcus.

C. Diplococcus.

D. Meningococcus.

E. Gonococcus.

CHAPTER 3

IMPORTANT COCCI

DISCUSSION FOR LEARNING

I. Gram positive cocci in clusters.

(1) Staphylococcus.

II. Gram positive cocci in chains.

(2) Streptococcus.

(3) Diplococcus or Pneumococcus.

III. Gram negative cocci.

(4) Gonococcus.

(5) Meningococcus.

Q. 3.1. Name the different pus producing bacteria ? Or Name the common pyogenic organism. [C.U. 1979]

Pyogenic organisms are:

I. Pyogenic cocci:

(1) *Staphylococcus aureus.*
(2) *Streptococcus pyogenes.*
(3) *Pneumococcus.*
(4) *Meningococcus.*
(5) *Gonococcus.*

II. Pyogenic bacilli.

(1) *Bacillus proteus.*
(2) *Escherichia coli.*
(3) *B. pseudomonas.*
(4) *B. pyocyanea.*
(5) *B. bacteroides.*

Q. 3.2. How they produce pus ?

They give rise to acute inflammatory reaction. As a result, destroyed tissues are autolysed and digested by ferments of pohymorphus. This leads to production of pus.

Q. 3.3. What is meant by bacterial endocarditis? What are the bacteria responsible for this disease ? Describe any one of them.

Bacterial endocarditis means affection of the endocardium by bacteria. It usually occurs during septicaemia and may be clinically divided into

(a) Acute and (b) Subacute.

In *Acute bacterial* endocarditis, the affecting organisms are of high virulence and healthy heart valves may be involved. The course of the disease is rapid, and requires very prompt therapy. It is caused by the *Staphylococuss aureus, Streptococcus pyogenes* (Group A) and occasionally gram negative bacili.

In *Subacute Bacterial Endocarditis* (SBE) the affecting organisms are of low or moderate virulence and already damaged heart valves are affected.

The causative agents of SBE include:

1. *Streptococcal species*:
   (a) *S. viridans*.
   (b) *Microaerophilic streptococci* (*S. mellen*).
   (c) *Non-haemolytic streptococci* (including S. facealis).
2. *Staphylococcus albus*.
3. *Neisseria species*.
4. *Hoemophillus* influenza.
5. *Gram negative bacilli, particularly* members of *Enterobacteriaceae* etc.

Q 3.4. Name some Gram positive cocci in clusters.

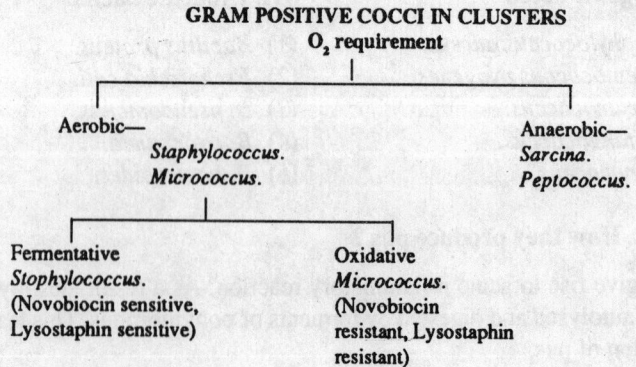

GRAM POSITIVE COCCI IN CLUSTERS

O_2 requirement

- **Aerobic—** ***Staphylococcus. Micrococcus.***
  - **Fermentative** ***Stophylococcus.*** **(Novobiocin sensitive, Lysostaphin sensitive)**
  - **Oxidative** ***Micrococcus.*** **(Novobiocin resistant, Lysostaphin resistant)**
- **Anaerobic—** ***Sarcina. Peptococcus.***

Q. 3.5. Why they are clusters ?

They are clusters as their cell division take place irregularly in different planes.

1. STAPHYLOCOCCUS

Q. 3.6. What is staphylococcus ? What are their morphological characters ? [D.M.S. 1974, 81, 84]

They are gram positive, catalase positive, aerobic, non-motile, non-sporic, spherical cocci and are arranged like a bunch of grapes.

Morphology *Shape* — Spherical.

Diameter — 0.8 to 1 m.

Arrangment — On solid media like bunch of grapes, in liquid media found singly, or in pairs, or in very short chains.

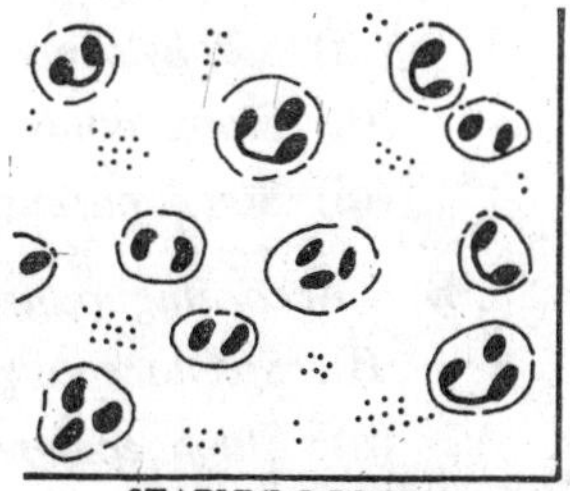

STAPHYLOCOCCUS

On stainin — Gram positive.

Motility — non-motile so non-flagelated.

Capsules — Not found in 18-24 hour old cultures but found in very young cultures of some stains. No spores.

Colonies: Colonies are circular discs, opaque and convex and may be pigmented white (*albus*), golden (*aureus*), or lemon (*citreus*).

Q. 3.7. What are the various species of staphylococcus seen in nature? Give their main characteristics ? How we can classify them? [D.M.S. 1974]

Generally the ***Genus*** **— Staphylococcus** contain the following species:—

(1) *Staphylococcus aureus.*

(2) *Staph. albus.*

(3) *Staph. citreus.*

(4) *Anaerobic staphylococci.*

1. *Staph. aureus* — Coagulase positive, Toxin forming pathogenic staphylococci, produces golden yellow colony.

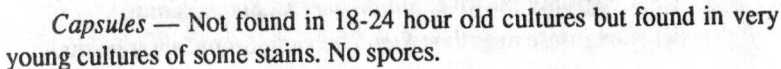

2. *Staph. albus* — Coagulase negatives, non-toxin forming, non-pathogenic staphylococci, produces porcelain white colony.
3. *Staph. citreus* — Coagulase negatives, non-toxigenic, non-pathogenic staphylococci, forms lemon yellow colonies.
4. *Anaerobic-staphylococci* — Capable of growth only under strict anaerobic conditions; common inhabitants of nose, throat and vagina.

Classification:

A. *According to their* **pigmentation:**
 (i) *Staphylococcus aureus* (golden).
 (ii) *Staph. albus* (white).
 (iii) *Staph. citreus* (lemon-yellow).

B. *According to the* **disease production:**
 (i). *Sphyloccous pyogens* (Pathogenic).
 (ii). *Staph. epidermidis* (Non-pathogenic).

C. *According to* **Bergery** (Scientist):
 (i) **Coagulase positive:** *Staph. aureus, Staph. albus.*
 (ii) **Coagulase negative:** *Staph. citreus, Staph. epidermidis.*

Q. 3.8. Briefly review Coagulase Test. [C.U. 1982]

It is useful test to identify pathogenic strains of staphylococci. It is performed in two ways. Tube method consists of adding 5 drops of overnight broth culture to 0.5 ml. of 1 : 10 dilution of citrated rabbit or human plasma and incubating the mixture 37°C for two hours. The plasma gets clotted in positive case. A mixture of 0.5 ml. saline and plasma, incubated at 37°C for two hours serves as control.

In slide method a microscopic slide is divided into 2 parts by a line with grease pencil and placing a drop of normal saline on each area suspension of organism is made in each of them. Now a drop of undiluted human or rabbit plasma is added to one and stirred gently with a platinum wire. In case of coagulase positive strain clumping takes place. To the second, a drop of saline is added with a view to have a control. Organism clump together due to precipitation of fibrinogen by bound coagulase present on the cell wall. The test tube technique measures free coagulase. The slide test is fairly reliable. But more reliable method is test tube method.

Q. 3.9. Describe the pathogenicity of staphylococcus.

Generally pathogenic lesions are produced by 2 types of staphylococci. They are *virulent type* and *non-virulent type or opportunistic pathogens.* The hallmark produced by staphylococci is **'focal'** or **circumscribed abscess.**

Generally staphylococcous enter the body through skin and mucous membrane where they are found as *commensals.* But they are also responsible for a large numbers of pyogenic infection in man like:—

Impetigo, Boils or Furuncles, Styes, Paranochia, Conjunctivitis, Carbuncles, Whitlow and Palmer space infections on subcutaneous and submucoustissues and Acute osteomyelities and Brodies' abscess in bones, Brochopneumonia in lungs; Pyelonephritis. Acute glomerulonephritis, Renal abscess and Perinephric abscess in kidney. Acute bacterial endocarditis in Heart; lymphangitis and lymphadnitis in lymphatics.

Some stains produce enterotoxin causing *gastro-enteritis* or *food poisoning.* Some strains also produce *Bacteremia, Septicemia* and *Pyemia* in generalised form.

N.B. Generally all Staphylococcal disease are due to toxins and enzymes produced by them. The important toxins are:

1. Alfa toxin —haemolytic
   —dermonecrotic
   —leucocidal
   —cytotoxic
   —antigenic
2. Beta toxin —Weak haemolysin
3. Delta toxin- Haemolytic
   —Cytotoxic
   —Leucocidal
   —non-antigenic
4. P-V leucocidin —Non-haemolytic
   —Leucocidal.

II. Enzymes—Coagulase, Hyaluronidase, Stephylokinase, Protease, Lipase, Penicillinase and Phosphetase.

Staphylococcal lesion is localised by the action of coagulase. Necrosis is due to a-*lysin*. Pus is formed due to death of leucocytes by a-lysin.

Diabetes melitus, Avitaminosis, Excess abrasions, Irritation of skin by chemical substances are conductive to the development of Staphylococcal infection suffering from smallpox, influenza, wounds, as well as operative trauma predispose to secondary infection by staphylococci. They are also found in infecting lesions of Diphtheria, Tuberculosis, Actinomycosis etc.

Q. 3.10. How staphylococcus are identified ?

Staphylococci are identified by their:—

(1) Morphological characters.

(2) Staining reaction in smear preparation.

(3) Cultural characters on nutrient agar.

(4) Pathogenic strains in coagulase test and DNAse test give:

(i) Positive-*Staph. aureus* (mostly manitol fermenter).

(ii) Nagative-*Staph. albus* (mostly manitol non-fermenter).

Q. 3.11. What is micrococci?

They are-(a) Gram positive cocci dividing in two planes at right angles (form tetrads).

(b) Non-pathogenic to man.

(c) Found as secondary invaders of skin and nasopharynx.

Q. 3.12. Show you aquaintance with Sarcina ?

They are — (a) Gram positive cocci dividing in three planes at right angles (form Cubical Packets).

(b) Non-pathogenic (but Sarcina ventriculi frequently found in the stomach).

(c) Found producing bright yellow colonies on solid media.

II. GRAM POSITIVE COCCI IN CHAINS

Q. 3.13. Name some Gram positive cocci in chains. (or Classify Streptococcous)

According to Brown:—

Gram Positive Cocci in Chains

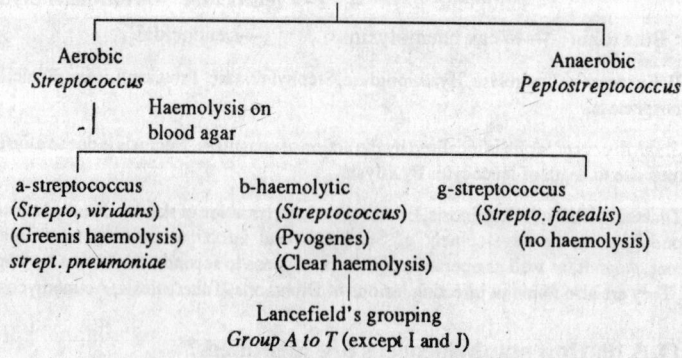

- Aerobic *Streptococcus*
  - Haemolysis on blood agar
    - a-streptococcus (*Strepto, viridans*) (Greenis haemolysis) *strept. pneumoniae*
    - b-haemolytic (*Streptococcus*) (Pyogenes) (Clear haemolysis)
      - Lancefield's grouping *Group A to T* (except I and J)
    - g-streptococcus (*Strepto. facealis*) (no haemolysis)
- Anaerobic *Peptostreptococcus*

2. STREPTOCOCCUS

Q. 3.14. What are the general characteristics of Streptococcus ?

Strepto means '*chain*' and chain formation is due to successive cell division along the same axis.

General characters:

(1) Generally streptococci are spherical or ovoid in shape.

(2) Form chains dividing in one axis (chain formation is best seen in liquid cultures and in pus, on solid media the cocci occurs as short chains, pairs or single cocci.

(3) Non-motile.

(4) Non-sporing.

(5) Growth scanty in medium devoid of native proteins.

(6) Produce characteristic haemolytic changes in media.

(7) Ferment carbohydrates producing only acid.

(8) Fail to liquefy gelation (often).

(9) Few are anaerobic.

(10) Produce extracellular products (some strains).

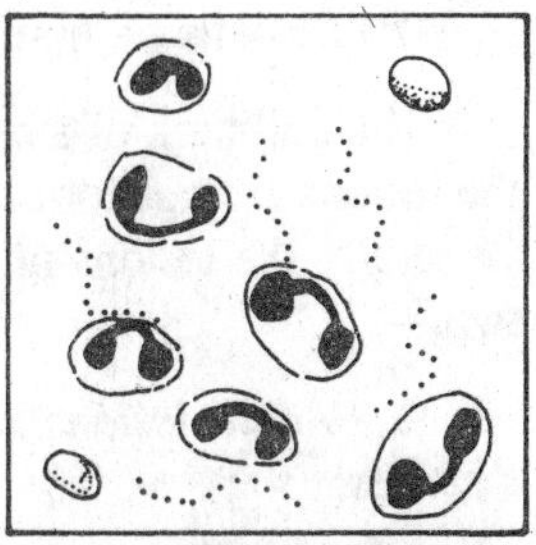
in pus. STREPTOCOCCUS

Q. 3.15. Describe the main characteristics of the bacteria streptococcus haemolyticus (Strept pyogenes) and also the lesions produced by them in man. [C.U. 1980 (Sup.)] [D.M.S. 1977 (Dec.)]

(A) Main Characteristics of Streptococcus Haemolyticus:—

1. Spherical in shape, Gram positive.
2. Arranged in long chains.
3. Aerobes and Pathogenic.
4. Optimum temperature for growth 37^0 C.
5. Luxuriant growth in slightly alkaline medium.
6. Small circular, discrete colonies, about 1 mm in diameter after 24 hours on glucose agar.
7. Clear zones of haemolysis round the colonies on blood agar.
8. Granular deposit at the bottom of tube in glucose broth.
9. Do not grow in bile broth medium.

10. Susceptible to Penicillin and Sulphonamides.
11. Form mucoid or matt colonies when recently isolated from lesions.
12. Glossy colonies formed by strains kept for sometime in the laboratory.
13. Group A strains produce erythrogenic toxin, Streptolysin S and O, Streptokinase, Hyaluronidase, DP Nase, Deoxyribonuclease, Ribonuclease, Amylase, Leucocidin etc.
14. Possess antigenic fractions such as M antigen, T antigen, C. substance.

(B) Lesions on man

The hallmark of streptococcal lesion is **spreading cellulitis**: Usually the lesions are pus forming; but the pus is watery and often blood stained. Generally the lesions produced by Strepto haemolyticus are divided into two:—

(a) *Acute lesions.* and (b) *Remote lesions* i.e. *post streptococcal diseases.*

a. Acute lesions:

(1) *In skin* — Impetigo contagiosa, Paronychia, Scarlet fever, Cellulitis, Erysipelas, wound infections.
(2) *In blood* — Septicaemia.
(3) *In Lymph vessels* — Lymphangitis.
(4) *In respiratory tract* — Sore throat, Acute Follicular Tonsilitis, Phrangitis, Peritonsilar abscess.
(5) *In lungs* — Broncho-pneumonia, Empyema.
(6) *In genital tract* — Puerperal Sepsis.
(7) *In heart* — Acute Bacterial Endocarditis.

b. Remote lesions:

(1) Acute Rheumatic Fever.
(2) Acute Glomerulo Nephritis (by Group A, Type 12.25, 4).
(3) Erythema Nodosum.

Besides these — *Mastoiditis, Otitis media, Meningitis* etc. are also caused by strept haemolyticus.

N.B.–Main characteristics of Strept. viridans:

1. Commensal of mouth, teeth, throat etc.
2. Gram positive, non-motile, non-sporing.
3. Produce short chains, aerobes.
4. Scanty growth on nutrient agar.
5. Greenish discolouration round the colonies or blood agar.
6. Resistance than streptococcus pyogenes.
7. Do not possess polysaccharide artigens.
8. Sensitive to penicillin when given for a long time in large doses.

Lesions in man: It produces Pyorrhoea Alveolaris, Apical abscess of the tooth, Chronic Pharangitis and Tonsilitis, Appendicitis, Peptic Ulcer (excites), Chronic Cholecystitis, Subacute bacterial endocarditis and its complications.

Q. 3.16. How can we diagnosis them ?

Generally test material is obtained from the pus of wounds, inflammatory exudate, tonsillar swabs, blood, urine and food stuffs. Tests include microscopy of pus, smear, inoculation of test material into blood agar plate, isolation of pure culture and its identification.

Virulence is tested on rabbits by injecting intracutaneously, the bacteria. The group and type of the isolated streptococcus and its resistance to an antibiotic are also determined. Serological diagnosis consists of demonstrating the specific Anti—O—haemolysin antibodies. Differential W.B.C. count shows *Polymophonuclear leucocytosis.*

Q. 3.17. Dick test is done for what and how ?

It is done in children to detect susceptibility to *Scarlet fever*. In this 0.2 ml. of 1:1000 dilution of toxin (erythrogenic) is injected intradermally in one forearm and control is also used by injecting the same quantity of toxin in the other forearm after antoclaving. After 24 hours reading is taken. Appearance of erythema of 1 cm. diameter characterises a positive result.

Q. 3.18. What is Schultz-Charlton reaction?

Blanc hing of the rashof Scarletfever (in 12-24 hours) in the area of intradermal injection of antistreptococcal serum, or serum from a convalescent case of Scarlet fever is called *Schultz-charlton reaction.* Previously it was used as diagnostic test for Scarlet fever.

3. DIPLOCOCCUS PNEUMONIAE

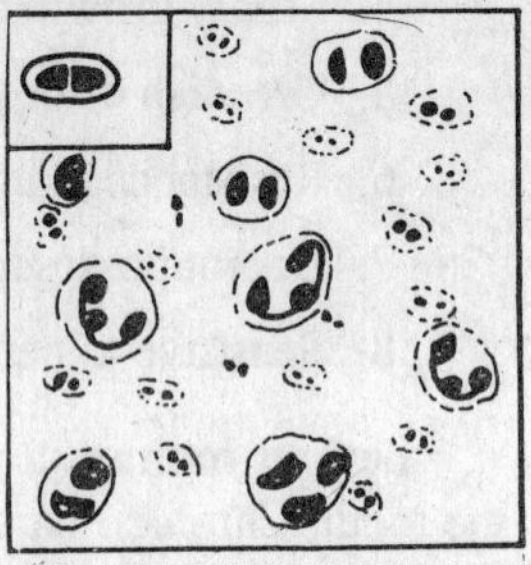

DIPLOCOCCUS PNEUMONIAE

Q. 3.19. Describe the main characteristics of Diplococcus Pneumoniae with Laboratory diagnosis ? [C.U. 1979, 82]

Streptococcus pneumoniae are also known as *Pneumococci* or *Diplococcus pneumoniae.*

Main characteristics:

(1) They are *Gram positive cocci,* oval or *lanceolate* in shape, *arranged in pairs* with long *axis in line with each other in tissue or in pus and in short chain in fluid media.* Each pairs is enclosed with a capsule which is typically seen in tissues. The capsule may be demonstrated by special straining methods. *They are also non-sporing* and *non-motile.*

(2) The opposite surfaces of cocci are either flat or concave.

(3) Best growth on media with blood or serum; culture tends to autolyse.

(4) Growth soluble in bile or bile salts; facultative anaerobe; optimum temperature 37°C.

(5) On blood agar the colonies are small, semi-transparent and surrounded by a zone of haemolysis (α-haemolysis). However, here colonies are plateau shaped and later develop elevated margin and concentric ridges (draughtsman colonies).

(6) Colonies round, smooth, semi-transparent and mucoid on solid media.

(7) No proteolytic activity but ferment specially insulin.

(8) Optochin inhibits growth.

(9) Capsular carbohydrate antigen, type specific and associated with virulence; nucleoprotein antigen common to all types.

(10) Capsular swelling reaction identifies the particular type of pneu-

mococcus. It is done by mixing a drop of appropriate antiserum with suspension of pneumococci or sputum or pus on a slide. Swelling is observed as enlarged halo round the organisms.

(11) White mice and rabbits susceptible (highly).

(12) Disease caused by this organisms are:

Lobar pneumonia, Broncho-pneumonia, Empyema, Otitis media, Meningitis etc.

Laboratory Diagnosis:

Laboratory diagnosis consists of *direct microscopic examination of pus or sputum for the organism or culture on blood agar of the test material for characteristic colonies.* Raised convex colonies exhibiting autolysis in the centre in few hours (*draughtsman appearance*) and α haemolysis (on blood agar), typing, insulin fermentation and sensitivity to optochin and bile salts. Capsular swelling reaction is done for quick diagnosis. Intraperitoneal injection of sputum sample into mice is done and the animal is killed later and autopsied to demonstrate the bacteria.

**[Peripheral blood count in Lobar pneumonia-Polymphonuclear leucocytosis. T.C. of WBC=above 10,000 per cu.ml. of Blood. Polymorphs are above 70%]

Q. 3.20. Describe the pathogenesis of Pneumococcus ?

The incubation period varies from a few hours to 48 hours, and Pneumococci may reach the lungs by way of the:—

(i) *Respiratory passages,*

(ii) *Lymphatics,* and

(iii) By *haematogenous route.*

The main avenue of infection to the lungs is by way of *Bronchial tree.* The bacteremia is secondary.

Pathology:

Pneumococcal infection causes an out pouring of filberinous oedema fluid into the alveoli followed by red cells and polymorphonuclear leucocytoces which results in consolidation of portions of the lung. There are four stages recongnised for purpose of description e.g. *stages of congestion, red hepatisation, grey hepatisation and resolution.* The process is progressive one, commencing from the hilum and quickly spreading towards the periphery involving one or more lobes and occasionally both lungs are involved. Many pneumococci are found throughout this exudate.

III. GRAM NEGATIVE COCCI

Q. 3.21. Name some Gram negative cocci with their characteristic features.

Gram negative cocci — These organisms may belong to any of the following genera *Neisseria.* These are aerobic gram negative cocci, usually arranged in pairs, bean shaped in appearance with long axis being parallel to each other. They are all oxidase positive. The pathogenic members include *N. meningitidis* (menigococcus) and *N. gonorrhoea* (*gonococcus*), and non-pathogenic are N. catarrhalis, N. pharangitis, N. flavescens.

**Veillonealla*—are strictly anaerobic, small gram negative cocci. They are potential pathogens and are isolated from mouth and alimentary tract.

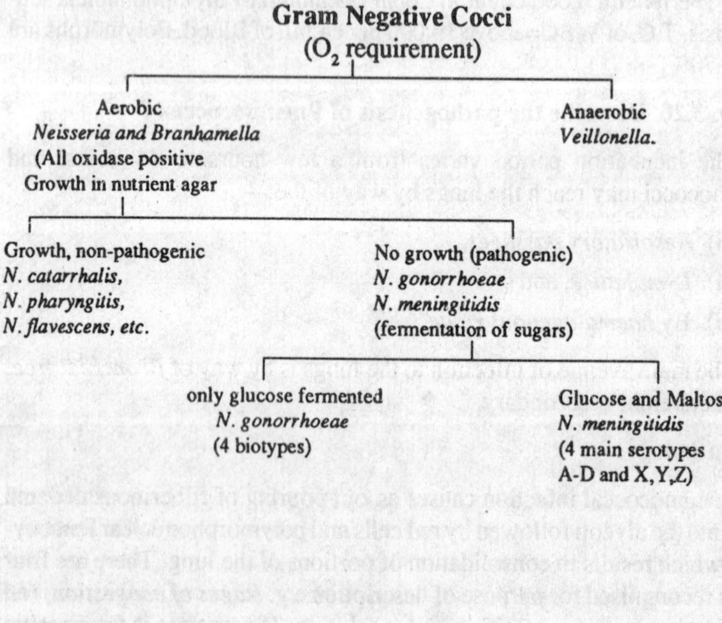

4. GONOCOCCUS

Q. 3.22. Describe the morphological characters of Gonococcus. What are the lesions formed by them ? How can we diagnosis a case of Gonorrhoea ? (D.M.S. 1977)

Morphology: The bacteria *Neissreia gonorrhoea* are known as *Gonococcus*. These are gram negative intracellular as well as extracellular diplococci, bean shaped or kidney shaped in appearance with their *concave* surface parallel to each other. Diameter 0.6-0.8 m.

In cultural media — small, greyish, transparent circular colonies are formed. No haemolysis is seen.

Lesions:

They produce — Gonorrhoea in males; Chronic cervicitis in female, Vulvo-vaginitis in female children, *Ophthalmia neonatoreum* in new borns.

As complication produce — Prostatitis, Epidymitis, Ulcerative endocarditis, Arthritis, Meningitis, Iritis, Uretheral stricture, Vesiculitis, Pyelitis in males.

In females — Bartholins abscess, Endometritis, Salpingitis, Pyosalpix, Oophritis, Pelvic peritonitis, Tubo ovarian abscess, Sterility and Abortion.

Laboratory diagnosis:

A. Direct method:

It consist of:

(1) *Microscopic examination of smear of pus stained by Gram's method.*

(2) *Culture of swabs from lesions.*

(1) Microscopic examination of stained smears show gram negative diplococci both intra and extracellular. In chronic male cases smear is prepared from material obtained after prostatic massage. In females, smear are prepared from urthral or cervical discharge or from exudate of Bartholin's gland.

(2) For culture, test material soon inoculated into fresh blood agar and chocolate agar at 37°C for 48 hours. Then colonies are studied. (Typical colony — circular, convex, translucent, glistening, greyish colour).

B. Indirect method:

(1) *Peripheral blood* — show Polymorphonuclear leucocytosis.

(2) *Serology* — by complement fixation test — This is positive only when the disease is present for serveral weeks or when pelvic complications have appeared.

5. MENINGOCOCCUS

Q. 3.23. Describe the morphological characteristics of Meningococcs. What are the lesions formed by this organism ?

(D.M.S. 1981)

The bacteria *Neisseria mengitidis* is known as *Meningococcus*. They are gram positive cocci, planoconvex in shape, non-motile, non-sporing and non-flegellated cocci; having a very thin capsule occurs in pairs — flattened surfaces opposite to each other, occasionally single or in tetrads usually they are intracellular (within polymorphs or pus cell), rarely extra cellular.

Size — 0.8 milimicron. *Ivolution forms* — frequent in older cultures, particularly alkaline media.

Colonies on solid media in 24-48 hours; smooth translucent, round (1-2 mm. diameter), bluish grey.

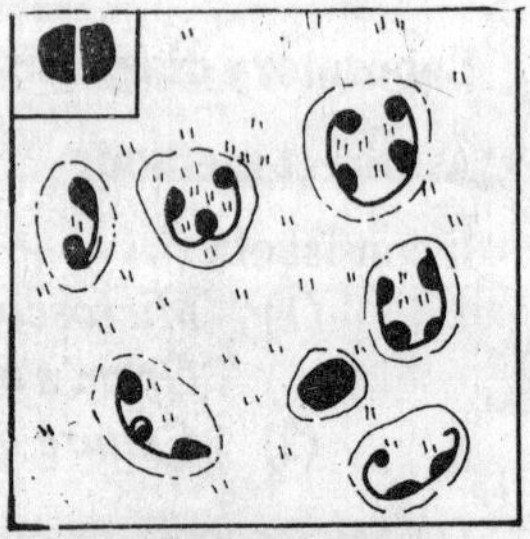

MENINGOCOCCUS

Pathogenic lesions:

In man produces:

1. Local Neso-pharyngitis.

2. Meningococcemia or Meningococcal Septicemia.

(a) Acute Septicemia or Spotted fever:

High fever, and petechial rashes due to acute vessculitis of small vessels causing petechial haemorrhages in skin serous membranes.

(b) Waterhouse-Friderichseen Syndrome.

An acute inflammatory condition due to meningococcemia- characterised by:—

(i) Sepsis.

(ii) Bilateral adrenal cortical necrosis and Haemorrhage due to extensive vascular damage.

(iii) Peripheral circulatory collapse.
(iv) Acute adrenal insufficiency.
(v) Death in 24 hours.

(c) Chronic Meningococcal Septicemia:

Characterised by Remitent fever, Recurrent maculopapular, skin rash, and Migratory arthralgia.

3. Acute meningococcal meningitis or Cerebrospinal meningitis.
4. Involvement of other tissues due to metastatic foci of infection.

e.g. Otitis media, Arthritis and Infective Endocarditis etc.

Q. 3.24. How will you diagnosis a case of Meningococcal Meningitis ?

Direct

It is done on finding the organism in Cerebro Spinal Fluid (obtained by Lumbar puncture).

Procedures for diagnosis include:—

(1) Physical, chemical and cytological examination of C.S.F. for characteristic findings.
(2) Smear prepared from centrifused deposit of the fluid (for studing morphology).
(3) Culture of the fluid for isolation and biochemical reactions.

C.S.F.

1. It is turbid under high pressure and in increased quantity. It contains more albumin than normal. Sugar is diminished or absent, chloride is diminished. It contains in large numbers polymorphs.

2. *Smear*: It shows Gram negative intracellular diplococci (sometimes extracelular).

3. *Culture*: It is made on blood or chocolate agar in an atmosphere of 10% CO_2. After isolation they are identified by fermentation tests and agglutination test (Ferment Maltose and Glucose).

Q. 3.25. Name the organisms which are responsible for meningitis.

These are:

Pneumococcus, Meningococcus, Staphylococcus, Streptococcus, Gonococcus. H. influenzae, Coliform bacilli, B. anthracis, Mycobacterium tuberculosis, Treponema pallidum, Streptothrix etc.

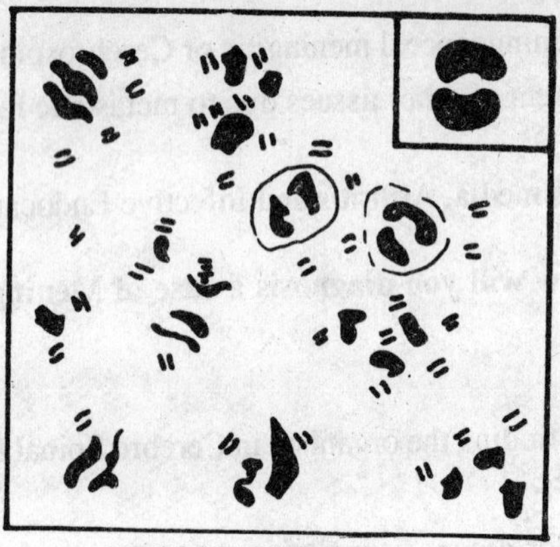

GONOCOCCUS

Q. 3.26. Describe the changes occur in C.S.F. due to meningo-coccal infections?

Collection of C.S.F. is generally done by Lumbar puncture; 3-4 samples, each of 2-4 ml. collected in sterile containers.

C.S.F. FINDINGS IN MENINGITIS

Test	In Normal	Findings during Meningitis	
		Acute stage	Sub-acute stage
1.*Physical*			
(a) Appearance	Clear	Turbid	Clear/Opalescent
(b) Pressure	50-150 mm. of H_2O	Raised	Raised
2.*Chemical*			
(a) Total protein	15-40 mg%	Greatly increased	Moderately increased
(b) Sugar	50-70 mg%	Greatly reduced may be nil.	Reduced
(c) Chloride	700-740 mg%	Reduced	Reduced

3. *Cytology* Cell count and cell types	0-5 cells/ cu. mm. and all lymphocytes	Greatly increased to about 20,000/ cu. mm. and mainly polymphos	Increased in hundreds mostly lymphocytes
4. *Culture*	*Sterile*	Causative organism	M. tuberculosis
5. *Blood*	Normal	Polymophonuclear leucocytosis and + ve meningococcemia.	

N.B.–Other findings: **In Bacteriological Examination:**

A specimen of C.S.F. is centrifused at 1500 RPM. The deposit is taken and subjected to:

(a) Smear and Gram stain-showing Gram-ve Cocci in pairs, bean shaped, some intra-cellular, some extra-cellular.

(b) Culture-on Chocolate Agar-incubation at 37°C, in presence of 5-10% CO_2, for 24 hours. Shows typical colonies.

For confirmation:

(1) Smear and *Gram stain.*
(2) Oxidase Test—*Colony turns black.*
(3) Biochemical Reaction—*Ferments Glucose and Maltose with production of acid only.*
(4) Agglutination with type specific antisera:—
Bordet — Durham Reaction.

Q. 3.27. What are the differences between N. meningitidis and N. gonorrhoea ?

	N. Meningitidis	N. Gonorrhoea
1. Occurrence of the disease.	Responsible for meningitis.	Responsible for gonorrhoea.
2. Habitat and mode of infection.	May occur in healthy carriers. This organism resides in the nasopharyx and goes to the meninges either directly through the ethmoid bone or commonly via haematogenous route.	No such. It is transmitted from one person to another through sexual contact.

3. Morphology	In clinical specimen these organisms are seen as gram negative intracellular diplococci. They are *bean shaped* in appearance with their long axis parallel to each other or concave surfaces opposed, non-motile, non-sporing cocci.	Same as meningococci. The characteristic diplococcal form is best seen in pus.
4. Cultural characters	Culture easy on chocolate agar at 37 °C in 5—10% CO_2, colonies are tranluscent, round, convex and with smooth glistening appearance after 24 hours of incubation.	Same as meningococcus.
5. Bio-chemical reactions	It ferments maltose and glucose in sugar tube with production of acid only.	Ferment only glucose.

CHAPTER 4

IMPORTANT BACILLI

DISCUSSION FOR LEARNING

I. Non-Spore forming gram positive bacilli

1. *Corynebacterium diphtheriae.*
2. *Schick test.*

II. Spore forming gram positive bacilli

3. *Bacillus anthracis.*

III. Clostridia

4. *Clostridium welchii*
5. *Clostridium tetani*

IV. Mycobacterium

6. *Mycobacterium tuberculosis.*
7. *Tuberculin test.*
8. *Mycobacterium leprae.*

V. Filamentous bacteria

VI. Enterobacteriaceae (Coliform bacteria)

9. *Escherichia coli.*
10. *Salmonella typhi*
11. *Widal test*
12. *Shigella.*

VII. Vibrionacae

13. *Vibrio cholerae.*
14. *Pasteurella pestis.*

VIII. Spirochates

IX. Riketisiae

X. Mycoplasma.

I. NON-SPORE FORMING GRAM POSITIVE BACILLI

1. CORYNEBATERIUM DIPHTHERIAE

Q. 4.1. What is meant by Corynebacterium ?

Coryne means (clubshaped), as the shape of the diphteria bacillus is clubshaped it is known as Corynebacterium diphtheriae. This shape is generally due to the presence of metachromatic granules at its body ends.

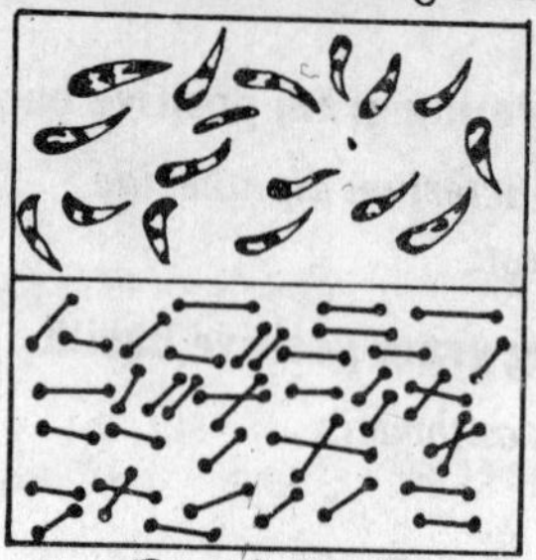

Cory. diphtheriae

The various species of the Genus-Corynebacteria are:

1. Pathogenic

(a) *Corynebacterium diphtheriae* (Types-gravis, intermedius and mitis)

(b) *Cory. ovis.*

(c) *Cory. pyogenes.*

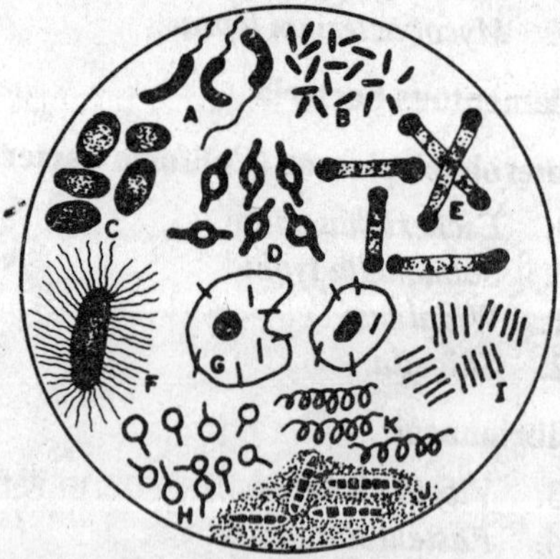

Fig:—3

A.	Vibrio cholerae	B.	Brucella abortus
C.	Pasteurella pestis	D.	Claustridium welchii
E.	Cory. diphtheriae	F.	Salm. typhi
G.	Myco. tuberculosis	H.	Claustridium tetani
I.	Myco. leprae	J.	Bacillus anthracis
K.	spirillum.		

2. Pathogenicity (doubtful)
(a) *C. acne*

3. Commensal
(a) *C. xerosis*
(b) *C. hofmanni*
(c) *C. renali*

Q. 4.2. What is the causative organism of the disease Diphtheria ? or What is meant by K.L.B. ?

The causative organism of diphtheria is *Corynebacterium diphtheriae.* This is also known as *Klebs-Loeffler Bacillus* (K.L.B.).

Q. 4.3. What is Sore Throat ? What are it causes ?

Sore throat refers to acute inflammation of the tonsils and faucial areas. This may be accompained by exduation leading to the formation of a pseudomembrane.

Organisms causing sore throat are:

Organisms Causing Sore Throat

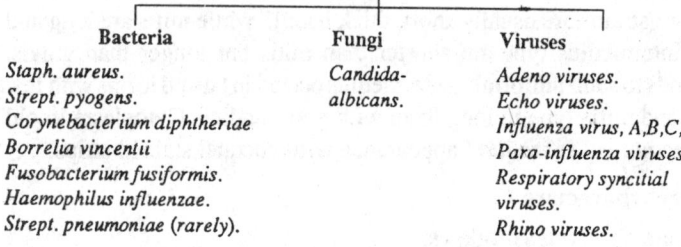

Bacteria	Fungi	Viruses
Staph. aureus.	*Candida-albicans.*	*Adeno viruses.*
Strept. pyogens.		*Echo viruses.*
Corynebacterium diphtheriae		*Influenza virus, A,B,C,*
Borrelia vincentii		*Para-influenza viruses*
Fusobacterium fusiformis.		*Respiratory syncitial viruses.*
Haemophilus influenzae.		*Rhino viruses.*
Strept. pneumoniae (rarely).		

Q. 4.4. What do you know about Cory. diphtheriae ? or Describe the morphological and cultural characters of Cory. diphtheriae.
[C.U. 1979, DMS. 75, 76 (Dec.) 71, 78, 79, 81]

In the genus-Corynebacterium, the species which are most pathogenic to man are ***C. diphteriae and C. ulcerans.*** The other species which of little clinical significance to man are collectively known as ***Diphtheroids.***

Corynebacterium diphtheriae is responsible for diphtheria. Three biotypes of C. diphtheriae are recongnised, viz. *gravis, intermedius* and *mitis.* All produce a powerful exotoxin which absorbs on to mucous surfaces, destroys epithelium and results in the formation of "Pseudomembrane" in the throat. *Gravis* is the most virulent type, followed by *intermedius* and *mitis* in that order. The treatment of the disease consists in early administration of antitoxin. Depending on the site of membrane formation, diphtheria may be pharyngeal, laryngeal or nasopharyngeal. Wound and skin diphtheria can also occur.

Morphology: These are aerobic, straight or slightly curved gram positive, bacilli, non-sporing, non-motile and non-acid fast. *Size*-3.5 x. 5 μ shows pleomorphism and beaded in appearance due to uneven staining. Morphologically they are best seen in smears made from growth on *Loeffler's slope.*

(a) In *Albert's stain* — The bacilli appear green and the metachromatic granules bluish black due to the volutin granules. The granules in gravis type are few or absent while mitis may show prominent granules.

(b) *In Gram's stain* —Gram positive slender rods, plomorphic, arranged in chinese letter ('L' and 'V') pattern. These peculiar arrangement of the organism is due to the method of division and incomplete separation during division. The organisms tend to decolourise rapidly, but granules retain their violet colour (so uneven in stained).

* *Gravis* strains are usually short, thick bacilli, while mitis are long and slander. Intermedius type are shorter than mitis but longer than gravis. Gravis tends to stain uniformly, intermedius occurs in barred forms with few granules and mitis type in long form with polar bodies. Cytoplasm in old cultures acquires '***Zebra like***' appearance with unequal stained strips.

Cultural characters

These are observed as follows:

(a) *In Loefflers Serum Slope*-Colonies are first small and circular, later become thick with crenated border.

(b) *In Tellurite blood agar*:—

(i) '*Gravis colonies*' are large, 5 mm in size, flat, greyish white, lustreless with friable consistency and '*daisy head*' appearance.

(ii) '*Intermedius colonies*' are small, 2 mm in size, lustreless with domed centre and irregular margin with '**frog egg**' appearance.

(iii) '*Mitis colonies*' are small, 3-4 mm in size, convex, grey to black, glossy colonies and butyrous consistancy with ***poached egg*** appearance.

(c) *In blood agar* — Matt colonies are produced. Gravis strain may show occasionally haemolysis. Intermedius strains are non-haemolytic. Mitis strains are usually haemolytic.

(d) *Broth culture* — Gravis produces granular growth. Intermedius and mitis produce uniform turbidity.

Q. 4.5. What is Babes-Earnst Bodies ? Or, Volutin granules.

Volutin granules of Cory. diphtheriae is known as "*Babes-Earnst Bodies.* These are metachromatic granules, which stain a different colour from the rest of the cell. These are stained dark purple with Albert's stain. Generally they are present at the polar end of C. diphtheria. Their number variable, usually less than size. They are inorganic polymerized polyphosphates, functioning energy storage. They can be seen by gram stain, but best demonstrated by Albert's stain.

Q. 4.6. What are the pathogenic effects of the bacteria C. diphtheriae ? [D.M.S. 1976 (Dec), 79)

Corynebacterium diphtheriae is responsible for diphtheria. Three biotypes of ***C. diphtheriae*** are recognised, viz. ***gravis, intermedius and mitis***. All produce a powerful exotoxin which absorbs on to mucus surfaces, destroys epithelium and results in the formation of "*pseudomembrane*" (made up of fibrin and leucocytes) in the throat. Gravis is the most virulent type, followed by intermedius and mitis in that order. Depending on the site of membrane formation, diphtheria may be pharyngeal, laryngeal or naso-pharyngeal. Wound and skin diphtheria can also occur.

N.B. * Generally children between 2-5 years of age are affected.
Site of infection—*Tonsil* or *Pharynx* or *Larynx* and *Nose*.

Colour — Dirty-greyish. Pseudomembrane composed of — Fibrinous exudates necrose epithelium, RBC and WBC.

** *Rapid multiplication* of bacilli occurs in the false membrane with production of toxin which on absorption gives rise to clinical symptoms; such as-toxaemia, fever, toxic myocarditis, heart block, acute cardiac failure, albumenuria, toxic nephrosis, fall in blood pressure (due to failure of suprarenals), palatalpalsy, polyneuritis, occular palsy.

*** *Complications* are brochopneumonia, mucosal haemorrhage in stomach, asphyxia, respiratory failure, diphtheritic paralysis (often transient, incomplete and localised).

*** *Local menifestations* are — aural, cutaneous, genital diphtheriasis and diphtheritic conjunctivitis.

Q. 4.7. How will we diagnosis a case of Diphtheria in Laboratory?
[C.U. 1971, D.M.S. 77, 78, 79, 81]

Laboratory Diagnosis of Diphtheria: It consists of— (i) Direct smear and culture, (ii) Test for Toxigenicity, (iii) Serological test, (iv) Schick test.

1. Smear and Culture

It consists of *smear examination and culture* of the material obtained from fauces, larynx or nose.

The specimen is collected with the help of strile swab. The swab is rubbed along the membrane, fauces, larynx or nose (turbinate bones) depending on the circumstances. Immediate inoculation gives best result. If delay in the examination is apprehended, swab is kept in contact with blood agar while in transit. Finding of the organism in smear or culture and determination of virulence in guineapigs complete laboratory procedures. Smear is examined after staining with *Neisser's or Albert's stain*. Culture is done on *Loeffler's inspissated serum and Potassium tellurite medium.*

N.B.

(a) In *Albert's stain* —The bacilli appears green with blue black beading due to the volutin granules.

(b) On *Loeffler's serum* —The colonies are small, circular, white and orange with thick centres and crenated borders.

(c) On *Tellurite medium*:

(i) *Gravis* —Relatively large, greyish black, flat lustreless colonies appearing like "*daisy heads*".

(ii) *Intermedis* —Relatively small, black, lustreless colonies with domed centres resembling "*frog egg*".

(iii) *Mitis* — Convex, smooth translucent colonies resembling "*Poached eggs*".

2. Test for Toxigenicity

(i) **In vivo**: *Inoculation of virulent stain in guinea pig causes*:—

(a) At the site of injection intense hyperaemia, necrosis and membrane formation.

(b) In adrenal glands — hyperaemia enlargement and haemorrhage (all visible on post mortem examination).

(ii) **In Vitro:** *Elek's gel precipitating* test for demonstrating the powerful exotoxin in the fauces.

A strip of filter paper is soaked in antitoxin, and placed on a serum agar plate. Test culture with diphtheria bacilli is streaked at right angles to long axis of filter paper. After incubation at 37°C for 48 hours, there will be precipitation of toxin by antitoxin along the strekes.

3. **Serology:— By Titration** — Estimation of antitoxin titre.

2. SCHICK TEST

Q. 4.8. What is Schick Test ? Describe it in details.

[C.U. 1981, D.M.S. 77, 79, 84]

Schick Test:

This is a test for knowing susceptibility to diphtheria toxin. Or it is an intradermal test:

(i) *To assess the immune status to diphtheria.*

(ii) *To determine the necessity for active immunisation. Children upto 12 years are assumed to be Schick Positive and immunized without testing.*

(iii) *As a retrospective diagnosis aid in case of suspected diphtheria.*

Principle

It is a test demonstrating presence or absence of antitoxin immunity i.e. presence or absence of circulating antitoxins in the host. If toxin is injected intracutaneously to a person with no antitoxin — there is local tissue damage and inflammation, indicating that the person is susceptible (Schick Positive).

If toxin is injected to person with fairly good level of antitoxin — no reaction will be there, due to neutralization of toxin by antitoxin; indicating that the person is immune (Schick Negative).

Procedure

Inoculum — Diphtheria toxin, diluted and stabilized (not toxoid). *Amount*-0.2 ml. *Route*-Intradermal. Site-Volar aspect of forearm. On the other forearm (control), injected the same amount of heated toxin (at 60°C at 15 minutes). Heat destroys toxin.

The test dose i.e. 0.2 ml. of the diluted toxin and the same dose of heated toxin is used as control. The skin of both forearms is washed with soap and swabbed with alcohol or ether. When dry, injection is made keeping the needle almost parallel with the skin and level upwards. When level is not in sight, injection of 0.2 ml. dilute toxin is made. The control (heated toxin) is injected into one forearm and the unheated toxin into the other.

Observation is made after 48 hours, and again after 1 week.

Observations and results

Test arm.	Local redness, erythema and oedema with in 24-28 hrs. Diameter—1—3 cm., persists for 4 days to 2 weeks.	No reaction.	Transient redness and swelling in 6-12 hours. (lasting for 72 hrs.) soon fades in both arms.	Local redness and swelling persists.
Control arm.	No reaction.	No reaction.		Transient redness. (in 24 hrs. and last for 72 hrs.), soon fades.
Inference.	Schick + ve.	Shick—ve.	Pseudo reaction Schick — ve.	Combined schick reaction.
Significance.	Susceptible or Frank diphtheritic.	Immune or Carrier.	Immune or Carrier.	Susceptible or tissue hypersensitivity.
Cause.	No antitoxin, so local tissue damage.	High level of antitoxin so toxin neutralized.	Tissue hypersentivity to non-toxic protein fraction of inoculum.	*

Interpretation of Schick Test and Throat swab test.

Schick Test	**Throat Swab**	**Inference**
+	+	Diphtheria

+	-	Susceptible
-	-	Immune
-	+	Carrier.

N.B. New born infant may be schick negative because of maternal antitoxin. In a few months the antitoxin disappears and they become schick positive. Children into 12 years are assumed to be schick positive.

Q. 4.9.How Immunization against Diphtheria is done ?

Active immunization of suceptible is done by formol toxoid, alum precipitated toxoid and Purified Toxoid Aluminium Phosphate (P.T.A.P). Formal toxoid is given in dose of 0.5 to 1 c.c. P.T.A.P is purified toxoid absorbed on to aluminium phosphate. It is stable free from bacteria and contaminants, and more potent in antigenicity. The advantage of this is that it gives little reaction.

Passive immunization is done by Anti Diphtheritic Serum (A.D.S). It protects the sufferer for only 2-3 weeks. To prevent diphtheria 1000 to 8000 units of antitoxin is injected within 24 hours of exposure to infection. Immunization with triple antigen (in three doses of one ml. at one month's interval) is an another way of achieving immunity against diphtheria.

II. SPORE FORMING GRAM POSITIVE BACILLI

Q. 4.10. Name some spore forming gram positive bacilli.

[D.M.S. 1977, 80]

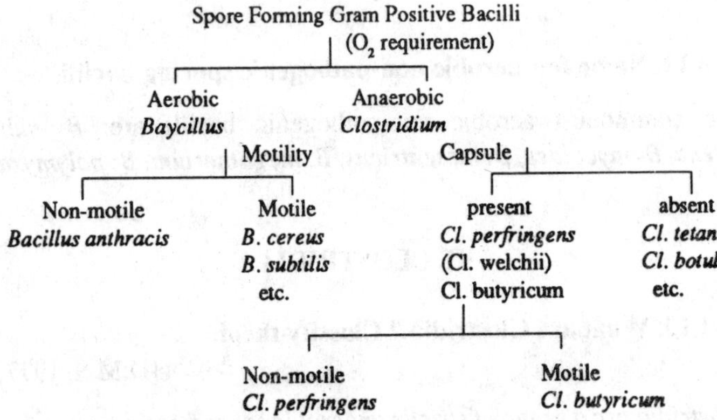

3. BACILLUS ANTHRACIS

Q. 4.11. What are the morphological characters and pathogenicity of the bacteria of B. anthracis (Anthax bacillus).

Morphology

(1) Gram positive, spore-bearing rods with truncated ends; aerobic, non-motile.

(2) Spores only formed in cultures and not in tissues (central, subterminal, but not bulging).

(3) Capsule (present in an animal body; lost in cultivation).

(4) Capsules stained by 1% solution (aqueous) of poly chromatic methylene-blue.

(5) *In culture* — (i) *On agar* — the colonies are white, granular and circular with waxy margins like, *medusa head.*

(ii) *Gelatin stab* — Shows an inverted fur tree growth appearance.

Pathogenicity

(1) Produces "*Splenic fever*" in cattle and sheep, from which man contracts infection.

(2) The bacillus enters in the human being through skin, respiratory tract, and alimentary tract and produces malignant pustule (skin), woolsorters disease (lungs) and intestinal anthrax.

(3) Complications are septicaemic or cerebrospinal meningitis.

Q. 4.12. Name few aerobic non-pathogenic sporing bacilli.

The commonest aerobic non-pothogenic bacilli are: *B. subtilis, B. cereus, B. mycoides, B. mesentricus, B. megatherium, B. polymyxa.*

III. CLOSTRIDIA

Q. 4.13. What are Clostridia ? Classify them.

[D.M.S. 1977, 80]

Clostridia are a group of strictly anaerobic spore forming, gram postive

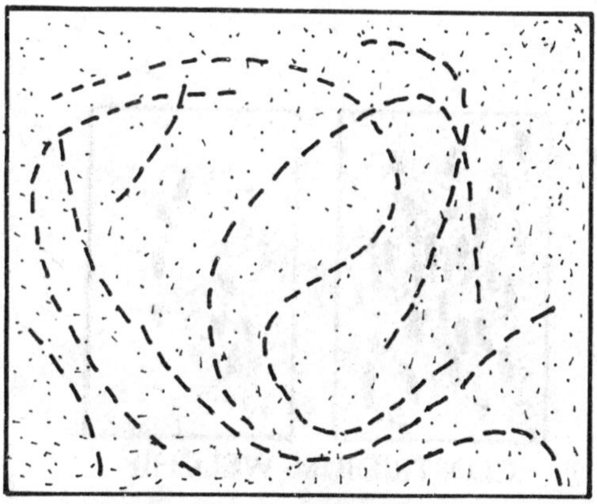

BACILLUS ANTHRACIS

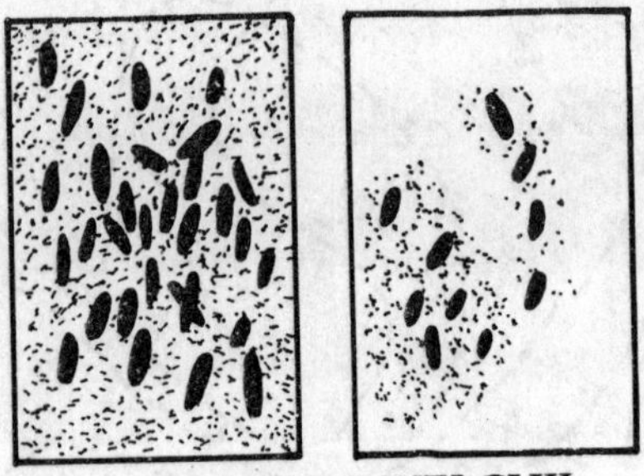

CLOSTRIDIUM WELCHII

Bacteria	Fungi	Viruses
Staph. aureus. *Strept. pyogens.* *Corynebacterium diphtheriae* *Borrelia vincentii* *Fusobacterium fusiformis.* *Haemophilus influenzae.* *Strept. pneumoniae* (*rarely*).	*Candida-albicans.*	*Adeno viruses.* *Echo viruses.* *Influenza virus, A,B,C,* *Para-influenza viruses* *Respiratory syncitial viruses.* *Rhino viruses.*

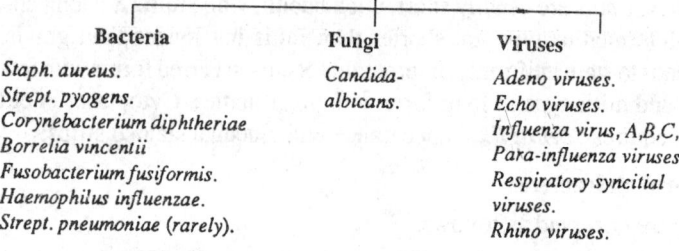

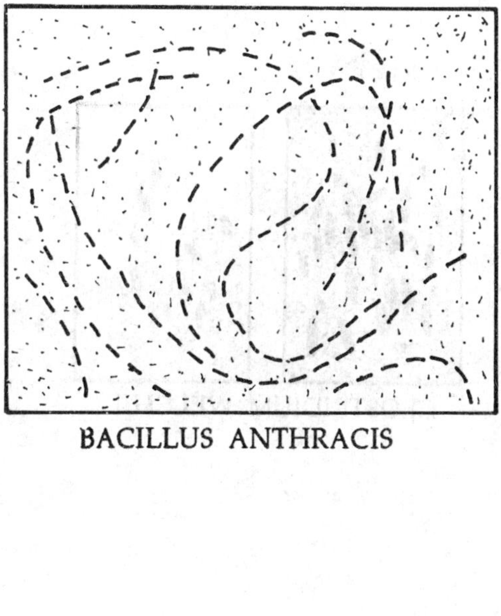

BACILLUS ANTHRACIS

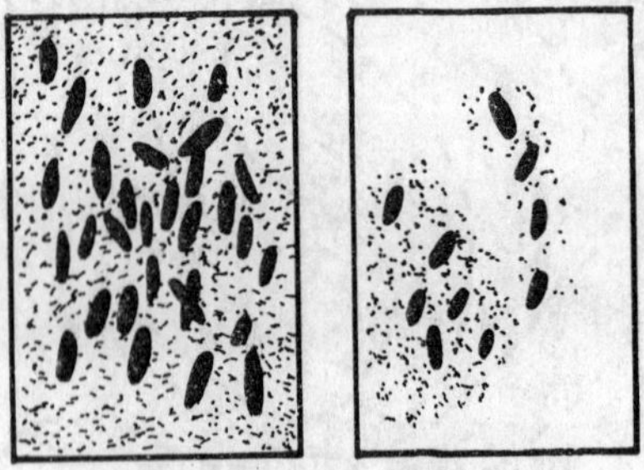

CLOSTRIDIUM WELCHII

bacilli. Generally the spores of these bacteria are wider than the other bacteria of the genus bacillus and produce a distinct bulge.

Generally they are classified on the basis of disease production, bio-chemical activity and morphological characteristics.

1. Based on disease production and bio-chemical activity:

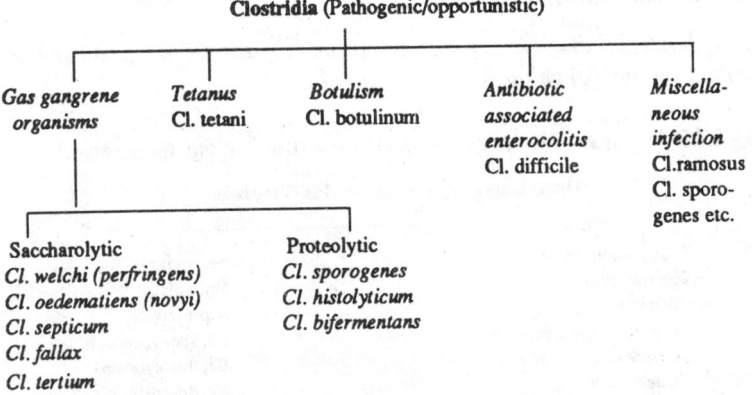

Clostridia (Pathogenic/opportunistic)

- *Gas gangrene organisms*
  - Saccharolytic: *Cl. welchi (perfringens)*, *Cl. oedematiens (novyi)*, *Cl. septicum*, *Cl. fallax*, *Cl. tertium*
  - Proteolytic: *Cl. sporogenes*, *Cl. histolyticum*, *Cl. bifermentans*
- *Tetanus* — Cl. tetani
- *Botulism* — Cl. botulinum
- *Antibiotic associated enterocolitis* — Cl. difficile
- *Miscellaneous infection* — Cl.ramosus, Cl. sporogenes etc.

2. Based on morphological characters:

(a) Thick rectangular gram positive bacilli—Cl. perfringens, Cl. fallax, Cl. bifermentans.

(b) Boat or leaf shaped pleomorphic bacilli with irregular staining — Cl. septicum.

(c) Slender bacilli with round terminal spores — Cl. tetani, Cl. tetanomorphum.

(d) Large bacilli with oval subterminal spores — Cl. oedematiens.

4. CLOSTRIDIUM WELCHII

Q. 4.14. What is meant by gas gangrene ?

Gas gangrene refers to the gangrene of tissues, associated with gas formation. The disease generally follows war injuries, road accidents and other types of injuries involving crushing of large muscle masses. The causative agent include *Clostridium perfringens* (60%), *Cl. odematiens, Cl. septicum* (20-40%) and *Cl. histolyticum* in that order, other species such as

Cl. sporogenes, Cl. fallax, Cl. bifermentans, Cl. sordellii, Cl. acrofoetida and *Cl. tertium* are only occasionally isolated.

In the *early stages*, gas gangrene may be clinically indistinguishable from anaerobic streptococcal myositis. In streptococcal myositis gram's stained smear show of large number streptococci and pus cells, but no bacilli. In contrast, smears made from gas gangrene tissue show diverse bacterial flora with scanty pus cells.

[*The bacterial diagnosis of gas gangrene is made by (a) direct smear examination and (b) culture*]

Q 4.15. What are the organisms responsible for gas gangrene ?

Organisms Responsible for Gas Gangrene

True pathogens or Saccharolytic clostridia
- *Cl. welchii (perfringens)*
- *Cl. oedematiens (novyi)*
- *Cl. septicum*
- *Cl. tertium*
- *Cl. fallax*

Secondary Proteolytic saprophytes
- *Cl. sporogenes*
- *Cl. histolyticum*
- *Cl. bifermentans*

Q. 4. 16. What are the morphological characteristics of the bacteria Clostridium welchii ?

Morphology

Gram positive spore bearing rod with ends truncated; Size — 5 μx1.5μ. Arranged singly or in pairs; capsulated, non-motile. Spores not found in the wound (tissues), but rarely seen in culture and when grow in special media. Spores are large oval, central or subterminal and non projecting. Size — 4-6μ x 1μ. Capsules are formed only in tissues, but not usually seen in culture.

Types

On the basis of toxin production *Cl. welchii* divided into type A, B, C, D, E and F.

Q. 4.17. What are the toxins produced by Cl. welchii ?

Clostridium welchii liberates different types of toxins and enzymes. Atleast 12 different toxins are produced by different types of *Cl. welchii* (types are A, B, C, D, E and F).

These toxins are:

Major Lethal Toxins	Minor Lethal Toxins
α—toxin	*Eta toxin*
β toxin	*Theta toxin*
Epsilen toxin	*Lambda toxin*
Iota toxin	*Nu toxin*
	Gamma toxin
	Delta toxin
	Kappa toxin
	Mu toxin

All toxins are antigenic. All stains produce alpha toxin.

Alpha toxin is a lecithinase and is demonstrated by the nagler reaction. The reaction is based on the fact that α— toxin of Cl. welchii will split lipoprotein of serum or egg yolk into an insoluble precipitate and produce an opacity in the culture media. The reaction is inhibited specifically by the antitoxin of *Cl. welchii*. The positive reaction indicates the toxigenic strain of *Cl. welchii*. The method is that an agar plate containing 20% human serum is at first dried. Few drops of alpha antitoxin are then spread over half the plate. Both halves are now inoculated with cultures and incubated overnight at 37°C in an anaerobic jar. An area of opacity surrounds the growth of *Cl. welchii* on the side of the plate without anti-toxin. On the side of antitoxin the reaction is prevented and so the surroundings of the growth remains clear.

Beta-toxin is lethal and necrotising effect.

Epsilen toxin is a prototoxin requiring for activation proteolytic enzymes.

Iota toxin has a lethal and necrotising effect. It is also activated by proteolytic enzymes.

Gamma and *Eta toxins* are minor lethal toxins.

Delta toxin is haemolytic to red blood cells of sheep, goats etc.

Theta toxin is a haemolysin (green).

Kappa toxin is collagenase and causes disintegration of muscles and connective tissue in gas gangrene.

Lambda toxin is proteinase and gelatinase.

Mu toxin is a hyaluronidase and helps in the spreading of infection.

Nu toxin is deoxyribonuclease.

Q. 4.18. What are the pathogenic effects of Cl. welchii ?

1. *Type A* (Cl. welchii) *chiefly responsible for gas gangrene in man.*

2. Also produces puerperal fever, cholecystitis, appendicitis, enteritis, peritonitis.

3. Factors which favour their multiplication in tissues are — crush injuries, blood clot (supply calcium), inadequate drainage, exudation in muscle fibres, contamination with soil, presence of secondary ogranisms (maintain anaerobic condition and pH for growth).

4. Pathological changes in gas gangrene are massive necrosis of the affected (subcutaneous tissue, muscles, blood vessels), gas bubble and haemorrhagic exudate.

5. The pathogenesis is that secondary infection of the wound with streptococci and staphylococci produce anaerobiasis and following this saccharolytic organisms grow on sarcolemma and break down muscle glycogen into CO_2, H_2 and lactic acid. Acidity which is not favourable for the saccharolytic organisms is overcome by multiplication of proteolytic group of organisms, profuse exudate and calcium salts. By this time, toxins are liberated and suprarenal glands are suppressed with a fall in blood pressure. Damage to the myocardium accounts for sudden heart failure.

Q. 4.19. How can we diagnosis a case of Cl. welchii infection in laboratory ?

Laboratory diagnosis consists of:—

(1) Microscopic examination of the exudate.

(2) Culture.

(3) Animal inoculation test.

However, isolation of clostridium form a wound does not always indicate gas gangrene. The diagnosis must take into a account clinical findings. Smears are examined after staining with gram's method. Thick rectangular bacilli suggest clostridium group of organisms. Spores are not seen in case of *Cl. welchii*. Culture is done on blood agar, nutrient agar, MacConkey's medium in tubes of Robertson's cooked meat medium and litmus milk tube. Nagler reaction is examined for knowing toxigenicity.

Pathogenicity test is done in mice or guineapig. For this five groups of mice are prepared — (i) *normal*, (ii) *immunized against Cl. welchii*, (iii) *immunized against Cl. septicum*, (iv) *immunized against Cl. oedematiens* and (v) *immunized against all these.*

Animals protected against the homologous organism survive, whereas control and those protected against other organisms are killed. If the case is of mixed infection, group five animals survive and others die. This, thus provides a method for isolating and identifying individual species from the mixture. On intramuscular inoculation into guineapig, Cl. welchii gives rise to massive *crepitant swelling with much gas*. Muscles are pale and necrotic and adrenals are congested.

5. CLOSTRIDIUM TETANI

Q. 4.20. What is Tetanus ? [D.M.S. 1977,78,80]

Tetanus is a disease characterised by tonic muscular spasms, usually commencing at the site of infection and later involving the whole of the somatic muscular system. (*Lock jaw* is quite frequently an early sign of tetanus in man.)

Q. 4.21. What is the Causative organism of the disease tetanus ?

Clostidium tetani is the causative organism of tetanus.

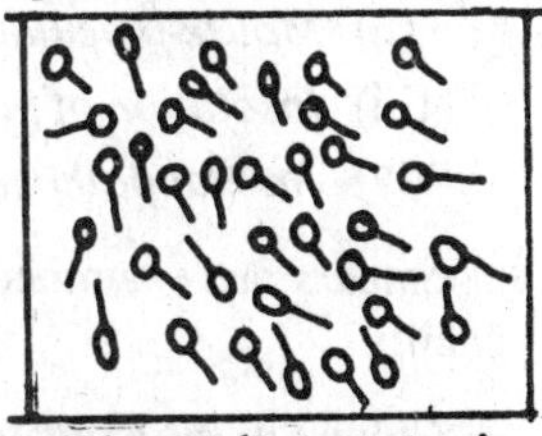

Clostridium tetani

Q. 4.22. Give its morphological characteristics and the name of the toxions produced by it. [D.M.S. 1977, 78, 80]

Morphology

(1) Gram positive long, slender rod, non-acid fast, motile (by peritrichae flagella). (2) Size 2-5μx 0.4μ; show involution forms. (3) Spores terminal, round and much wider than the organism giving a *drumstick appearance*.

Toxions

Produces *fibrinolysin, haemolysin, exotoxins* (e.g *tetanospasmin, tetanolysin*). *Tetanospasmin* is toxic to the motor end plates and hence called *neurotoxin*. *Tetanolysin* has haemolytic effect.

Q. 4.23. What are its pathogenicity ? [D.M.S. 1978,80]

1. It causes *tetanus* in animals (mices, guineapigs, rabbits) and man.

2. The tetanic spasm starts at the site of injection. However, it may be negligible. This is followed by lock jaw (*tismus*). Spasm in facial muscle, jaw and neck gives rise to a characteristic facial expression called *Rhisus Sardonicus*. Spasm gradually spreads to other skeletal muscle and during

spasmodic attack *opisthotonus* (resting on head and heel) is found. Spasms are both tonic and clonic. There is high fever. Death comes on account of exhaustion, asphyxia or heart failure.

3. The toxin from the site of infection reaches CNS through nerve trunk. It interferes with the vital enzyme system here, probably, choline metabolism of nerve cells is disturbed and so avilability of acetylcholine is impaired.

Q. 4.24. How can we diagnosis a case of tetanus infection ?

Laboratory diagnosis:

It consists of:

(i) *Smear preparation from wound exudate.*
(ii) *Mouse inoculation.*
(iii) *Insolation of pus culture.*
(iv) *Animal pathogenicity test.*

Smears are examined after staining by Gram's method for drumstick bacilli.

Culture of the exudate is made in cooked-meat medium (anaerobically). Then it is injected (0.2 ml. of 5-10 days culture) at the base of mouse's tail. Stiffness of the tail indicates the bacillus. Following this there is generalised involvement of muscles.

For isolation, the test material is heated to 80°C for 10 minutes. This destroys spreaders like proteus. Now the specimen is inculcated in Filde's peptic blood agar slope and incubated anaerobically. Edge of the culture in Cl. tetani case, shows after 24—48 hours fine filamentous growth above the matter of condensation in motile strains (on hand lens examination).

Final identification requires animal pathogenicity test in mice or guineapigs.

Q. 4.25. What are its main Bio-chemical activities ?

[D.M.S. 1978, 80]

1. It produces no change in milk media.
2. Does not liquefy coagulated serum.
3. Liquefies gelatin.

4. Does not ferment any carbohydrate such as glucose, maltose, lactose, salicin, sucrose etc.

Q. 4.26. How immunization are done against tetanus ?

Immunization in Tetanus is of three types:

1. **Active**
2. **Passive**
3. **Combined—Active and Passive.**

1. Active immunization is done by *formol toxoid* or *Alum Precipitate Toxoid (A.P.T).*

The dose schedule is as follows:

1st Injection —1 ml. I.M.

2nd Injection —1 ml. I.M. (after 6 weeks)

3rd Injection —1 ml. I.M. (after 9 months)

4th Injection when sustained injury after a year.

It is indicated in cases of deep punctured wounds, stab wounds animal bite, lacerated wound, children, road accident, wounds of farm-workers etc. Substantial immunity is achieved after the 2nd Injection. The immunity gained after 3rd injection lasts for about one year.

2. Passive immunization—Immunising agent—*Antitoxin or Anti-Tetanus Serum* (A.T.S.)

Passive immunization is indicated in non-immune person liable to suffer tetanus. It provides protection of short duration and can give rise complications like anaphylatic reaction during administration. The prophylactic dose of antitoxin is 1500 I.U. ½ I.M. or S.C. as soon as possible after injury. The dose is repeated at weekly intervals when wound is not heated. A large dose (3000-10,000 I.U.) advocated in case of severe wound. The antitoxin should never be given I.V. for prophylaxis.

3. Combined active and passive immuunization—Simultaneous injection of horse A.T.S. (A.T.S. 1500 units) or A.T.G. (Human antitetanus immunoglobulin) 250 units in one arm, and A.P. Toxid (0.5 ml.) in the other arm. This is followed after 6 weeks, by another dose of 0.5 ml. of A.P.T.

IV. MYCOBACTERIUM

6. MYCOBACTERIUM TUBERCULOSIS

Q. 4.27. What are the basic characteristics of mycobacterium ?

The basic characteristics of mycobacteria are:

(i) Gram positive, non-sporing, non-motile, strictly aerobic bacilli.

(ii) They are acid fast.

(iii) Cell wall contains a special waxy material-mycolic acid.

(iv) They grow very slowly in artificial culture media.

(v) They have a tendency to branching.

(vi) Their lesions are characteristically granulomatous type (in chronic cases).

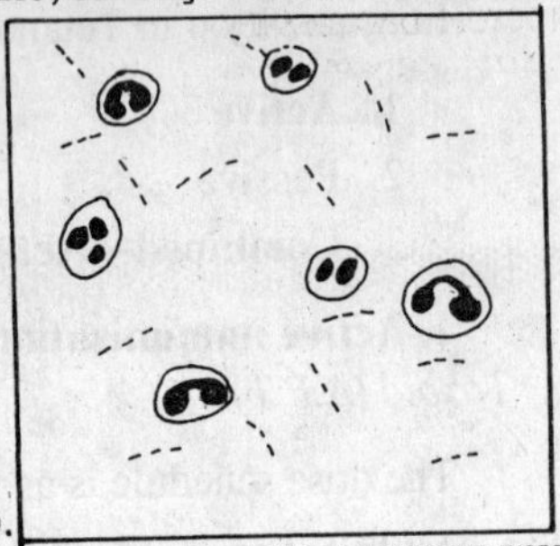

MYCOBACTERIUM TUBERCULOSIS

Q. 4.28. What is meant by atypical or anonymous or opportunist mycobacteria ?

These are a group of mycobacteria resembling tubercle bacilli morphologically, and produces lesions in man indistinguishable from tuberculosis.

But atypical mycobacteria give positive results in any two or more of the four screening tests i.e. they either:

1. Grow at 25° C

or, 2. Grow in presence of P-Nitro Benzoic Acid (P.N.B.A).

or, 3. Poduce pigments

or, 4. Grow in presence of thiacetazone.

Q. 4.29. What is acid fast stain ?

It is a type of differential staining, meant for bacteria which are impermeable and resistant to simple and usual stains (e.g. gram stain), due to their rich lipid content.

Synonym—*Ziehl-Neelsen Stain.*

Q. 4.30. What is the principle of acid fast stain ? [C.U. 1979]

Acid fast bacteria are those which retain a concentrated dye (Carbol fuchsine) and resist decolorisation by strong (20%) sulphuric acid, thus being stained-red and are the basic principle of acid fast staining. Non acid fast are those which are decolorized by strong (20%) sulphuric acid, and stained-blue (i.e. they take up the colour of the counter stain-methylene blue). Some bacteria, e.g. *Mycobacteria*, with lipid rich cell wall, prevent staining by ordinary dyes; but on forced staining with concentrated hot dyes like carbol fuchsine, they remain the dye and resist decolorisation with strong sulphuric acid. Such bacteria, are acid fast. *Acid fast organisms are also alcohol fast.*

Q. 4. 31. Name of the common acid fast bacilli pathogenic to man.
[C.U. 1979, D.M.S. 78, 79]

Name of the Acid fast bacilli which are pathogenic to man, are:

1. Parasitic Mycobacteria

(a) *Mycobacterium tuberculosis* (i) Human type, and
(ii) M. bovis causes tuberculosis.

(b) *M. leprae*—Causes leprosy.

2. Saprophytes

(a) *M. ulcerans*—Produces indolent skin ulcers.
(b) *M. balnei*—Causes swimming pool granuloma.

3. Atypical Mycobacteria—Produce lung lesions indistinguishable from tuberculosis.

(a) *M. kansassii*
(b) *M. intracellulare*
(c) *M. xenopii*
(d) *M. fortuitum etc.*

Q. 4.32. Name some Non-pathogenic Mycobacteria.

1. *Mycobacterium butyricum.*
2. *M. stercoris.*
3. *M. Pheli* are non-pathogenic mycobacteris.

Q. 4.33. Mention the Salient morphological features of Mycobacterium tuberculosis. [D.M.S. 1976 (Dec.), 78, 79)

Morphological features of M. tuberculosis:

(**Types**—*Human, bovine, avian, murine, and cold blooded*),

Morphology—Slender, straight or slightly curved, rod-shaped organisms, sometimes rounded or expanded ends. They are weakly gram positive, occurs singly, or in pairs, or in clumps. *Size*—3 x 0.3 microns. Non-motile and non-sporing. Their special staining property is their ***acid and alcohol fastness***. They do not grow on ordinary media, but grow on media like *Low enstein—Jensen medium, Dorset egg medium, Petroff s medium, Dubois medium or Tween 80.*

Generally in the *cultural media* their colonies are dry, irregular tough and tenacious, wrinkled, initially white and later buff coloured. Virulent strains characteristically from "Serpentine cords" in culture.

* *In Human type*—Organisms are slender, slightly curved, and granular.

** *In Bovine type*—Straight, short stubby or stumpy, uniformly stained.

Q. 4.34. Describe the Pathogenicity of Mycobacteria ?

[D.M.S. 1978]

1. The *human types* are pathogenic to man, and mammalian animals.
2. The *avian types* are pathogenic to birds, rabbits and pigs.
3. *Cold-blooded type* produces lesions in cold-blooded animals and fish.
4. *The bovine type* is pathogenic to man and other mammal and causes often lesions of lymph nodes, bones and joints.
5. The human type has predilection for pulmonary lesions is man.
6. The human and bavine types cause tuberculosis in man which is a chronic inflammation with features of tubercle formation, caseation, ulceration, healing with calcification and fibrosis or death.
7. Sources of infection are sputum (of patient with pulmonary tuberculosis), milk (infected with bovine type) and discharge from tuberculosis lesion of breast (causes infection is suckling baby).
8. Organisms gain entry into the body through ingestion, inhalation skin and genitourinary tract (sometimes) and conjunctiva (rarely).
9. The disease spreads by direct extension, lymphatics, blood streams, tubes (such as bronchus, gastro intestional tract, genitourinary tract, serious cavities, meninges).

Q. 4.35. How can we diagnosis a case of tuberculosis ?

[C.U. 1979, D.M.S. 78 (Dec.), 79]

Laboratory diagnosis of tuberculosis consists of *direct* and *indirect methods.*

In direct method an attempt is made to find out the tubercle bacillus by subjecting the test materials (*sputum, laryngeal swab, pleural effusion, gastric lavage, faeces*), depending on the circumstance, to smear and cultural examinations and animal inoculation tests.

Indirect method utilises allergic reaction and consists of ***tuberculin tests and complement fixation test.***

VARIOUS METHODS OF DIAGNOSIS

1. Direct Methods

(a) *Smear and acid fast staining of sputum.*
It reveals acid fast bacilli, slender and beaded.

(b) *Culture*—Directly or after concentration of material, inoculation into low enstain Jensen medium or Dubo's media.
Typical colony in 4+8 weeks. Culture should not be discarded as negative for 8 weeks.

(c) *Animal inoculation* (In Guineapig).
This is confirmatory for diagnosis.

2. Indirect Methods

(a) *Blood picture*—Lymphocytosis and Monocytosis.
(b) *E.S.R.*—High.
(c) *Tuberculin test.*
(d) *Complement fixation test.*

1. Tuberculin Test

This test is based on the fact that tissues of infected person become sensitized to *tuberculin*. Now-a-days it is done by intracutaneous method of ***Mantoux***.

In Mantoux Test—0.1 C.C. of 1 in 10,000 dilution *'old tuberculin'* is injected intradermally into the skin of one forearm. A control is produced on the same forearm with normal saline similarly.

A positive reaction is characterized by the development within 48-72 hours of an area of erythema and infiltration, 10 mm. or more in diameter, at the site of the injection of the tuberculin. If test is found negative after 48 hours, a dilution of 1 in 10,000 is injected and if this is also negative test showed be repeated with 1 in 1000 dilution.

The value of tuberculin test is limited. It is because more and more persons give the test positive in the absence of infection with ageing. In young children a positive test has greater significance. At all other ages a negative reaction is of value as proof against a diagnosis of tuberculosis. It is pertinent to remember that in the earliest stages of the disease the test may be negative, and in very acute cases or in the last stages of the disease, a positive test may be obtained.

2. Complement fixation test

Complement fixation test with WKK antigen gives positive results in 70 to 80% cases of pulmonary tuberculosis but it is positive in chronic cases. Microscopic examination (for histo-pathology) of tuberculosis granuloma shows a central caseation with giant cells, epitheloid cells and lymphocytes. Surrounding these are fibroblasts. The tuberculous exudate shows preponderance of lymphocytes.

Q. 4.36. What is tubercle ?

The characteristic lesion of tuberculosis is the tubercle which is visible in naked eye like millet seed.

Microscopically—There is a central area of necrosis or caseation of tubercle. Generally the central parts is avascular, and bacilli being aerobic cannot grow in avascular central area with low PO_4. Highly fatty acid content in the caseous central area also inhibits the growth of bacilli. This is surrounded by nodular collection of epitheloid cells and scattered Langhan's type of giant cells. The epitheloid cells are modified mononuclear cells with a clear cytoplasm and pale vesicular nucleus. A zone of lymphocytes is present around the epitheloid cells. The zone of lymphocytes is surrounded by a zone of fibroses tissue and granulation tissue.

Q. 4.37. Are bacilli always found in the tubercle ?

In full formed tubercle by the time the epitheloid cells are formed, most of the bacilli are disintegrated. So it is difficult to isolate the bacilli.

Q. 4.38. What are the fate of a tubercle ?

Fate of a tubercle

1. Healing of lesion.
2. Spreading of lesion.

1. Healing of Lesion:

(a) *Spontaneous resolution*—Usually in experimental tubercles.

(b) *Fibrosis*—It is the hallmark of healing. Fibrosis takes place by proliferation of fibroblasts from the periphery, thus forming a fibrous capsule. Ultimately, the central caseous area is replaced by a solid fibrous nodule.

(c) *Calcification*—There may be dystrophic calcification of casous mass. Calcified mass may harbour living bacilli and may lead to relapse.

(d) *Osification.*

2. Speading of Lesions

Bacilli are carried by macrophages to surrounding tissue spaces; where new tubercle are formed. Finally tubercle coalase to form a large lesion.

Q. 4.39. What do you mean by primary focus or Gohn's focus in lung ?

Primary focus or Gohn's focus is a primary parenchymal lesion of a lung due to primary effects of Myco. tuberculosis. It is situated in any part of lung and subpleural in distribution. It measures about 8 mm. in diameter. In majority of cases, it is arrested and encapsulated by fibrous tissue. It may even be calcified thus healing may occur. Such healed lesion is known as *Gohn's body*. Primary focus in lung may be accompanied by involvement of lymphatics and the regional lymph nodes i.e. mediastinal group of lymph glands, tonsil with cervical lymph glands, bowel with mesenteric group of lymph glands.

Q. 4.40. What are the characteristics of primary type of tuberculosis ?

1. Occurs in childhood.
2. Lung (any part) is involved under the pleura.

3. Hilar lymph nodes show caseation (definitely involved).
4. Spread is rapid along the lymphatics.
5. Lesion exudative.
6. With little or fibrosis.
7. Healing by resolution or calcification and fibrosis.

Q. 4.41. What does characterise a post-primary tuberculosis ?

1. Usually affects young adult.
2. Area near the apex is involved.
3. Spread is slow often along the tissue spaces.
4. Lesion proliferative.
5. Fibrosis is a marked feature.
6. Hilar-lymph nodes may or may not be involved.
7. Lesion leads to, often, cavitation.
8. May heal by fibrosis and scar formation.

Q. 4.42. How can we diagnosis a case of tubercular meningitis ?

Laboratory diagnosis of Tubercular Meningitis:

Examination of C.S.F. is the main way to diagnosis a case of tuberculosis meningitis.

In tubercular meningitis (Suspected case) C.S.F. is secured by lumbar puncture and observed it.

1. Examination of C.S.F.

(a) Physical:

(i) Pressure—Increased.

(ii) Colour—Crystal clear, but on standing for sometimes, a fine 'cobweb coagulum' is formed.

(b) Chemical:

(i) Protein—Increased—60—100 mg. per 100 ml.

(ii) Sugar—Diminished less than 50 mg. ml.

(c) Cytological:

(i) Cell number—Increased (Pleocytosis) 200—400 cells per cubic mm.

(ii) Cell type—Lymphocytes.

(d) Bacteriological:

(i) *Smear*—With *cobweb cagulum* or with CSF centrifuge acid fast stain, shows acid fast bacilli.

(ii) *Culture*—By inoculation into Low-enstein-Jensen media. Positive result obtained after 6 weeks.

(iii) *Animal pathogenicity*:

By inoculation of C.S.F. into Gunineapig-Result obtained after 6 weeks.

(e) Coloidal gold curve—Meningitic.

2. Examination of Blood

(a) Monocytosis with relative lymphocytosis.

(b) E.S.R.—High.

Q. 4.43. What do you know about B.C.G. ?

The abbreviation stands for *Bacilli, Calmete, Guerin*. It is a vaccine.

Bovine strain of living attenuted tubercle bacilli are in suspension form in the vaccine. The organisms are rendered avirulent (attenuted) by prolonged subcultures in *glycerine bile potato medium*. The vaccine is used for active immunisation against tuberculosis only in those who show negative tuberculin test. It is administared subcutaneous and intracutaneously. The intraderma dose is 0.05—0.1 mg. of bacillus in 0.1 ml. It is stored at 3—6°C away from sunlight. B.C.G. makes tuberculin negative subjects, tuberculin positive with in two months. The positive reaction remain for 4 years. Subjects voccinated with B.C.G. should be kept away from the tuberculosis for at least 6 weeks. This contra indicated in tuberculin positive cases, and in individuals suffering from eczema, furunculosis measles, mumps whooping cough etc.

7. TUBERCULIN TEST OR MANTOUX TEST

Q. 4.44. What is tuberculin test ? Give in details.

Tuberculin test—*This is a test to delayed hypersensitivity of tissue in response to tuberculo-proteins.*

1. Principles

Tuberculin (the extract from tubercle bacilli; containing tuberculo-protein and other constituent) when injected in small amount:—

(a) In a normal healthy animal—results a negligible inflammatory response.

(b) In an animal who has a previous tubercular infection 4-6 weeks earlier; leads to *induration, oedema, erythema* and *pseudopodia* formation at the site of injection with 48-72 hours. This is positive tuberculin reaction, indicating existence of hypersensitivity to tuberculo-protein.

2. Material

(a) *Old Tuberculin* (O.T.):

Used by *Koch.* A concentrated filtrate of tuberculous broth culture (steamed killed) 6 weeks old on synthetic media.

(b) *Purified Protein Derivative* (P.P.D.)

Obtained by precipitation of proteins from O.T. by trichoroactic acid or half saturated solution of ammonium sulphate.

N.B. (i) Strength of tuberculin:

(a) Old tuberculin:
0.1 ml. of 1 in 10.000 dilution = 1 T.U. (Tuberculin Unit).
0.1 ml. of 1 in 1.000 dilution = 10 T.U.
0.1 ml. of 1 in 100 dilution = 100 T.U.

(b) P.P.D.=0.0001 ml. = 5 T.U.

(ii) Types of tuberculine test :

(a) *Intradermal method* (Mantoux test)—Most commonly used, most accurate and reliable.

(b) *Multiple puncture*—A layer of concentrated P.P.D. (100,000 T.U. per ml.) is applied to skin and six intradermal picks are made by a "Heaf gun". It is more rapid test, but not so easily standardised as mantoux test.

(c) *Tine test*:— A test disc containing P.P.D. is pressed on the forearm and a positive result is indicated by papules with induration of 2 mm. or more.

(d) *Others* :—(i) *Subcutaneous* (Koch).
(ii) *Cutaneous scarrification* (Von-pirquit).
(iii) *Patch or jelly* method (Volmer).
(iv) *Ophthalmic* (Calmette).

3. Procedure of Mantoux Test :

(a) 0.1 ml. of 1 in 10,000 dilution of O.T. in normal saline (or an equivalent amount of P.P.D.), is injected intradermally on flex or surface of one forearm. A similar dilution of normal saline is injected into the other arm as control.

(b) The results are read after 48-72 hours.

(c) *The negative test* is indicated by no change or negligible inflammatory change at the site of inoculation, (Tuberculin negative).

(d) *A positive test* is indicated by:

INDURATION (not less than 10 mm. in diameter), *with or without erythema, oedema and pseudopodia formation.*

These local reactions may be accompanied by focal reactions (flaring up of already present tuberculous lesions) or general reactions-fever, malaise, prostration etc.

Reading :

Longitudinal Diameter or induration:

less than 10 mm—Test is negative.
10 mm or more—Test positive.
more than 15 mm—Strongly positive.

** **An immediate reaction which passes off within 48 hours is considered negative.**

(e) If the test is negative after 48-72 hours, the test is repeated using 1 in 1000 dilution (10 T.U.) and if this is negative, a further test with 1 in 100 dilution (100 T.U.) is attempted. If this too, gives a negative result the patient is considered to be mantoux negative. A repeatedly negative result for a period of six weeks even on using gradually higher concentration of tuberculin, usually rules out the diagnosis of tuberculosis.

4. Interpretation of the tuberculin test + ive and - ive :

(a) Tuberculin positive :

1. It indicates presence of tuberculous infection in the body, either past infection at least 4-6 weeks old or active disease.
2. In a child below three years age-indicates active tuberculosis.
3. In a serial study, if there is conversion from tuberculin negative to positive; it indicates active tuberculosis.
4. It indicates a potential state in the host, in which active disease can

be caused without further exposure.

5. It indicates delayed hypersensitivity to tubercle bacilli.
6. *False positive test:*
   (a) Transient positive reactions, which disappear within 48 hours.
   (b) In warm climates, shows presence of other mycobacteria.

(b) Tuberculin negative:

1. It means that the individual has never had any contact with tubercle bacilli, past or present.
2. Individual has got no immunity to tuberculosis, so that there is more susceptibility to infection.
3. The test may be considered negative, if results are repeatedly negative for a period of six weeks, even on using higher concentration of tuberculin.
4. *False negative reactions*:
   (a) Due to loss of ability to express cell mediated immunity e.g. Acute miliary tuberculosis or overwhelming tuberculosis, sarcoidosis, hodgkins disease, lepromatous leprosy, Immunosupressive drugs like corticosteroids and cytotoxic agents, old age, gross malnutrition, intercurrent infection like measles, whooping cough and rheumatoid disease.
   (b) Last trimeter of pregnancy—due to interaction of placental hormones.
   (c) If the test is done too early (before 4 weeks of infection).
5. *Significance of tuberculin test:*
   (a) Early diagnosis particularly in children.
   (b) Mass surveillance.
   (c) Before giving B.C.G. (Screening Test).
   (d) After giving B.C.G. (to test efficacy of B.C.G.).
   (e) Deffential tuberculin test with antigens from the other mycobacteria helps in distinguishing tubercle bacilli from atypical mycobacteria.

Q. 4.45. Why the tuberculin test is done from lower dilution to higher dilution ?

In highly sensitized persons, or on using a very high dose of tuberculin or by giving tuberculin I.V., there may be anaphylactic reaction—associated with necrosis of the area, prostration, fever, sometimes hypothermia and death. This indicates a hypersensitive status to tuberculin. This is why,

it is customary to begin the test with lower dilution i.e. I.T.U. of old tuberculin and then gradually increase the dose.

8. MYCOBACTERIUM LEPRAE
(Hansen's bacillus)

Q. 4.46. What are the morphological characteristics of Hansen's bacillus ?
Give its pathogenesis and laboratory diagnosis ?

Mycobacterium leprae is commonly known as *Hansen's bacillus* and is one of the few organism which does not yet fulfil the Koch's postulates. It has not yet been grown on artificial culture medium though there are several reports claiming success.

Morphology

They are slender, straight or slightly curved rods with a beaded appearance, found in '***Cigar bundle***' patterns. It is slightly less acid fast than M. tuberculosis.

Length 1.5-8 μ (Arrangement like bundles of cigarettes), non-motile, non-sporing, non-capsulated and difficult to stain, show pleomorphism.

Pathogenesis

1. Causes a chronic infective granulomatous disease called *leprosy*.
2. Skin and nerves are affected.
3. Leprosy occurs in two forms namely, *lepromatous* and *tuberculoid.*
4. *Lepromatous type* is characterised by large number of bacilli in smear from skin and nasal mucosa and negative lepromin test.
5. *Tuberculoid type* is characterised by scanty bacilli in the skin lesion and absence of bacilli in the nasal mucosa and positive allergic test.
6. Nerve involvement early in tuberculoid type and late in other type (i.e. lepromatous).
7. Incubation period 2-3 years.
8. Children more susceptible than adults.
9. Lepromatous cases highly infective whereas tuberculoid type relatively non-infective.
10. Source of infection—*Sick person.*

11. Transmission through nasopharynx and injured skin. Intimate and prolonged contract with the leprosy patient is main mode of infection.
12. One more type of leprosy is undifferentiated type. In this type bacilli are not always found and allergic tests are often negative.

Laboratory diagnosis

It is done by demonstrating the acid fast bacilli inside the lepra cells in smear preparation (stained by the Ziehl—Neelsen technique). In case of doubt, tissue containing the organisms is ground up and injected into guineapigs. Absence of lesions suggest the leprosy bacilli. Specimens for examination are scrapings from nasal mucosa and skin suips from affected area.

Lepromin test is not of much help as many healthy persons give positive reactions.

Q. 4.47. Describe the Lepromin test.

In this test intradermal reaction to antigen of lepra bacilli is observed. The antigen used is lepromin which is a suspension prepared from leproma after trituration and prolonged boiling. The method is simple.

0.1 C.C. lepromin is injected intradermally. In a positive reaction an erythema and a small papule are produced at the site of injection in 48-72 hours. The reaction either disappears totally at the end of first week or changes to the late reaction. The late reaction is characterised by a nodule at the site of injection in 10-14 days. The nodule increases to a diameter of 1-2 cm. with necrosis in the centre. Positive reaction indicates allergic tissue response against invasion by bacilli. The test is negative in lepromatous but positive in tuberculoid cases. It is not definite in indeterminate and border line groups. The test is of help in classifying cases of leprosy and in assessing the prognosis.

It is not of much (to) help in the diagnosis of leprosy.

V. FILAMENTOUS BACTERIA

Q. 4.48.What are the bacteria in the sputum of a normal individual ?

The sputum of normal individuals may contain *Streptococci, Pneumococci, Diphtheroid bacilli, Micrococcus catarrhalis* and *Haemophilus influenzae.*

Q. 4.49. What is the name of the causative organism of the disease whooping cough ? Give its morphological characters.

The name of causative organism of the disease whooping cough is *Bordetella pertusis.*

It is gram negative, Ovoid rods, smooth form encapsulated.

Size—0.3 μ x 1.2 μ (short chains) in liquid media. Non-motile, non-sporing and non-acid fast.

Q. 4.50. Name some filamentous bacteria ?

Actinomyces and *Nocordia* are filamentous bacteria.

Actinomyces — Gram positive, non-acid fast, non-motile, micro-aerophilic or anaerobic bacilli. They are pathogenic to men and animals.

Nocardia—Gram + ve, branching filamentous rods, aerobic, weakly acid fast and no culture produce aerial hypha. The organisms are found mainly in soil.

VI. ENTEROBACTERIACEAF
(Coliform Bacteria)

Q. 4.51. What do you mean by Coliform bacteria or Entero bacteria ?

The lower intestinal tract contains a vast number of organisms belonging to genera:

Escherichia,	*Proteus,*
Klebsiella,	*Pseudomonas,*
Citrobacter,	*Shigella,*
Itafnia,	*Salmonella,*
Serratia,	*Alkalescens,* and
	Arizona.

These are called ***Coliform bacteria***. Instead of doing harm some of these produce useful components of the vitamin B complex.

Enterobacteria *is synonym of* ***coliform bacteria***. Those which are pathogens are mostly non-lactose fermenters in contrast to the saprophytes. However at times saprophytes are found as secondary invaders infections.

Generally member of Enterobacteriaceae consists of gram negative, non-sporing bacilli with the following characteristics:

(i) Can grow on very simple media.
(ii) Are either motile with peritrichate flegella, or non-motile.
(iii) Ferment glucose with or without gas production.
(iv) Reduce nitrates to nitrites.
(v) Are catalase positive.
(vi) Are oxidase negative.

These organisms differ from other gram negative bacilli like members of Vibrionaceae and Pseudomonadaceae is being oxidase negative and motile with peritrichus flagella.

9. ESCHERICHIA COLI

Q. 4.52. What is E. coli ? Give its morphological characters, cultural characteristics and bio-chemical activities. [C.U. 1981 (Sup.)]

E. coli (Escherichia coli) *is a commensal of gestro-intestinal tract frequently causing urinary tract infection and infantile diarrhoea.*

Morphology

They are gram negative bacilli, non-sporing, non-capsulated and there is no particular arrangement. Feebly motile with 4 to 8 peritrichate flagella.

Cultural characteristics

1. Grow in simple media.
2. Produce colonies—circular, raised, smooth and with faecal odour.
3. Lactose fermenters; so produce pink colonies on Mac- Conkey's plate.
4. Haemolysis on blood agar by pathogenic strains.
5. Gas at 44°C in MacConkey broth by faecal E. coli (Eijkman's test).
6. Haemolysis of human red cells by strain isolated from urine.
7. Produce uniform turbidity in broth.
8. Facultative anaerobe.

Biochemical activities

1. Ferment lactose, glucose, manital, sucrose (sometimes) to acid and gas.
2. IMVIC reactions are + + - -.
3. Does not liquefy gelation.
4. Does not split urea to NH_3.

5. Give positive ONPG test.

Q. 4.53. What are the pathogenic lesions produce by E. coli ?

Pathogenic Lesions

In man these are—Pyelitis, Pyelonephritis, Perinephric abscess, Cystitis, Hydronephrosis, Pynephrosis, Prostatitis, Epididymitis, Ureteritis, Renal failures; Wound infection, Ostomyelitis, Arthritis, Rarely Septic Endocarditis, Acute and chronic Cholecystitis, Cholangitis, Appendicitis, Peritonitis, Diverticulitis etc.

The pathogenicity of Esch. coli depends upon the presence of O and K somatic antigens. E. coli produces endotoxins. Modes of infection are—Direct extension, lymphatics and haematogenous.

Q. 4.54. What do you mean by U.T.I. ?

Urinary Tract Infections (U.T.I.) implies infections of the kidney, ureter and bladder. When the infection involves kidney or ureters only, it is referred to as upper U.T.I., whereas infection from bladder downwards (excluding urethra) is considered as lower U.T.I. The diagnosis of U.T.I. cannot be made an clinical features alone since some patients with signs and syumptoms of U.T.I. may not show significant bacteriuria ($\geq 10^5$ organism/ml) whereas asymptomatic patients may yield significant growth.

Therefore laboratory investigations are essential for confirmation of diagnosis U.T.I.

Q. 4.55. What are the main causes of U.T.I.? [C.U. 1981 (Sup)]

Organisms causing U.T.I.

Common	Uncommon	Rare
E. coli *K. Pneumoniae* *P. mirabilis* and *other Proteus sp.* *P. aeruginosa* *S. faecalis* *S. aureus.*	*Enterobacter-* *providence* *Serratia,* *Micrococcs type 3* *Alcaligenes.* *faecalis etc.*	*Candida-albicans* *Streptococci* other than group A & B.

Q. 4.56. How can we diagnosis a case of E. coli infection ?

[C.U. 1981 (Sup.)]

Diagnosis is made by finding the organism in urine sample or discharge. *Catheter specimen of urine is secured from females. In male mid-stream urine collected with aseptic precaution suffices.* Centrifused deposit of urine is cultivated in MacConkey's and blood agar plates. The growth is studied for its morphological, staining and biochemical characters.

Purulent discharge is examined after Gram's staining for the characteristic morphology of the organism. It is also cultured in suitable media to carry biochemical tests with the pure growth.

N.B. 1. **Direct smear** from sediments shows E. coli.

2. **Culture specimens**—(a) In blood agar show a zone of haemolysis.

(b) On MacConkey's medium after inoculation for 24 hours., Rose pink colony, metallic sheet, flat, non viscous, circular with distinct edges.

Biochemical test :

(a) Fermentation of glucose, lactose and dextrose with gas production.

(b) Indole reaction positive.

(c) Mannite motility positive.

10. SALMONELLA

Q. 4.57. What are the causative organisms of Enteric Fever and Food Poisoning ?

Salmonella groups of organisms are pathogenic for man and responsible for Enteric Fever and Food Poisoning. These are :

Salmonella

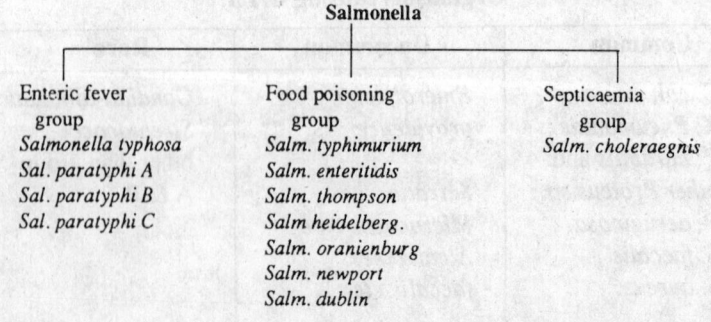

Enteric fever group	Food poisoning group	Septicaemia group
Salmonella typhosa	*Salm. typhimurium*	*Salm. choleraegnis*
Sal. paratyphi A	*Salm. enteritidis*	
Sal. paratyphi B	*Salm. thompson*	
Sal. paratyphi C	*Salm heidelberg.*	
	Salm. oranienburg	
	Salm. newport	
	Salm. dublin	

Q. 4.58. What are the causative organism of the disease Typhoid or Enteric fever and Paratyphoid fever ?

[C.U. 1979, 80, 82, D.M.S. 77, 80, 82, 84]

Salmonella typhi and Salmonella paratyphi A, B, C, are the causative organisms of typhoid or Enteric fever and Paratyphoid fever respecttively.

Q. 4.59. What are the main differences between S. typhi and para-typhi ?

Salm. typhi is anaerogenic. Ferments glucose and mannitol with production of Acid only and no gas.

Salm. paratyphi—Ferments Glucose and Mannital with production of acid and gas. No fermentation of lactose and sucrose. Indole reaction— Ve, Gelatin liquifaction—Ve.

Q. 4.60. What are the morphological, cultural and serological characteristics of Salmonella Typhi ? [D.M.S. 1972, 80, 82, 84]

Morphology:

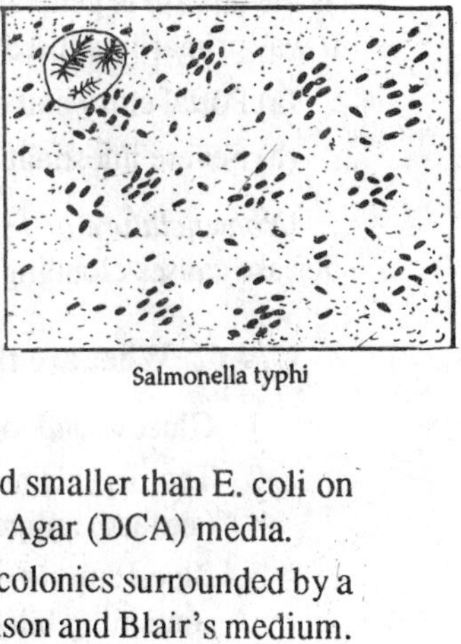

Salmonella typhi

They are (i) Gram-negative, Non-sporing bacilli, (ii) Actively Motile by pertrichate flagella of 2.5 by 0.5 μ size.

Cultural characters :

1. Facultative anaerobe or aerobe.
2. Optimum temperature for growth, 37°C.
3. Grows in nutrient agar.
4. Colonies colourless, translucent, pale and smaller than E. coli on MacConkeys and Desoxycholate Citrate Agar (DCA) media.
5. Round, jet black, about mm. in diameter colonies surrounded by a blackish zone with metallic sheet, on Wilson and Blair's medium.

Serological characters :

Salmonella typhosa *possesses a flagellar*—H antigen and *theremostable somatic 'O'* and *'Vi'* antigens. All these lead to the production of specific antibodies in the body, i.e. H, O, and Vi—agglutinins. Vi and O—antigens are located on the surface of organism. Presence of Vi-antigens hinders agglutination of Salmonella by O-sera. Vi-antigen disappears from cultures Phenel is added to the medium and also when the temperature is low

(20°C) or high (40°C) in the medium. Other antigens are located deeply in the organism. These are non-specific. Later Salmonellae were found to possess *M-mucous antigen* (Pohysaccharide). *Vi-antigen content* of cultures varies much. Immunization with H-and O-antigens are done for obtaining the corresponding sera.

N.B. H—German '*Houch* means flagella.

O—German '*Ochne*' means body.

Vi—Stands for virulence.

Q. 4.61. What do you mean by Enteric fever ?

Enteric fever includes typhoid and paratyphoid fevers caused by *Salmonella typhi* and *paratyphoid*, A, B *and* C.

Enteric fever is also a generalised septicemic infection with wide spread involvement of all the body tissues.

It is not a mere intestinal lesion. So the term "*Enteric fever* is a misnomer, as the disease is generalised. It was named Enteric fever with the idea that it was primarily a disease of intestinal evidenced by :

(a) Portal entry and exit of infecting bacilli—being intestinal tract.

(b) Severe intestinal lesions—like Haemorrhage and perforation.

[*Nomenclature of Typhoid*—The word *Typhus* means *cloud*. Since the disease causes clouding of consciousness, it is called Typhoid.]

Q. 4.62. What are the significant reactions of Salmonella typhi ?

1. Glucose and mannital are fermented without gas production.
2. The organisms contain "*C*" (somatic), "*H*" (Flagellar) and "V" (surface) antigens.
3. Blood culture within the first 7 to 10 days must be ideally in media containing bile salts.
4. Faeces culture ideally during second to third week (DCA is a good selective medium).
5. Urine culture.
6. Widal reactions—Arising titre is significant.
7. Bile culture also for carrier detection.
8. Slide agglutination of colonies.

9. Does not produce indole.
10. Does not liquefy gelatin.
11. Produces hydrogen sulphide (variable).
12. V.P. negative.
13. Citrate positive.
14. Urease negative.
15. K. C. N. negative.
16. O. N. P. G. Test negative.

Q. 4.63. How can we diagnosis a case of Typhoid fever ?
[C.U. 1979, 80, 82, 84, D.M.S. 71, 80, 82, 84]

Laboratory diagnosis :

Typhoid fever refers to a febrile illness causes by *Salm-typhi* and *paratyphi* A,B and C. *Salm. Paratyphi* C. is not common in India.

The laboratory diagnosis of typhoid fever is made by:

(a) *Isolation of the causative agent from clinical specimens.*

(b) *Demostrations of antibodies in patients serum.*

The following investigations are usually performed :

1. *Blood culture*—This is positive in 90% cases in 1st week, 75% of cases in 2nd week, 60% of cases in 3rd week and 25 of cases there after.

2 *Stool culture*—This is positive through out the course of the disease.

3. *Urine culture*—This is less valuable than stool culture and blood culture, as the organisms are irregularly shed in urine. Only in 25% of cases, it is positive in the 3rd and 4th week of illness.

4. *Widal agglutination test*—This becomes positive from 2nd week onwards and the titre steadily rises upto 3rd or 4th week after which it declines.

***1. IN FIRST WEEK OF ILLNESS**

The diagnosis is based mainly on the Isolation of organisms by *blood and clot cultures.*

(a) Blood culture :

About 5 ml of blood is collected aseptically by venepuncture and inoculated into 50 ml of 1% glucose citrate broth or 0.5% bile broth. After inoculation at 37°C for 48 hours, subcultures are made on MacConkey agar and blood agar. These are incubated at 37°C for 18-24 hours. Non lactose fermenting colonies from MacConkey's agar are tested for motility and biochemical reactions. *Once organisms biochemically resemble Salmonella*, its confirmation and species identification is performed by slide agglutination tests, according to *Kauffman* and White Scheme using O and H antisera.

(b) **Clot culture :**

This is an alternative to blood culture. About 5 ml of patient's blood is collected and allowed to clot. The serum is separated out and used for the WIDAL TEST. The colt is lysed by the enzyme *Streptokinase* (100 units per ml) and used for culture in a blood culture bottle as before. Clot culture is prefered because both culture and widal test can be performed from the same specimen. Clot culture is also said to yield a higher positivity than blood culture.

*** 2. IN SECOND WEEK ONWARDS**

The diagnosis of Enteric fever (typhoid) from second week onwards depends on the isolation of organisms from stool, urine and sometimes blood and on demonstration of antibodies in patient's serum.

(a) **Stool culture** : This is probably more informative than blood culture as treatment which chloramphenicol does not eliminate the organisms from stool as rapidly as it does from the blood. Organisms are isolated from using enrichment media (Selenite F broth and tetrathionate broth) and selective media (DCA, SSA, XLD, Wilson-Blair).

(b) Urine culture—Clean voided urine samples are certrifuged and the deposit inoculated into selective and enrichment media as for stool culture.

(c) Blood culture—Same as *1st week.*

(d) Widal test (in short).

12. WIDAL TEST OR TUBE DILUTION AGGLUTINATION TEST

When *Blood cultural method fails*, unequivocal evidence of infection is obtained from the *Widal Reaction* in about 90% of cases.

Vi-antibodies do not appear with any regularity early in the disease and are, therefore, of more importance in detecting persistence of infection or a carrier state in a healthy individual than in diagnosis. Antibodies begin to appear in patients serum in between the seventh and tenth days of illness. In the uninoculated and in those who have not previously suffered from typhoid, 'O' agglutinins appear first. Most typhoid patients show a four fold rise of titre in 'O' agglutinins with 4 to 5 days. In a *virgin case a titre of 1: 200 'O' agglutinins is highly suggestive of typhoid fever.*

A four fold rise of titre is diagnostic. 'H' agglutinins appear more slowly and tend to persist for longer than 'O' agglutinis both after the disease and inoculation. A low 'O' and high 'H' titre suggests an anamnestic reaction. A level of antibodies in the serum bears constant relationship to the severity of illness.

Procedure: (*Widal Test.* synonym—Tube dilution agglutination test).

Patient serum is diluted with normal saline. Dreyer's agglutination tubes are placed in *Widal* rack. After serial or paralled dilutions, the standard suspension of 'H' and 'O' antigens are added to the tubes. The rack with tubes is placed in a water-bath at 56°C for 4 hours and then it is kept overnight at room temperature or in refrigerator at 4°C. Readings are taken next morning. *'H' agglutination appears a* **snow flakes** and *'O' agglutination appears as* ***fine granular deposites at the bottom of tubes.***

Q. 4.64. What are the Limitations of Widal Test ?

For interpretation of the test following facts should be taken into consideration :

(1) The local tire of the place should be known and the results interpreted accordingly.

(2) Tests done within 7 days of illness and after 4 weeks are usually negative.

(3) Demonstration of four fold rise in tire by testing paired sera samples is diagnostic. A single titre unless very high, may be difficult to interpret.

(4) Other infections non-enteric febrile conditions may also cause an increase in agglutinins (anamnestic reactions).

(5) Previous TAB vaccination, carried out within 6 months test, tend to increase the titre of antibodies against H antigens.

(6) Non-specific antigens like fimbriae, present in antizen suspension may cause false agglutination.

(7) Cases treated with chloramphenicol may not show a significant rise in the test.

Q. 4.65. How can you detect a Typhoid carrier ?

This may be done as follows :

(1) Widal test may show raised antibody titres.
(2) Vi-agglutination test is positive in a titre of 1/10 or more.
(3) Several stool cultures (3-6) may help in isolation of causative agent.
(4) Organism may be cultured from bile obtained after duodenal incubation.

Q. 4.66. Mention the different Relationship of Laboratory diagnosis with reference to the stages of Enteric fever.

Order of Importance

First week	*Second week*	*Third and 4th week*
1. Leucocyte count	1. Agglutination +++	1.Agglutination ++
2. Blood culture+++	2. Stool culture±	2. Stool culture +
3. Agglutination ±	3. Blood culture±	3. Urine culture +
4. Stool culture ±	4. Urine culture ±	4. Blood culture -
5. Urine culture ±	*	*

In short:

Order of Importance

Weeks	(i)	(ii)	(iii)	(iv)
1st	B	A	S	U
2nd	A	S	B	U
3rd	A	S	U	—
4th	A	S	U	—

N.B. B = Blood culture, S = Stool culture,
A = Agglutination, U = Urine culture.

Q. 4.67. What are the factors responsible for the pathogenesis of Salm. typhi and paratyphoid A, B & C ?

Various factors responsible for the pathogenesis of Salm. typhi and paratyphoid A, B & C.

(1) Ability of the bacilli to survive and multiply inside phagocytes.

(2) Toxicity of Endotoxins ('O' antigen).

(3) Presence of Vi-antigen in Salm. typhi and paratyphi C; protects organisms from lytic action of antibody and complement.

12. SHIGELLA

Q. 4.68. What are the causative organism of Bacillary dysentery in man? Give their main characteristics.

Various species of the genus—**Shigella** are the causative organisms of bacillary dysentery on man. Generally the severity of infection of this disease is to some extent related to particular group or species of the organisms.

There are four species or groups, which are :

Group A—**Shigella dysenteria** (consists of 10 sero types).

A_1—**Shigella shigae.**

A_2—**Sh. schmitozii.**

$A_{(3-10)}$—**Sh. arabinotarda.**

Group B—**Sh. flexneri** (consists of 6 sero type).

Group C—**Sh. boydii** (consists of 15 sero types).

Group D—**Sh. sonnei** (consists of only one sero type).

Generally **Sh. dysenteria** causes severe illness whereas *Sh. sonnei* infection is usually mild. Other species are *Sh. Flexneri* and *Sh. boydii.*

Main characteristics:

1. *Shigella species* are gram negative, aerobic, non-motiles, non-flagellated, non capsulated, non-lactose fermenting, non-gas forming bacilli, but ferment glucose with liberation of acid only.
2. They parasitize man and primates only.
3. Give positive ONPG Test.
4. Ferment mannite (Sh. flexneri, Sh. boydii, Sh. sonnei).
5. Do not produce H_2 (Sh. flexneri, Sh. boydii).
6. Produce indole (Sh. dysenteriae type 2, 7, 8 and some mannite ferments).
7. Possess fimbriae (some serotyps of Sh. flexneri).

8. Do not grow in citrate agar.
9. Isolation done in desoxycholate citrate agar.
10. Aerobes or facultative anerobes.
11. Optimum temperature for growth 37°C.
12. Grow in nutrient agar broth.
13. Sh. dysenteriae produce an exotoxin called paretic toxin. It causes polyneuritis in man.
14. Produces an endotoxin called marasmic toxin which causes diarrohea and collapse with fall of temperature.

Q. 4.69. How can we diagnose a case of Shigella infections (Dysentery).

The causative organism is isolated from stools by the method of culture, for recognition. Cultivation may be made of material obtained from rectal swabbing. Only fresh faecal matter is utilised. Where delay is indispensable, a suitable piece of bloody mucus is selected from stool and placed in 30% glycerine in isotonic saline. Cultures are made on DCA, MacConkey's medium and S Agar within 24 hours circular, convex non-lactose fermenting colonies appear except in the case of *Shigella sonni*, which is a late lactose fermenter. Colonies obtained are utilised now for studing morphological and biochemical characters of the organism and for type determination. *Serological tests are not of great significance.*

Q. 4.70. What are the causes of Food Poisoning ?

The causes are:

1. Salmonella group:

(i) *Salmonella typhimurium.*
(ii) *Salm. enteritidis.*
(iii) *Salm. newport.*
(iv) *Salm.* montevideo.
(v) *Salm. oranienburg.*
(vi) *Salm, thompson.*
(vii) *Salm. choleraesuis.*

2. **Staphylococcus aureus** : Phase group III and IV, Phase type 42D or 6/47.

3. **Clostridium groups:**

(i) *Clostridium welchii.*
(ii) *Cl. botulinum.*
(iii) *Cl. perfringens.*

4. **Paratyphod B.**
5. **Bacillus cereus.**
6. **Shigella.**
7. **Enterococci.**

Q. 4.71. Which Organisms are associated with dysenteric disorders ?

These are :

1. *Shigella dysenteriae.*
2. *Sh. flexneri.*
3. *Sh. boydii.*
4. *Sh. sonnei.*
5. *Salm. typhosa.*
6. *Salm. paratyphi* (A, B and C).
7. *Pr. morgariri.*
8. *Arizona dispar group.*

Q. 4.72. Enumerate the non-lactose fermenting intestinal organism.

These are :

(i) *Salmonella typhosa.*
(ii) *Salm. paratyphi A, B & C.*
(iii) *Salm. typhimurium.*
(iv) *Salm. enteritidis.*
(v) *Shigella shiga.*
(vi) *Sh. flexneri.*
(vii) *Sh. boydii.*
(viii) *Sh. sonnei.*
(ix) *Proteus* (pathogenic).

VII. VIBRIONANCAE

13. VIBRIO CHOLERAE

Q. 4.73. What is the Causative organism of the disease cholera? Give its morphological characteristics and laboratory diagnosis.

[D.M.S.1978]

(*Cholera* was discovered by *Robert Koch* in Calcutta.)

Vibrio cholerae—*Cholera vibrio is the causative organism of the disease cholera.*

1. They are Gram negative, *comma shaped* (curved) rods.
2. Length 1.5 to 3 μ; breath 0.2 to 4 μ.
3. Single or in pairs.

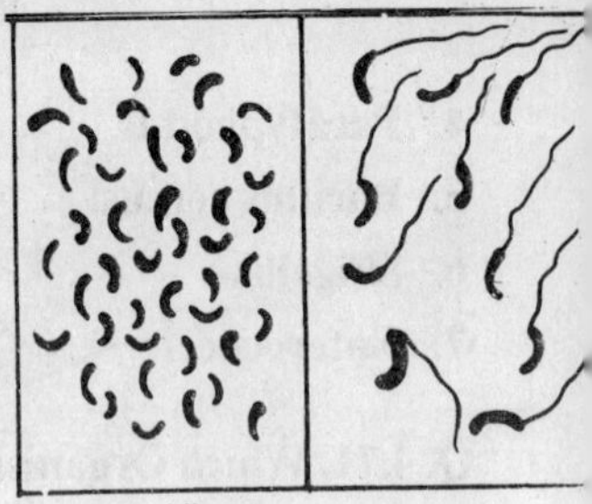
VIBRIO CHOLERAE

4. Motile by monotrichate flagella (darting or scintillating movement).

5. 'S' or spirillum (involution) form in old culture.

6. Non-sporing and non-capsulated.

Antegenic structure :

They possess both 'O' (Somatic) and 'H' (Flagellar) antigns, 'H' antigen is heat labile, non-specific and non-protective. 'O' antigen is heat stables and protective. It contains two factors, on specific for V. cholerae and other non-specific. Agglutinins are found after recovery in the serum and faecal. Faecal agglutinations are more protectives than humoral antibodies. Other antibodies produced by this organisms are vibriocidal antibody and precipitin.

Laboratory diagnosis :

It consists of:

(1) *Isolation of the organisms from faeces or vomitus.*

(2) *Detection of agglutinins or bactericidins in the blood serum.*

Direct smears from stools may be examined after staining with Ziehli's fuchsin for typical "*fish in stream appearance*".

(i) For isolation bile salt agar, bile gelatin agar, *Monsur*'s medium etc. are used. Medium is inoculated with test material or growth, in enrichment (alkaline peptone water) media.

Isolated pure colonies are studied for morphological, cultural, and bacteriological characters of the organism. Phase sensitivity agglutination with specific 'O' sera are also carried with pure cultures. For immediate diagnosis the organism is examined under dark ground illumination for motility like that of a swarm of gnats or mosquitos. Another way of arriving at the rapid diagnosis is to adopt fluorescent antibody method.

(ii) Serological diagnosis comprises of agglutination reaction. It is based on the presence of agglutinin in the serum of subject suffering from cholera. It is of little diagnostic value before the sixth day. A titre of 1/100 or more is generally taken *as diagnostic*.

Q. 4.74. Why the stool has "rice water" appearance in cholera ?

Large number vibrios and flakes of mucous membrane ascribe it that appearance.

Q. 4.75. What constitutes the most important part of treatment in cholera?

As the disease is a self-limiting one and the problems are dehydration and circulatory collapse, fluid replacement and prevention of shock receive major attention in the treatment.

Q. 4.76. What is Receptor Destroying Enzyme (RDE) in cholera vibrio ?

This very enzyme destroys receptors for virus particles on the surface of red blood cells.

Q. 4.77. What is Pfeiffer's phenomenon in case of cholera vibrio?

Lysis of the organism in the presence of antiserum and complement is called *Pfeiffer's phenomenon.* It is demonstrated by injecting intraperitonerally *V. cholerae* in guineapigs, already receiving the antiserum and the organisms.

Q. 4.78. Can Vibrio cholera ferment arabinose, xylose and dulcitol ?

No fermentation of these sugars.

Q. 4.79. What do you know about El Tor Vibrio ?

They have the following characteristics :

(1) Morphology and cultural characters same as cholera vibrio.
(2) Produce haemolysis (also non-haemolytic variants).
(3) Give positive V-P reaction.
(4) Cause agglutination of chicken red cells.
(5) Spreads rapidly over much wider area than classical cholera.
(6) Resistant to phase.
(7) Resistant to polymyxin B.
(8) Produces infection indentical to classical cholera.

Q. 4.80. What is 'cholera red' reaction?

A drop of H_2SO_4 or HCI (Conc.) to a 24 hours peptone water culture of Cholera vibiro gives red colour. The same is referred to as cholera red reaction. The reaction is not specific, for it is given by many other vibrios. The red colour is due to the action of acid on indole and nitrates produced from peptone by the Cholera vibrio.

14. PASTEURELLA PESTIS

(Yersinia pestis)

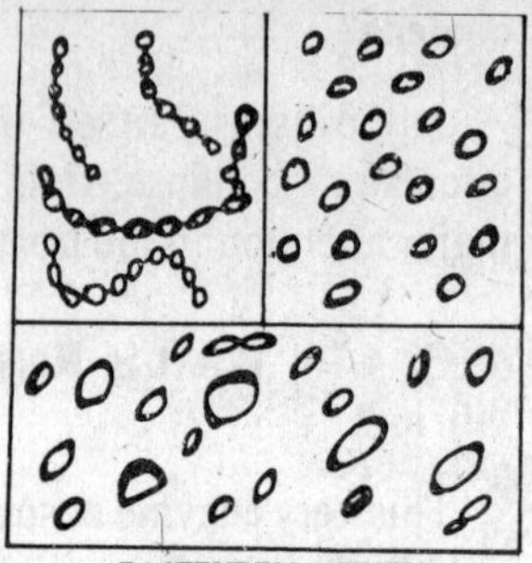

PASTEURELLA PESTIS

Q. 4.81. What is the causative organism of the disease plague? Why is it called Yersinia Sp.? Give its morphology.

The causative organism of the plague is *Pasteurella pestis* bacillus. The genus Pasteurella is now a new genus *Yersinia* within the family Entero-bacteriacea, according to the discoverer *Yersinia* who described the plague bacilli.

So the causative organism of plague is *Yersinia pestis.*

Morphology : These are short, ovoid rods, showing bipolar staining in animal tissues resembling '*saftypins*' with a denser or darker stain at two ends, and almost clear in the centre, when stained with Methylene blue or Leishman's stain. They are also non-motile and non-sporing. In liquid cultures they are common in chains.

VIII. SPIROCHAETES

Q. 4.82. What are Spirochaetes ?

Spirochaetes are slender, flexous, non-flagellate filaments, having an intrinsic active bending movement. They are structurally more complex than ordinary bacteria. They stain poorly with ordinary dyes, but all of them are Gram negative if they can be stained at all.

Q. 4.83. What are the diseases produced by spirochaetes ?

Relapsing fever: Borrelia recurrentis.
B. carteri.
B. duttoni.

Vincent's angina: Borrelia vincenti.
Weil's disease: Leptospira ictero haemorrhagiae.
Syphilis: Treponema pallidum.
Yaws: Treponema pertenue.
Piuta: T. carateum.

IX. RICKETTSIAE

Q. 4.84. What is Rickettsiae bodies ?

Rickettsiae bodies are minute forms of bacteria and represent a stage of evolution intermediate between bacteria and viruses. They have following characteristics:

(1) Small rod shaped bodies (non-motile and difficult to stain).
(2) Gram negative.
(3) Show bipolar staining and pleomorphism.
(4) Cannot grow on ordinary bacteriological media.
(5) Not filtrable through L_3 bacterial filters.
(6) Can be demonstrated in tissue cultures or in the chorioallantoic membrane of chick embryo (as they grow and multiply in the cell).
(7) Are intestinal parasites of certain arthopods like lice, fleas, ticks and mites.
(8) Susceptible to bactericidal agents.
(9) Possess antigens specific for each species.
(10) In man cause **typhus and typhus like fevers.**
(11) Can be isolated by inoculating susceptible laboratory animals such as guineapig.
(12) These cause typhus fevers and a group of similar disease; transmitted by arthropods lice, fleas, ticks and mites. All pathogenic rickettsiae release a soluble CF antigen when shaken with either.

Pathogenicity :

Rickettsia prowazeki enters the human body with the dust of dried faeces of louse and causes *typhus fever* in which roseolouspetechial eruptions are found.

Rickettsia rikettsi produces *Rocky* Mountáin spotted fever. *Rickettsia burneti*-Q *fever* and *Rickettsia tsutsugamushi*-scrub typhus, *Rickettsia quintana* causes trench fever, Rickettsia mooseri causes endemic or urine typhus.

Q. 4.85. What are Actinomycetes?

They are gram positive, filamentous micro-organisms, occupying an intermediate position between '*true bacteria*' and '*fungi*' and are known as '*higher bacterta*' or mycelial bacteria. This heterogenous group of organisms characteristically form branching mycelium which tends to fragment into coccal and bacillay forms. They are anaerobic or microaerophilic in nature. e.g. Actinomycetes israisli, A. bovis, etc.

X. MYCOPLASMAS

Q. 4.86. What is Mycoplasmas ?

This is a group of very small highly, pleomorphic organisms, lacking a rigid cell wall and enclosed by a thin cytoplasmic (limiting) membrane only. These occupy in *intermediate* position between **bacteria** and **rickettsial** organisms. Mycoplasmas are known are *Pleuro-pneumonia-like organisms or PPLO* because one of the members of the group, *Mycoplasmas pneumoniae* was the agent of bovine pleuropneumonia.

Morphology : They range from 0.1 micron to 1 micron. The smallest granules easily pass through coarse bacterial filters, and are called elementary corpuscles. **Shape**—Extremely pleomorphic and fragile (due to lack of a rigid cell wall), may show coccoid forms, clubs rings and filaments. They are gram negative but stain poorly, best stained with **Giemsa stain**. Electron microscopy reveals—doubled layered plasmamembrane, granular nuclear material and ribosomes.

CHAPTER 5
VIRUS

Q. 5.1. What is virus? Give its nature ? [D.M.S. 1978, 79, 81]

The word "*virus*" has a long history in the English language, coming from a Latin word meaning "*slime*" or "*poison*". It was considered to be word always associated with some disease or harmful influences without really knowing what a virus was. It has acquired its present, biological meaning, only duirng this century.

Viruses are a biological enigma as they exhibit characters that are typical as of the inanimate as well as of animate. It is difficult to give a precise definition of such a thing. So four definitions are given serially.

(1) *Virus may be defined as an ultramicroscopic disease producing nucleo-protein particle that can multiply only within living organisms.*

(2) *A virus is a non-cellular infectious agent that can only multiply within the host cell.*

(3) *A virus is a protobiotic entity that has no ability for autonomous growth outside a living cell.*

(4) *Viruses are sub-microscopic (electron-microscopic) particulate, antigenic, amphoteric, obligatory parasitic, infectious entities endowed with genetic continuity and mutability and capable of entering into and multiplying only in specific living plant, animal or human cells.*

Nature of Virus :

1. Viruses are very small, acellular or non-cytoplasmic organisms which can easily pass through the bacterial filter.
2. They are obligate parasite i.e. can live only as parasite within the cell of other organisms.
3. They have two phases in their life-cycle; one is intracellular i.e. within the cell of other organisms, the other is extra cellular i.e. outside the body of other organisms.

4. In extracellular phase: they behave like inaminate object and form crystals.
5. Intracellular phase: they reproduce like other living organisms.
6. During intracellular phase: they synthesize their structural material with the help of the enzymes of host organism.
7. Their reproduction is like the replication of gene or chromosome.
8. Reproduction and mutability are their living characters.

(A) Non-living Characters of Virus:

1. Viruses are noncellular bodies.
2. They do not respire and show no metabolism.
3. They can form crystals and their crystallized forms retain capacity of infection.
4. They cannot be grown in artificial culture media.
5. They do not have any independent existence i.e. they can be grown only with living cells.
6. They do not respond to any change of environment.
7. They have no reproduction and growth in extra-cellular environment.
8. They possess high specific gravity.
9. During reproduction they do not grow and divide but rather new viruses are formed by the assembly of their constituents.

(B) Living Characters of Virus:

1. Viruses are disease producing particles.
2. They live as obligate parasite.
3. They multiply enormously within living organisms.
4. They can undergo incubation period in certain cases.
5. They show mutability.
6. They can infect other organisms.
7. They can be inactivated by treatment with pepsin.
8. They possess the genetic material DNA like other living organisms.

Q. 5.2. What are the differences between Virus and Bacteria?
[D.M.S. 1979, 81]

Virus	Bacteria
1. Body non-cellular	1. Bacteria are non-chlorophylous unicellular plants.
2. Cell absent, but outer covering present.	2. Bacteria posses — definite Cell wall surrounding the inner protoplasm.
3. Cytoplasm absent	3. Cytoplasm present
4. Nucleus absent	4. Protoplasm is without a true nucleus i.e. nucleus with unclear membrane, nuclear reticulum etc.
5. Chromosome absent, only nucleic acid present.	5. Protoplasmic organelles are absent, except ribosome and mesosome.
6. Genetic material is either DNA or RNA.	6. Genetic material is only DNA.
7. Protein and nucleic acids are the only organic material.	7. In addition to protein and nucleic acid various other organic substances are present.
8. Enzymes present are incapable of synthesizing new virtal parts.	8. Many enzymes are present within the cytoplasm and are capable to synthesize new cellular material.
9. Cell division absent	9. Cell division is without mitosis.
10. New viruses are formed only from the nucleic acid.	10. Reproduces generally by cell division and spore formation.
11. New virus particles are formed, within the host cell, by the union of protein sheath and nucleic acid, synthesized separately.	11. Special types of sexual processes like congugation, transformation and transduction, are also present.
12. Viruses lives as inanimate non-living object outside the host cell.	12. A few bacteria are chemosynthetic i.e. utilize the energy produced during Oxidation of some inorganic salts.
13. It is obligate parasite	13. Bacteria are both anaerobes and aerobes.
14. During reproduction it synthesizes its structural components with the help of host's enzyme system.	14. They are capable of synthesizes their structural components within their own enzyme system.

Q. 5.3. Classify Virus. [D.M.S. 1981]

Classification of Virus or Types of Viruses.

(I) According to *Professor Andre Lwoff* (1966)

Phylum-Vira (non-cellular)

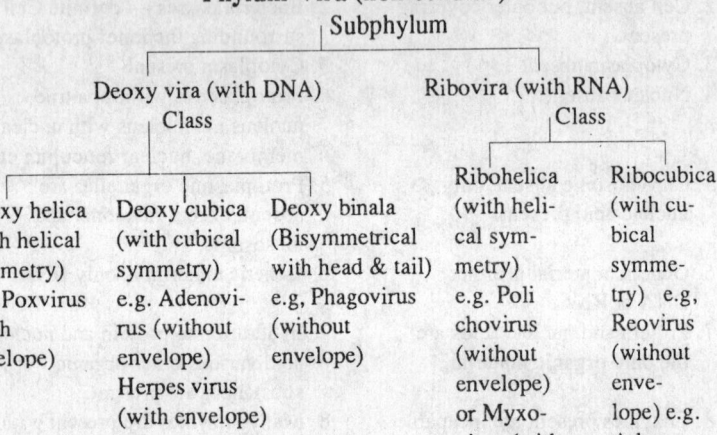

Subphylum

- Deoxy vira (with DNA)
  - Class
    - Deoxy helica (with helical symmetry) e.g. Poxvirus (with envelope)
    - Deoxy cubica (with cubical symmetry) e.g. Adenovirus (without envelope) Herpes virus (with envelope)
    - Deoxy binala (Bisymmetrical with head & tail) e.g, Phagovirus (without envelope)
- Ribovira (with RNA)
  - Class
    - Ribohelica (with helical symmetry) e.g. Polichovirus (without envelope) or Myxovirus (with envelope)
    - Ribocubica (with cubical symmetry) e.g, Reovirus (without envelope) e.g. Arbovirus (with envelope)

(II) BASED ON TISSUE SPECIFICITY

Viruses are :

1. *Dermotropic* — Infective wart, Mulluscum contagiesum, Trachoma, Lymphogranuloma inguinalae and mouth diseases etc.
2. *Neurotropic viruses* — Rabies, Polimyelitis, Viral Encephalitis, Landry's ascending myelitis etc.
3. *Neuro–dermotropic* — Smallpox, Chickenpox, Herpes zoster, Herpes ferbrilis etc.
4. *Respiratory* — Common cold, Influenza, Atypical pneumonia, Psittacosis, Measles, Mumps etc.
5. *Viscerotropic* — Dengu, Yellow fever, Infective hepatitis, Homologous serum, Jaundice, Sandfly fever etc.

Q. 5.4. What are the various parts present in a virus ?

Electronmicroscopic Structure

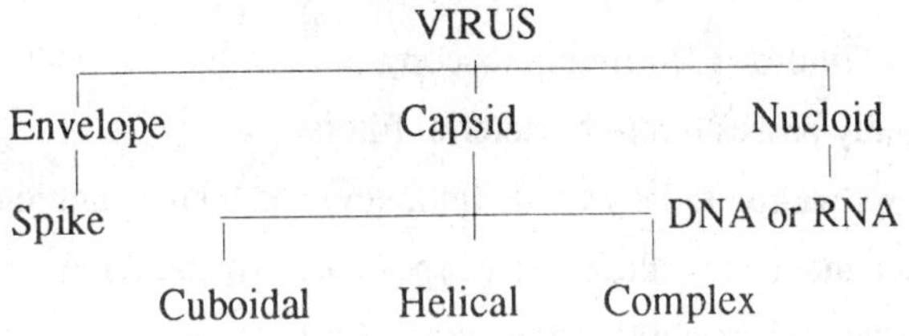

Q. 5.5. Name some viral diseases with their main symptoms.

[D.M.S. 1978, 79]

Viral diseases	Main symptoms
1. *Measles*	Fever, sore throat, rash
2. *Smallpox, Chickenpox*	Fever, bodyache, external lesions.
3. *Poliomyelitis*	Paralysis of limbs.
4. *Rabies*	Spasmodic contraction of muscle, difficulty in swallowing.
5. *Influenza*	Fever, chill, bodyache.
6. *Encephalitis*	Fever bodyache.
7. *Herpes*	Vesicular eruptions of the skin and mucous membrane in clusters.
8. *Infective Hepatitis*	Jaundice, necrosis and autolysis of hepatic cell.

Q. 5.6. How can we prevent and control a viral disease ?

Prevention and control of virus disease :

Prevention of viral disease is done firstly by keeping the patient in a "**quarantine**" place, secondly "**immunization**" with the help of vaccination, and thirdly by isolation of the '**vectors**' carrying the virus. Various methods have been employed from time to time to control viral disease. Chemotherapy or chemical control of viral disease is one of them. Various chemical agents which prevent viral growth are termed antiviral chemical agent. They act both as prophylactic and as therapeutic to control viral disease. These drugs have got some selective retarding effect on the synthesis of nucleic acid and protein of the virus and thus they effect the production of virus progenies.

Q. 5.7. Notes on :

1. POLIOMYELITIS VIRUS

(i) Size 27mμ on Electronmicroscopy.

(ii) Rapidly passes through bacterial filters.

(iii) Grows well in kidney tissue (monkey) and human amnion.

(iv) Three main antigenic types (Types one, two and three isolated).

(v) Resistant to freezing, drying pure glycerine etc.

(vi) Destroyed by oxidising agents and heat over 45°C.

(vii) Can be conserved for many years in nervous tissue at 0°C in 50% glycerine.

(viii) Causes poliomyelitis or infantile paralysis involving the nerve cells of spinal cord and medulla, primarily in children.

(ix) Provides high degree of immunity to the person who has recovered from polio.

(x) Laboratory diagnosis constitutes of isolating the virus from :

(a) *nervous tissue at autopsy or*
(b) *from faeces or*
(c) *throat washings.*

For isolation organisms are cultivated in cerebrum of monkey. Cerebrospinal fluid of a polio case is devoid of polioviruses but they change the composition of C.S.F. Increased protein content, increase number of lymphocytes, no alteration in sugar or chloride contents are features of C.S.F. in Polio.

2. ARBOR VIRUS

Viruses : this group are transmitted by mosquitoes, ticks and sandflies, all belonging to arthropod. The virus multiplies in the insects without producing any disease. These are divided into antigenic groups, namely A, B and C. Spherical in shape and 22-50mμ in diameter, they contain RNA. Characteristically they possess haemagglutinating activity. They are unstable at room temperature. Infection with arborvirus results in encephalistis, aseptic meningitis. The virus is isolated from blood in the early stage of infection.

Mice inoculation (intracerebral or intraperitoneal) and egg inoculation are also employed in laboratory diagnosis.

3. ONCOGENIC VIRUS

Virus that produce tumours in natural host or in experimental animal or that induce changes in cultured cell are called **oncogenic virus.** Properties of cells transformed by viruses are loss of parallel orientation and chromosomal aberrations in fibroblasts; increased growth rate, increased production of organic acids and acid mucopolysaccharides loss of contact inhibition, capacity to divide indefinitely in serial culture, appearance of new virus specified antigents (Tantigen, TSTA): loss of surface antigens capacity induce tumours in suceptible animals.

Oncogenic viruses are :

(i) *Leucovirus* — cause leucosis or sarcoma in the hosts and develop by budding through the host cell membrane.

(ii) *Papilloma* — viruses cause benign tumours in their natural hosts but some of them (e.g. condyloma acuminata) may turn malignant in man.

(iii) *Pox virus* — such as molluscum contagiosum contagiosum and the yaba virus induce benign tumours.

(iv) *Adenoviruses* — human types 12, 18 and 31 are most oncogenic for many species of new born.

(v) *Herpes virus* — called the *Epstein-Barr virus* is found regularly in cultured lymphocytes from Burkitt's lymphoma patients.

(vi) *Herpes simplex* — type 2 infection and Cancer of cervix are strongly associated but their aetiological relationship has not been proved. It is also suggested that herpes simplex type 1 infection may be associated with Cancer lip.

4. ECHO-VIRUSES

They are found in the faeces of normal individuals. They may be responsible for acute diarrhoea in children and acute fever of short duration. The abbreviation ECHO stands for *Enteric-Cytopathogenic-Human-Orphan*. Lastly, they may also cause aseptic meningitis.

5. BACTERIO-PHAGE (or PHAGE VIRUS)

Q. 5.8. What is Bacteriophage or Phage Virus? Give its morphology.

Bacteriophages are viruses that are parasitic on bacteria. They exhibit a marked specificity of action. Each phage attacks only groups of closely related bacteria. There are certain phages which attack only particular strains of a species. In such cases susceptibility to a particular bacteriophage forms an easy basis for species subdivision. The same principle is applied in bacteriophage typing of bacteria. Such typing of bacteria is of considerable value in epidemiological studies. *Bacteriophages are subdivided into 2 main groups*—the **lytic** or **virulent** and the **symbiotic** or **temperate**. Lytic phages produce lysis of the infected bacteria, e.g. T_1 to T_7 coliphages (lyse certaine stains of E. coli). Symbiotic phages do not lyse the infected bacteria. They are transferred from parental to daughter bacteria at cell division. Lysogenic cultures are those cultures which carry symbiotic bacteriophages. Symbiotic bacteriophage is also called **prophage.**

Morphology : They are filterable bodies found multiplying within the growing bacteria. They ultimately lyse the bacteria. They are active in high dilutions. Their size varies from 10-100mμ. They are like **tadpole** possessing a polygonal **head** and a **tail.**

The head is a mass of DNA covered with protien. The tail is also covered by a protein. The distal protion of tail is composed of fibrils which help attachment of phase to the bacterial cell. After attachment DNA of head is injected into the bacterial cell. This sets in replication of phage. Thus huge number of phage particles are produced with the bacterium. The latter then bursts releasing the phage.

Two types of changes may be responsible for the multiplication of phage :

(1) The phage DNA so alters the metabolism of the host cell that the latter starts synthesizing page particles.

(2) The phage RNA becomes dormant (prophage) and divides with each division of bacteria. Only young living culture are attacked by phage. Dead organisms do not undergo lysis even when they absorb the phage. Phage is destroyed by ultra violet rays and heat over 70°C. They are resistant to glycerine, alcohol etc.

Phages occur in faeces, sewage water and soil. They are antigenic.

Organisms possessing identical biochemical and scrological reactions are different by means of selected phages.

Q. 5.9. What are the Importance of phage virus ?

Phages are used to trace the source of infection in epidemics. They are of help in the investigation of cross infections and identification of bacteria. Phage studies are significant in appreciating the genetic variations in bacteria.

Q. 5.10. How can we demonstrate a phage virus ?

Phages are demostrated in 2 ways :

(1) By inoculation of material containing phage into a young broth culture of sensitive strain. The culture undergoes lysis within an hour of inculation if the phage is lytic. This is evidenced by clearing of the culture. A partial clearing occurs in case of symbiotic phage.

(2) By spreading bacteria on the surface of an agar plate and depositing, subsequently the phage on it. A patch of clearing is seen in the part of culture attacked by the phage (lytic). The plaques produced by symbiotic phage shows a central area of growth surrounded by a ring of lysis.

Q. 5.11. What is meant by Street Virus and Fixed Virus?

Rabies virus found in brain and spinal cords of dogs in street of **Paris** *was called by* **Pasteur** *by Street Virus.*

It had longer incubation period and when injected subdurally into râbbits, the incubation period was found to be 12 to 14 days. The virus has the power to invading cells of salivary glands and it could produce **Negri bodies**, specially in nerve cells.

Fixed Virus :

By serial subdural inoculation and successive transfer into rabbits, the virulence of street virus could be enhanced and by this street virus could be adopted into a fixed virus. This virus kills rabbit regularly in 6 to 7 days and its virulence cannot be increased further. But it has not lost its pathogenecity for dog and man when injected subcutaneously. It is so because the incubation period was reduced to and fixed at 4 to 6 days.

So Fixed Virus :

1. When injected — Infectivity for man is minimised.

2. It could not produce Negri bodies.

3. It could not multiply in salivary glands.

Q. 5.12. What is meant by Inclusion bodies ?

These are abnormal structures found in Cytoplasm or nucleus of a cell infected with virus. They are acidophilic or basophilic granules. In Cytoplasm, they are found in Vaccinia, molluscum contagiousm, rabies etc. In varicella, herpes and yellow fever they are intranuclear. They are also found in poliomyelitis, trachomo, lymphogranuloma venercum and adeno virus infection. Inclusion bodies vary much in nature. If in an instance, it appears to control the development and growth of a virus, in another it represents either a remnant of virus multiplication or a mass of virus particles. However, they are of diagnostic significance. For example, demonstration of intracytoplasmic inclusion body (Negri body) in case of rabbit is pathogenic of the disease.

PART-II

PARASITOLOGY

CHAPTER 1

PROTOZOA

DISCUSSION FOR LEARNING

(I) PARASITES OF PUBLIC HEALTH IMPORTÂNCE

(II) PROTOZOA

1. *Entamoeba histolytica.*
2. *Gardia intestinalis.*
3. *Leishmania donovani.*
4. *Plasmodium.*

(I) PARASITES OF PUBLIC HEALTH IMPORTANCE

Q. 1.1. What are Parasites ?

Parasites are those animals who live in the body of another; man or animal host, to derive nourishment.

Commensal parasites do not produce any disease in their hosts, whereas disease producing parasites are *pathogenic*.

The animals parasites can be broadly divided into two categories: viz. **Protozoa** and **Helminths.**

The most important Parasites are:

PARASITES

- **Protozoan**
  1. *Entamoeba histolytica*
  2. *Giardia intestinalis*
  3. *Trypanosoma gambiense, T. Cruzi .*
  4. *Plasmodium vivax, P. falciparum. P. ovale, P. malarae.*
  5. *Leishmania donovani, L. tropica: etc .*
- **Arthopoda (Not in the syllabus)**
  - Insecta
  - Arachnida
  - Crustacea
  - Chilopoda
  - Diplopoida
- **Helminthic Groups**
  - *Platyhelminthes (Cestodes)*
    1. *Taenia Solium*
    2. *T. saginata*
    3. *T. echinococcus.*
    - *Trematodes (flukes)*
  - *Nemato-helminthes (Nematodes)*
    1. *Ascaris lum bricodies.*
    2. *Ankylostoma duodenale.*
    3. *Wucheria brancrofti.*
    4. *Vrmicularis etc.*

Q. 1.2. What is Host?

Organism infected by a parasite is a host. Definitive host is that in which an animal parasite attains sexual maturity.

Intermediate host in one which is essential for the life cycle of an animal parasite, but in which does not become sexually mature.

Q. 1.3. Describe the different relationship between host and parasite.

The parasite develops some kind of relationship with the host. Their mode of reproduction within the body of the host varies. Some reproduce themselves within the host and pass from host to host while others require more than one host to complete their life cycle. The host in which the sexual cycle takes place or which harbours the adult stage of the parasite is called the **definitive host,** whereas the one that harbours the non-sexual cycle or the stage of growth other than the adult is called **intermediate host** or **biological carrier**. Man plays the role of definitive host in case of most of the parasite disease affecting man except that in malaria and hydatid Cyst (Ecchinococcus granulosa infection) he is intermediate host.

Viewed in another way the parasite may be pathogenic or non-pathogenic. In the former case the process is called **infection** and when a macro-parasite like a helminth establishes on the superficial tissues of the host the condition is referred to as **infestation**.

The student should, however, understand that ultimate goal of the parasitism is symbiosis, because the interest of the parasite is to live upon the host for its own survival and propagation without any disturbance, as much as possible, and not kill him with the disease, as it indirectly means death to the parasite itself, which is obviously not to its advantage. This happens when a new association is established or the association is not of long duration. On the other hand infection always follows an attempt on the part of both to adjust themselves to each other and to live as commensals, e.g., *B. Coli*, *E. coli* and some helminths. Again, the parasite may be host specific as in threadworm and roundworm or it may affect more than one host, e.g., *Trichinella spiralis* affecting pigs and man and *Leptospira ictrohaemorrhagica* and *Pasteurella pestis* both rat and man.

(II) PROTOZOA

AN ACELLULAR, HETEROTROPHIC, OFTEN MOTILE EUKARYOTE.

Q. 1.5. What is Protozoa ?

Protozoa are primitive unicellular units in the lowest state of evolution of animal kingdom, complete morphologically (with cytoplasm and nucleus) with powers of digestion, nutrition, locomotion and reproduction etc. *Dobel* preferred to call it **noncellular** or **acellular**.

Intestinal protozoa of man affect a human being all over the world. **Haemosporozoa** and **haemoflagellates** have restricted endemic areas in relation to temperature, humidity and altitude.

Q. 1.6. What are the important features of Protozoa ?

Or, What are the morphological characteristics of Protozoa ?

1. *Protozoa* are usually **microcopic** and **unicellular**.
2. Their bodies may be elongated, oval or spherical and the shape remain constant.
3. Their bodies also consist of a cytoplasm, nucleus and nucleoplasm.
4. The cytoplasm has two parts: **ectoplasm** and **endoplasm**. The former is concerned with locomotion, ingestion of food, excretion and protection. Some of the species have **periostome** and **cytosome** corresponding to mouth and oesophagus respectively.
5. The locomotion is derived from **Pseudopodia** (in amoeba), **flagella** (in trypanosomes) and **hair-like filaments** (incili-ata).
6. The endoplasm, the inter-granular portion of the cell contain foodvacuoles which helps digestion of food, various granules, glycogen, fat globules, protein (chromatoidal bodies), bacteria, pigments etc. and mitochondia.

7. The nucleus contains a chromatic substances (nuclear membrane, Karyolymph, reticulum and plastin or nucleolus), and has the following functions:
   (a) Governing the vital activities of the cell including nutrition.
   (b) Controls metabolism.
   (c) Takes part in the fertilisation of the cell and its division, growth and reproduction and maintains the hereditary channel.
8. Reproduction commonly by **fission** (binary or multiple). In certain forms sexual reproduction may occur either by **conjugation** or **fusion of gametes.**

Q. 1.7. Name some protozoa which are non-pathogenic to man.

Protozoal Parasites Non-Pathogenic to Man

Phylum-PROTOZOA

Subphylum

PLASMODROMA

Class	Order	Genus	Species	Habitat
RHIZOPODA	**Amoebida**	Entamoebe	*E.coli*	Large intestine
			E. gingivalis	Mouth
		Endolimare	*E. nana*	Large intestine
		Iodamoeba	*I. butschlii*	Large intestine
		Dientamoeba	*D. fragilis*	Large intestine
ZOOMASTIGOPHORA				
		Chilomostix	*C. mesnili*	Caecum
		Trichomonas	*T. hominis*	Ileocecal region.
		Enteromonas	*T. tenax*	Teeth and gum
		Embadomonas	*E. hominis.*	Large intestine
		Trypanosoma	*E. intestinalis*	Large intestine
			T. rangchi	Blood

Q. 1.8. Name some Protozoal parasites which are Pathogenic to man [C.U. 1981)

Protozoal Parasites Pathogenic to Man

		Phylum-PROTOZOA Subphylum Plasmodroma			
Class	**Order**	**Genus**	**Species**	**Habitat**	**Pathogenic Effects**
RHIZOPODA	Amoebida	*Entamoeba*	*E. histolytica*	Large intestine	Dysentery, liver abscess.
MASTIGOPHORA		*Trichomonas (genital flagellate)*	*T. vaginalis*	Vagina.	Vaginitis
	Protomonadida	*Trypanosoma (Blood and tissue flagellate)*	*T. brucei*	Blood, lymphnode CNS	Sleeping sickness
			T. cruzi	Heart, Nervous system	Chagas's disease
		Leishmania	*L. donovani*	R. E. System	Kala-azar and Dermal leish monoid orientalsore.
	Diplomonadida (intestinal flagellate)		*L. tropica*	Skin oral-nasal	
			L. brasiliensis	mucus membrane.	Espunda.
		Giardia	*G. intestinalis*	Small intestine	Diarrhoea
			P. vivax	RBC	Benign tertian
SPOROZOA		*Plasmodtum*	*P. falciparum*	RBC	Malignant tertian malaria and pernicious malaria.
	Coccidiida		*P. malariae*	RBC	Quartan mala
			P. ovale	RBC	Ovale tertian malariae
		Isopora	*I. hominis*	Ep. cells of intestine	Diarrhoea
			I. belli	Ep. cells of intestine	Diarrhoea
		Toxoplasma	*T. goduddi*	R.E. system, Parenchyma cell.	Encephalo myelitis, Choroidoreti mitis etc.
CILIATA	Heterotrichida	*Balanatidium*	*B.Coli*	Large intestine	Dysentery.

(I) ENTAMOEBA HISTOLYTICA

Q. 1.9. What is Entamoeba histolytica ?

Entamoeba histolytica is a parasite that inhabits in the mucous and submucous layers of the large intestine of man producing a disease called '**Amoebic dysentery**'.

The genus *Entamoeba* was established in 1879 by **Leidy**. *Entameoba histolytica* was first described as **Amoeba** coli by **Losch** in 1875 but **Schaudium** established the species *Entamoeba histolytica* in 1903 and differentiated the pathogenic and non-pathogenic types.

Q. 1.10. What are the morphological characteristics of E. histolytica ?

Entamoeba histolytica is a motile protozae having two forms, namely :

(I) **Trophozoita or Vegetative Form.**

(ii) **Cystic Form** i.e. **a resting phase** of trophozoite encysted by a resistant membraneous wall.

(I) TROPHIC

The **trophozoites** vary in size from 15 to 40 micra, the average being 18 to 25 micra. **Dobell** (1919) and others have shown that the parasite has got two races: one large i.e. **magna form** and the other small i.e. **minuta form**. The trophozoite of *Entamoeba histolytica* in living condition shows two distinct portions: **ectoplasm** and **endoplasm**.

The **ectoplasm** is clear and translucent while the **endoplasm** is granular. The endoplasm often contains injested RBCs. The **pseudopodia** may be long, finger-like or short and rounded in shape. In freshly passed stool the parasite is very active and moves rapidly in a straight line with a single clear pseudopod at the anterior end. This is known as '**directional movement**'. The movement becomes slaggish when the faeces cool down and in this condition the amoeba throws out pseudopodia at various directions and remains stationary.

The **neucleus** is indistinct in living condition but, when stained with haematoxylin it shows a small dot like **central karyosome** or **endosome**, a uniform ring of small peripheral **chromatin granules** and at times some chromatin granules in between them. Sometimes there may be traces of linin network in the form of fine fibils in between karyosome and nuclear membrane. The nuclear membrane is very delicate. The size of the nucleus is about 4 to 6 micra in diameter.

(II) CYSTIC

The cysts of both races of *E. histolytica* vary in size from 20 to 30 micra (average 12 micra) in diameter. In haematoxylin stained preparation a matured cyst looks **spherical** and **quadrinucleate.**

Its cytoplasm is clear and often contains black rod-like **chromatid bars** or **bodies with rounded ends.**

The young cysts are uninucleate or binucleate and their nuclear structure is just like that of the trophozoites. But the nucleus of a matured cyst is very small and its detailed structure is difficult to differentiate, particularly of the small race. It shows a very small central karyosome and a delicate nuclear membrane.

Presence of chromatoid bodies is the characteristic of the cysts of E. histolytica. They occur either singly or in multiples of two or more. About the exact nature of these bodies there is a controversy. Some authorities consider it as nutrient material of the cyst while others believe them as excess of chromatin thrown off during nuclear division. The chromatoid bodies occur in the early stages of the cysts but they disappear in the mature quadrinucleate cyst.

In young cysts glycogen is present in a diffused state forming a **glycogen vacuole** which is most noticeable in the mononuclea cyst, and in the course of time, as the cyst matures, the vacuole diminishes in size. Generally the presence of glycogen can be demonstrated in preparation with Lugol's iodine solution producting a brownish colour.

Q.1.11. How can we diagnosis a case of Amoebic dysentery ?

Examination of Stool for the Parasite

Principles: (a) 1. Freshly passed stool is ideal.

2. Earlier the examination made better is the result.

(b) Coverslip preparation is passed once or twice over the flame so that we can see brisk motility of the vegetative forms.

Methods:

Preparations — 1. Saline coverslip preparation.
2. Iodine preparation (Lugol's Iodine).

Comments:

*The iodine preparation is made for the identification of the cystic form of the parasite —*Nuclei are seen better*.

**Saline preparation is made for the cellular exudate. (RBC, pus-cells, and macrophages) the vegetative form the parasite actively moving about and to see the chromidial bars within the cyst.

Q. 1.12. Describe the life history of Entamoeba histolytica.
[D.M.S. 1976 (Dec.), 78 (Dec.)]

Entamoeba histolytica is parasitic to man and is responsible for amoebic dysentery. The life cycle of E. histolytica completes in only one host i.e. **in the man** and is the parasite of the large intestine of man, penetrates the intestinal submucosa and produces ulcer.

It has *three phases* of development in its life cycle, viz:

(i) *Trophozoite form with a transitory phase of Precystic form.*
(ii) *A resistant Cystic form with encystation of the parasite.*
(iii) *A metacystic form which develops after ex-cystation.*

In acute amoebic dysentery, the **Tropic** or **Vegetative forms**, are found in the patient's stool. Each tropic form has a clear ectoplasm, a nucleus with central karysome and a granular endoplasm containing RBC. It moves in a definite direction, by throwing out finger-like pseudopodium. As the vegetative forms do not survive in the environment when voided with the faeces, they are unable to transmit infection.

Cysts are found in a chronic carrier. The cysts have a definite cell wall, clear cytoplasm with 1, 2, or 4 nuclei, containing central karyosome. There may be chromatoid bars and glycogen mass.

Transmission: Only matured 4 nucleated cysts are infective and they can trasmit disease through water, food and drinks, as well as, through soiled hands.

LIFE CYCLE

When the mature *quadrinucleate cysits* i.e., the *infective forms* of the parasite, are swallowed along with the contaminated food and drink by a susceptible person, they further develope inside the gut. Generally the fully developed cysts, gaining entrance into the alimentary canal, pass unaltered through the stomach, as the cyst-wall is resistant to the action of the gastric juice; but as it is digested by the action of the trypsin in the intestine, the **excystation** occurs and the cyst reaches the caecum or the lower part of the ileum (neutral or slightly alkaline medium).

(A) EXCYSTATION

During this process, the cytoplasmic body retracts and loosens itself from the cyst-wall. Vigorous amoeboid movements cause a rent to appear in the cyst-wall through which at first a small mass of cytoplasm and then ultimately the whole body comes out. Each cyst liberates a single amoeba with four nuclei, a **tetranucleate amoeba** which eventually forms eight *amoebulae* (**metacystic trophozoites**) by the division of nuclei with successive fission of cytoplasm. The young amoebulae being actively motile, invade the tissues and ultimately lodge in the submucous tissue of the large gut, i.e. in their normal habitat. Here they grow and multiply by binary fission.

*[*It is to be noted that the trophozoite phase of the parasite is responsible for producing the characteristic lesion of amoebiasis.*]

**During growth, *Entamoeba histolytica* secretes a proteolytic ferment of the nature of *histolysin* which brings about destruction and necrosis of tissues and thereby helps the parasite in obtaining nourishment through absorption of these dissolved tissue juices. The tissue invading amoebae gradually recede from the dead tissues towards the margin of healthy ones and in this way the trophozoites of *E. histolytica* often wander about in the tissue of the gut-wall,

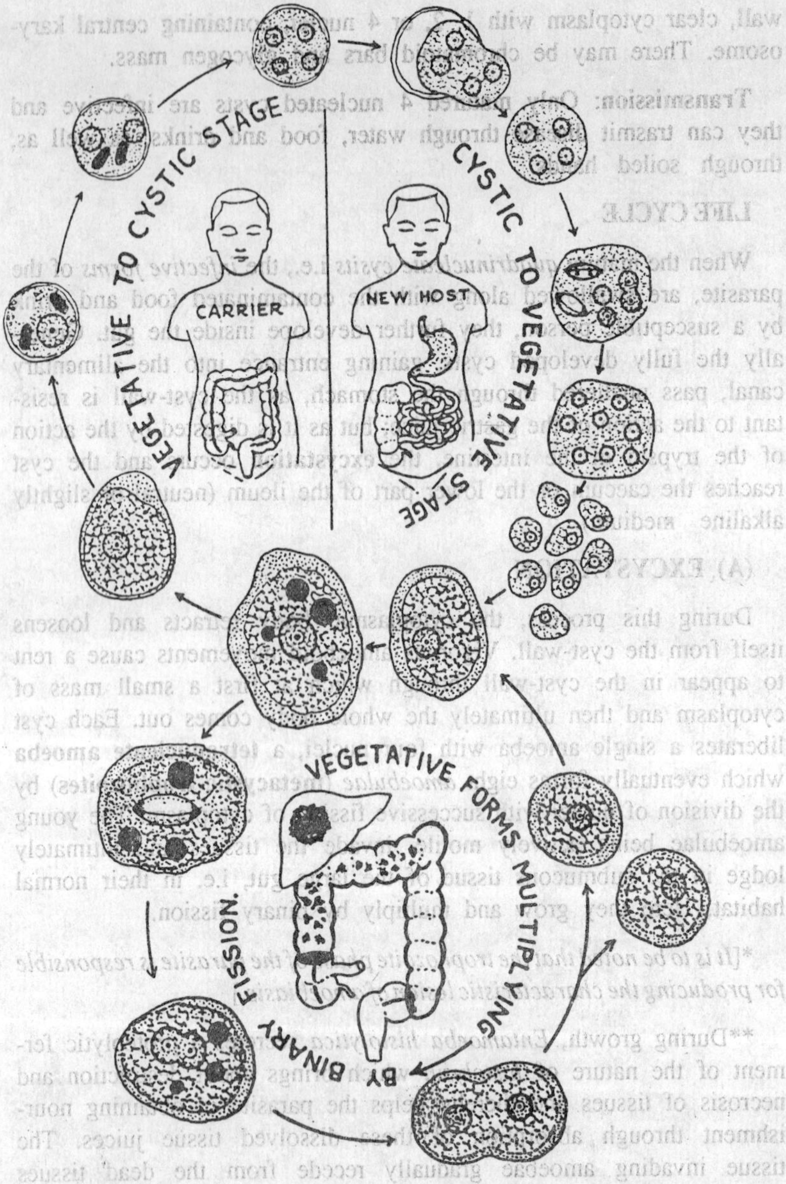

Fig 1. Method of reproduction of *Entamoeba histolytica*, showing excystation, encystation and multiplication of trophozoites (vegetative forms).

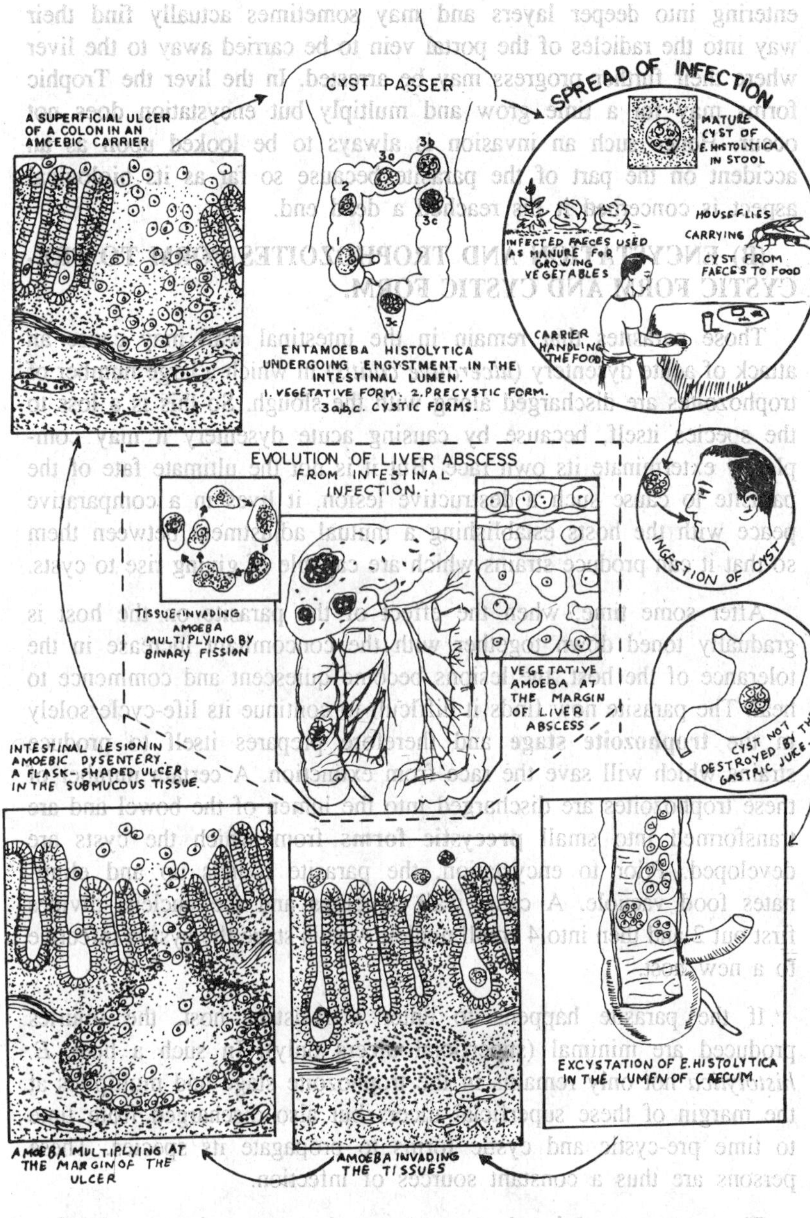

Fig 2. Life cycle of *Entamoeba histolytica*

entering into deeper layers and may sometimes actually find their way into the radicles of the portal vein to be carried away to the liver where their further progress may be arrested. In the liver the Trophic forms may for a time grow and multiply but encystation does not occur. Hence such an invasion is always to be looked upon as an accident on the part of the parasite because so far as its biological aspect is concerned it his reached a dead end.

(B) ENCYSTATION AND TROPHOZOITES FORM TO PRE-CYSTIC FORM AND CYSTIC FORM.

Those parasites that remain in the intestinal wall may cause an attack of acute dysentery (*ulcerative colitis*) in which a large number of trophozoites are discharged along with the slough. So this is a loss to the species itself, because by causing acute dysentery it may completely exterminate its own race. But it is not the ultimate fate of the parasite to cause such a destructive lesion, it lives in a comparative peace with the hosts establishing a mutual adjustment between them so that it can produce strains which are capable of giving rise to cysts.

After some time, when the effect of the parasite on the host is gradually toned down together with the concomitant increase in the tolerance of the host, the lesions become quiescent and commence to heal. The parasite now finds it difficult to continue its life-cycle solely in the **trophozoite stage** and therefore prepares itself to produce strains which will save the race from extinction. A certain number of these trophozoites are discharged into the lumen of the bowel and are transformed into small **precystic forms** from which the cysts are developed. Prior to encystation, the parasite rounds up and eliminates food vacuole. A cysts wall develops and the nucleus divides first out 2 and then into 4 small nuclei. At this stage the cyst is infective to a new host.

If the parasite happens to enter a resistant host, the injuries produced are minimal (superficial ulcers only). In such a host, *E. histolytica* not only remains in the trophozoite stage and multiplies at the margin of these superficial ulcers but also discharged from time to time pre-cystic and cystic forms to propagate its species. These persons are thus a constant sources of infection.

The mature **quadrinucleate cysts** are the most resistant and infective forms of the parasite and are particularly developed a state of equillibrium has been established between the host and the parasite. But the cysts produced in an infected individual are unable to develop in the host in which they are produced and therefore necessitate a transference to another susceptible host where they can grow and continue their life cycle as stated above.

Q. 1.13. (a) How they are transmitted?

Cysts of Entamoeba are transmitted from one individual to another in a variety of ways. The cysts are generally transmitted with food or drink. House flies and cockroaches may transmit cysts mechanically. Raw vegetable is also another source of infection. In many countries human faeces are used as fertilizer and thus roots and leaves of plants remain contaminated with viable cysts. Food handlers are also sometimes responsible for the spread of infection owing to imperfect personal sanitary measures.

Q. 1.13. (b) What is the infective form of the E. histolytica ?

It is the **cystic form** which is infective because due to the resistant cyst wall it is not destroyed by acid (gastic juice) and secondly the cysts can remain alive in the soil even upto 8-10 days. Cysts present in 2 places Lumen of intestines and soil.

Q. 1.13. (c) Which form of the parasite cause the lesion ?

Lesions are caused by the **vegetative forms** and these are always present in the tissue, because of histolysin liberated by then destroy tissue.

Q. 1.14. What are the pathogenic effects of E. histolytica ?

Entamoeba histolytica produces ulceration of the large intestine of man, and also, in a percentage of infected cases, abscess of the liver and rarely of other organs. The unencysted amoebae pass into the simple tubular glands, Lieberkiihns glands, of the intestinal wall and multiply there, often penetrating through the muscularis mucosae into the submucosa. The deeper cells of the glands degenerate owing to pressure by the parasites, or toxins produced, or both, and small ulcers, with undermined raised edges, result. These ulcers become larger individually or by coalescing with others adjacent to them. During the process of ulceration, amoeba, blood cells, tissue debris, and mucous are liberated into the lumen of the intestine and owing to the irritation and dirrhoea, they are quickly discharged in the faeces. Later, the ulcers heal and cicatrize, but in many cases the infection persists for years in a chronic condition.

Q. 1.15. What are the differences between Amoebic and Bacillary Dysentery ? [C.U. 1982]

Differences between Amoebic and Bacillary Dysentery

ITEMS	AMOEBIC	BACILLARY
(A) PATHOLOGY		
1. Nature of lesion	Necrotic due to proteolytic ferment.	Suppurative due to diffusible toxin.
2. Depth of ulcer	Usually deep	Shallow
3. Margin of ulcer	Ragged and undermined.	Uniform, clear-cut (sharp).
4. Intervening mucosa	Normal	Inflamed
5. Organisms in lesions.	Ent. histolytica	Sh. shiga
6. Type of necrosis (at cellular level).	Pyknosis (Pyknotic body and Mouse eaten cells).	Karyolysis (Ghost cell and Ring nucleus)
7. Liver abscess	Common	Rare
8. Cellular response	Mononuclear	Polymorpho nuclear.
(B) STOOL		
1. Macroscopic :		
(a) *Number*	6 to 8 motions a day	Over 10 motions a day
(b) *Amount*	Relatively copious	Small
(c) *Odour*	Offensive	Odourless
(d) *Colour*	Dark red	Bright red
(e) *Nature*	Blood and mucus mixed with faeces	Blood and mucus; no faeces.
(f) *Reaction*	Acid	Alkaline

(g) *Consistancy*	Not adherent to the container.	Adherent to the bottom of the container.
2. Microscopic		
(a) *Cellularity*	Poor	High
(b) *RBC*	In clumps, reddish-yellow in colour.	Discrete or in rouleaux; bright red in colour.
(c) *Pus cells*	Scanty	Numerous
(d) *Macrophages*	Very few	Large and numerous, many of them contain RBC, hence mistaken for E. histolytica.
(e) *Eosinophil*	Present	Scarce.
(f) *Pyknotic bodies*	Very common	Nil
(g) *Ghost cells*	Nil	Numerous
(h) *Parasites*	Trophozoites of E. histolytica.	Nil
(i) *Bacteria*	Many motile	Nil
(j) *C.L. crystals*	Present	Nil

Q. 1.16. What are the main differences between the vegetative forms and cystic forms of E. histolytica and E. Coli? [C.U. 1980]

(A) [VEGETATIVE FORMS OR TROPHOZOITES]

	E. Histolytica	**E. Coli**
(a) **Size**	Range from 10 to 40μ	Usually 20 to 30μ
(b) **Nucleus** :		
Unstained	Rarely visible	Usually visible
Stained	Peripheral chromatin thin.	Peripheral chromatin coarse.
Karyosome	Small and central	Larger and usually eccentric.
(c) Pseudopodia	Active	Sluggish
(d) Ectoplasm	Clearly differentiated from endoplasm.	Not clearly differentiated from endoplasm.
(e) Contents of food vacuoles.	Red blood cells present in acute amoebic dysentery.	Yeast and other particles present, no red cells.

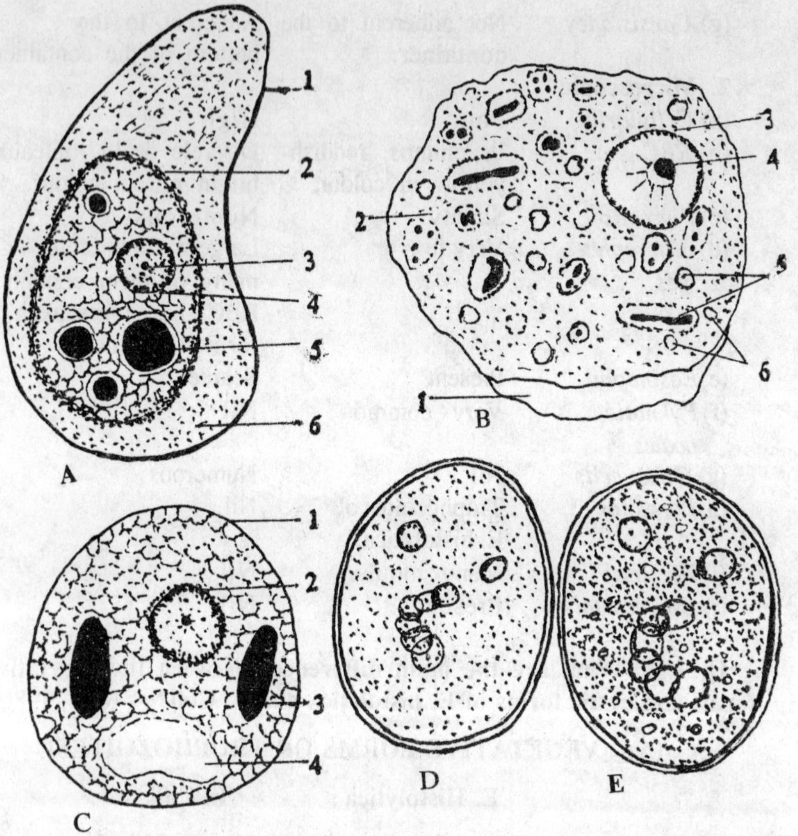

Fig. — 6

1. Trophozoite of E. hystolytica :

1. Pseudopodium, 2. Endoplasm, 3. Karyosome, 4. Nuclear membrane, 5. Ingested red blood cells, 6. Ectoplasm.

2. Uncysted E. coli.:

1. Ectoplasm, 2. Endoplasm, 3. Nucleus, 4. Karyosome, 5. Vacuoles, 6. Ingested bacteria.

3. Cyst of E. histolytica:

1. Cyst wall, 2. Nucleus, 3. Chromotoid body, 4. Glycogen vacuole.

4. Cyst of E. coli (Unstained, nuclei can be seen usually).

5. Cyst of E. coli (Stained with iodine, nuclei stained).

(B) CYSTIC FORMS

	E. Histolytica	E. Coli
(a) **Size**	6 to 15 μ m. (12μ)	15 to 20 μ m. (18μ)
(b) **Unstained** *chromidial bars*	Rounded, usually present.	If present fine and pointed.
(c) **Stained with Iodine**		
(i) Glycogen mass.	Light brown and diffuse if present.	If present light brown and diffuse.
(ii) Number of nuclei.	1 to 4	1 to 8
(iii) Chromatin of nuclei.	Many regular fine dots on nuclear membrane, and small central karyosome.	Many regular coarse dots on nuclear membrane, and large central karyosome.

Q. 1.17. Name some flagellated Protoza parasitic to man.

Flagellated parasite or Protoza parasitic to man are:

(1) *Giardia intestinalis.*
(2) *Trypanosomas gambiense.*
(3) *Leishmania donovani.*
(4) *L. tropica.*
(5) *Trichomonas hominis etc.*

2. GIARDIA INTESTINALIS

Q. 1.18. Describe the morphological characteristic of Giardia intestinalis ?

Giradia intestinalis is a flagellated Protozoa and lives as a parasite in the intestine of man and causes a disease called **'giardiasis'**. Generally they are found in the intestine in 2 forms, viz: **trophozoites** and **cystic.**

(a) Trophozoites :

It is a pear shaped structure of 12 x 9μ diameter. There is a sucking disc in its border end, by which the parasite is attached to the intestinal wall of the host. It is a *bilaterally symmetrical parasite*, which contains two nuclei, in between the nuclei, there are a pair of slender axostyles. At the anterior end of the axostyles there are two basal granules, from which anterior pair of flagella arise to cross each other. There are also other 3 pairs of flagella. Generally the flagella are arranged in the following pattern— *right, 1, left-1, anterolateral-1, posterolateral-1, ventral-2 and caudal-2.*

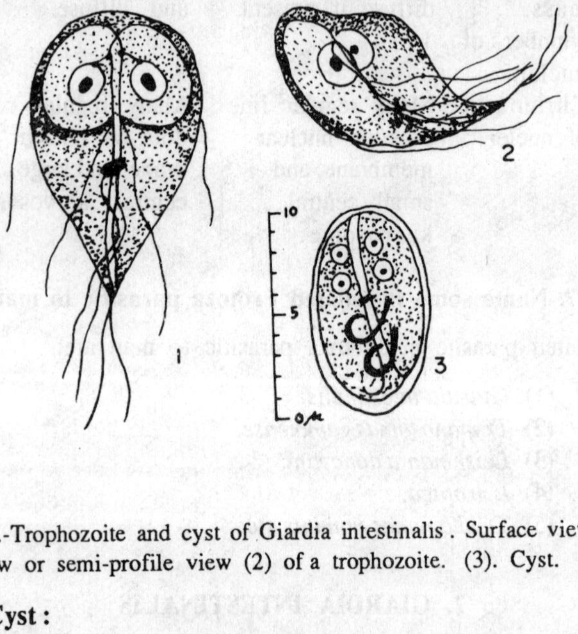

Fig.3.-Trophozoite and cyst of Giardia intestinalis. Surface view (1) and side view or semi-profile view (2) of a trophozoite. (3). Cyst.

(b) Cyst :

It is oval, double contoured of 12 x 5μ diameter, with crescentic fibrils situated at its middle. At one pole of the cyst there are two or four nuclei.

**Generally infection occurs through contaminated drink and food. The cyst when swallowed with contaminated food liberated the trophozoites in the intestine by a process of excystation and trophozoites are liberated and multiply.

Diagnosis : Microscopical examination of stool.

3. LESHMANIA DONOVANI

Q. 1.19. What is Kala-azar ? What are the Leishmanias? Describe their life history? [C.U. 1979, D.M.S. 77, 80, 82, 84]

Kala-azar or **Visceral leishmaniasis** is characterised by a slow onset of fever, of alternating remittent or intermittent type, leading rapidly to a cachectic condition with first enlargement of spleen followed by that of liver.

Inspite of persistent fever the patient has a clear tongue and good appetite. Later on there is extreme emaciation and anaemia. The bleeding from the gums and teeth, dark pigmentation of the skin, cancrum oris, dysentery, and tuberculosis are associated sequle of the untreated cases.

Leishmania donovani is the causal agent of *Kala-azar* and other two species are *L. tropica* and *L. brasileinsis* which are close remsembles to *L. donovani,* but they are responsible for *cutaneous leishmaniasis* or *oriental boils* and *Espunda*, a serious disease of buccal and nasal cavities respectively. *Leishmanias* are member of the genus '*Leishmania*' which are parasitic to man and other vertebrats occur in **Leishmanial forms** (non-flagellates forms) and in the intermediate hosts they are seen in **leptomonad forms** (flagellated forms).

Fig.-4

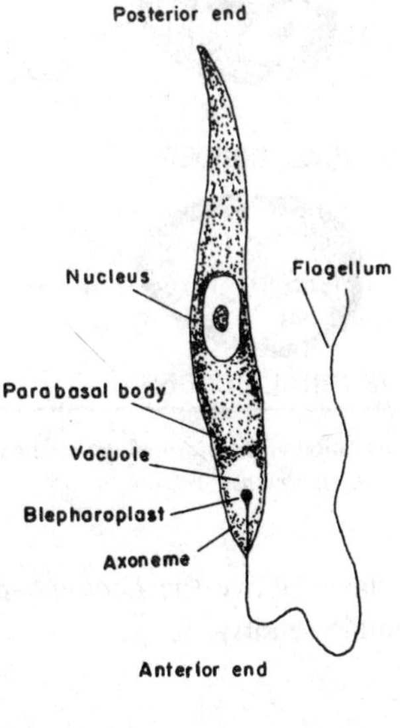

—Diagrammatic representation of the morphology of leptomonad form of *L. donovani*.

In man the leishmanias are intracellular parasites of the reticuloendothelial system namely, the endothelial cells, large *mononuclear leucocytes* and *Kupffer cells* of *liver*. In case of heavy infection they have been found to invade ectodermal cells and polynuclear leucocytes.

LIFE HISTORY

The parasite i.e. Leishmania donovani undergoes two forms in its life cycle viz, *Leishmania* and *Leptomonad* forms.

1. Leishmania Form :

It is found in the reticulo endothelial cells of the human host in liver, spleen and bone marrow of a kala-azar patient. It is an aflagellated parasite with a round body of 2 to 4 x 2μ, with a nucleus and a kinetoplast. The kinetoplast consists of a rod—like parabasal body and a dot—like blepharoplast. The axoneme or rhizoplast is a delicate membrane extended from the (future) root of the flagellum, along side of which there is an unstained vacuole.

When tissue juices, e.g. liver, spleen and bone marrow containing leishmania forms are cultured in NNN medium, the parasites assume leptomonad forms in the culture.

Fig.-5/6.

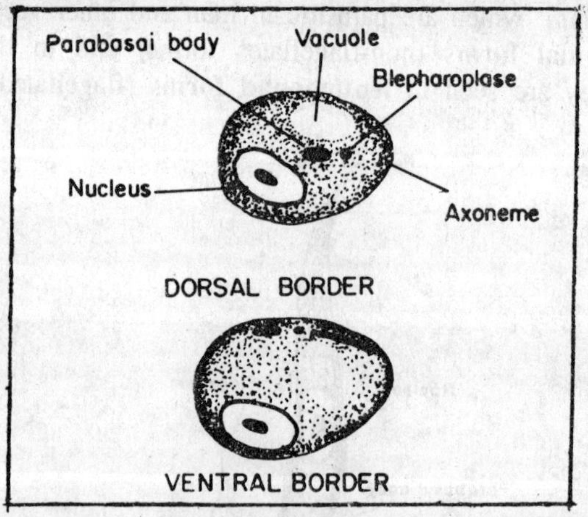

Figs.5 & 6—Diagrammatic representation of the morphology of leishmanial form of *L. donovani*.

2. Leptomonad Form :

Apart from the culture as stated above the *Leptomonad form* is also formed in the midgut of the female sandfly.

LIFE CYCLE OF L. DONOVANI

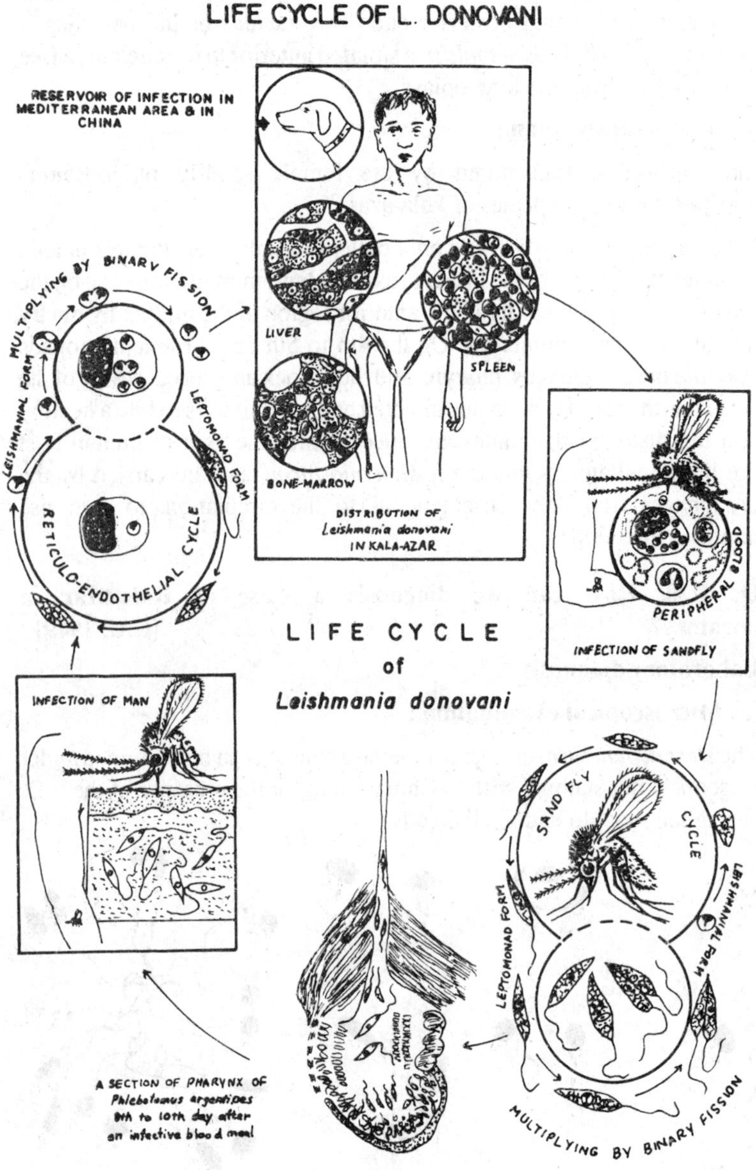

Figs.7—A composite diagram to show the developmental stages of *L donovani* in man and sandfly.

In this form the parasite has a leaf — like body of 5 to 15μ, with a round anterior end and pointed posterior end. The *nucleus* of the parasites is centrally placed and the *kinetoplast* is situated anterior to the nucleus, a free flagellum arises from the kinetoplast.

Mode of Transmission :

The disease is transmitted by the female sandfly **phlebotomus argentipes** the vector species of kala-azar.

When a female sandfly feeds on a patient of kala-azar, the leishmania forms enter the midgut of the insect to assume leptomonad forms and on the 3rd day they multiply rapidly in the anterior region of the midgut by binary fission and becomes numerous. On the 4th to 5th day these leptomonads ascend into the oesaphagus, pharynx and they block and buccal cavity of the insect. Thus the sandfly becomes infected and when it tries to bite a healthy person the disloged flagellates are injected into the skin of human host where the flagellate assume the *leishmania forms* and are carried by the macroaphages from the subscutaneous to the circulation, to give rise generalised infection.

Q. 1.20. How can we diagnosis a Case of Kala-azar in Laboratory? [C.U. 1979]

Laboratory diagnosis

(a) Microscopical examination :

The *sternal puncture*, or *splenic puncture* smears, can be examined under microscope, after staining with Leishman stain for the presence of the L.D. bodies in the reticulo endothelial cells.

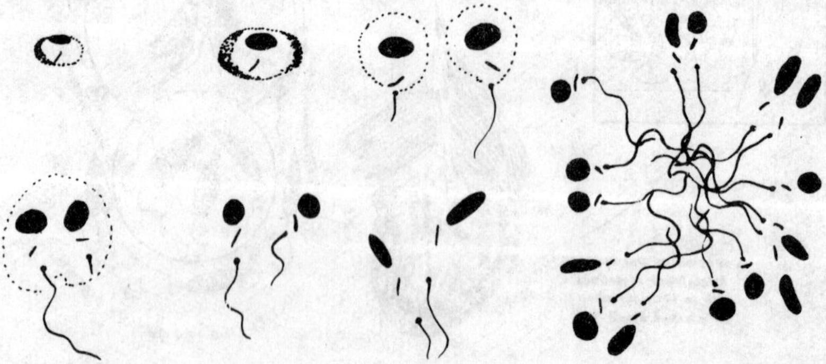

Fig.8—Stages of development of *L. donovani* in N.N.N. medium. Stained with Leishman's stain.

(b) Culture :

The splenic or the bone marrow juices obtained by the puncture can be cultured in N.N.N. Medium at 22°C for 1 to 4 weeks for the presence of leptomonad forms.

(c) Aldehyde test :

(i) *Aldehyde test* — 1 drop of 40 percent formalin is added to 1 ml of patient's serum placed in a test tube. If positives, there will be a milky white *opacity with jellification* within 20 minutes.

This Napier's aldehyde test is not positive before 3 months duration of kala-azar.

(ii) *Antimony test* — It is less reliable than the Aldehyde test and it is positive only after 6 weeks of illness. In this test 4 percent solution of Ureastibamine (in distlled water) is mixed with 1 to 10 diluted patient's serum in distilled water. In positive case, there will be formation of flocculent precipitate at the junction of the two fluids.

(iii) *Complement fixation test* — This test is positive within 3 weeks of illness. The W K K antigen used in this test is prepared from human tubercle bacilli.

(d) Blood examination :

Progressive *leucopenia* —Total count is low. D.C. SHOWS — Lymphocytosis and Eosinophil is absent.

4. PLASMODIUM

Q. 1.21. What is meant by Malaria parasites? Who has been discovered them? [D.M.S. 1978 (Dec.)]

Members of the genus—**Plasmadium** are collectively known as **Malaria Parasites**, because they cause a febrile disese called **malaria**.

In the **man** i.e. in the intermediate host they invade the reticuloendothelial system and in the **female Anopheles** mosquito i.e. in definitive host, they reside in the salivary glands.

Charles Laveran in 1880 discovered the presence of some amoeba like organisms in the *Red blood cells* of patient suffering from chill and fever and he termed these organisms **plasmodium**.

He injected the blood of a malaria patient into the blood stream of a healthy man observed that fever develops in the injected man. Later on, many observed like **Golgi** and **Celli** confirmed the observations of

Laveran. But its connection with the intermediate host and modes of transmission were experimentally worked out in *Calcutta* by **Sir Ronald Ross in 1889.**

It is to the credit of **Grassi** (1890) who provided absolute scientific proof of the specific relationship between *Anopheles* mosquito and the human malaria parasites.

LIFE CIRCLE OF PLASMODIUM IN MAN

Q. 1.22. Give an illustrated account of the life cycle of Plasmodium in man.

Or

Soon after sporozoites of malarial parasite are injected in man by mosquito they are not found in the Red blood corpuscles. Where do they go and what happen to them? Which stage is the sign of their presence in the blood? [C.U. 1979, D.M.S. 74,80, 82,84]

The life cycle of malarial parasite is completed in two phases :

(1) Asexual or Endogenous phase.
(2) Sexual or Exogenous phase.

A sexual phase takes place in man. It is divided into three phases :

(a) *Pre-erythrocytic phase.*
(b) *Exo-erythrocytic phase.*
(c) *Erythrocytic phase.*

(a) Pre-erythrocytic phase :

When an Anopheles mosquito (where main food is the blood of man) in which malaria parasites are present. bites a healthy man, it leaves some sporozoites in the blood of man with the saliva of mosquito. Each sporozoite is sickle-shaped and about 14 micra long. These sporozoites come into the blood stream of man. After about half an hour they leave the circulatory system and reach parenchymatous cells of the liver.

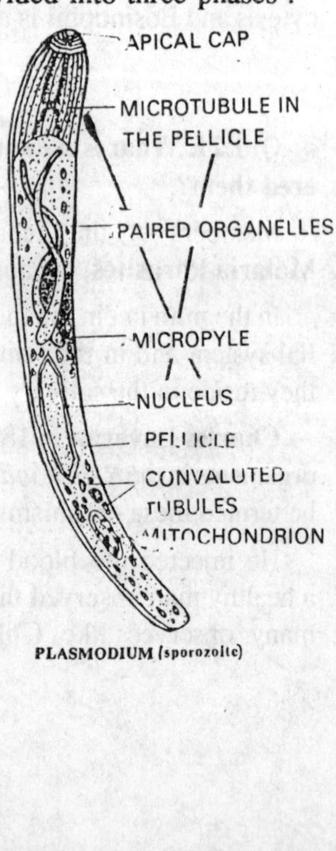

PLASMODIUM (sporozoite)

Liver Schizogony :

In parenchymatous cells of liver they grow and form **schizonts.** After some time the nucleus of **Schizont** divides into about 1,000 small nuclei. A little **cytoplasm** around each nuclei and thus 1,000 **merozoites** are formed which are also called **cyptozoites.** The nucleus of schizont divides by multiple fission. This division is known as **liver schizogony.** Now the wall of schizont and liver cell bursts due to great number of cryptozoites in them, and all the cryptozoites go into the sinusòdies of the liver. There is no effect of medicines on these merozoites which also remain uneffected by the resistance of the host.

(b) Exo-erythrocytic phase :

The *cryptozoites* of the pre-erythrocytic phase which are released in the liver sinusoides attack new liver cells and they again form **schizonts.** These again undergo multiple fission and form many cryptozoites which are called **metacryptozoites.** This phase is know as **exo-erythrocytic phase.** After two or more such phases some metacryptozoites come into blood circulation and attack the red blood corpuscles.

(c) Erythrocytic cycle :

Meta-cryptomerozoites start growing in the RBC's obtaining their food from them. They are round in shape and soon a non-contractile vacuole is formed in them. This stage is called **signet-ring stage** with further growth the vacoule disappears and it assumes *Amoeba* like form. It starts feeding on haemoglobin and grows rapidly. This is know as **trophozoite stage.** After feeding on haemoglobin they form a yellowish brown substance called **Haemozoin.** As the trophozoite increases in size, it becomes round and completely fills red blood corpuscles. This is known as **schizont.** The red blood corpuscles become weak and loses its normal shape due to the growth of the schizont within it. It swells in size and becomes light in colour with its regular shape. In its remaining cytoplasm several small, orange or yellow coloured granules are formed which are known as **schuffier's dots.** Multiple fission takes place in schizont and its nucleus divides into many small nuclei around each of which a little cytoplasm gathers. In this manner 6 to 36 **merozoites** are formed in each schizont. After sometime schizont bursts liberating the merozoites in the blood. These merozoites attack fresh red blood corpuscles. This process is repeated many times and innumerable red corpuscles destroyed.

***Haemozoin** is a toxic substance formed as a waste product in R.B.C. When it is released in the red blood it dissolves in the plasma due to which Malarial fever starts with chills and shiverings.

LIFE CYCLE OF PLAMODIUM IN MOSQUITO

Q. 1.23. What are the different stages of sexual phase of malaria parasite?

Or

Give an account of the life history of plasodium vivax in mosquito.

[D.M.S. 1975, '78]

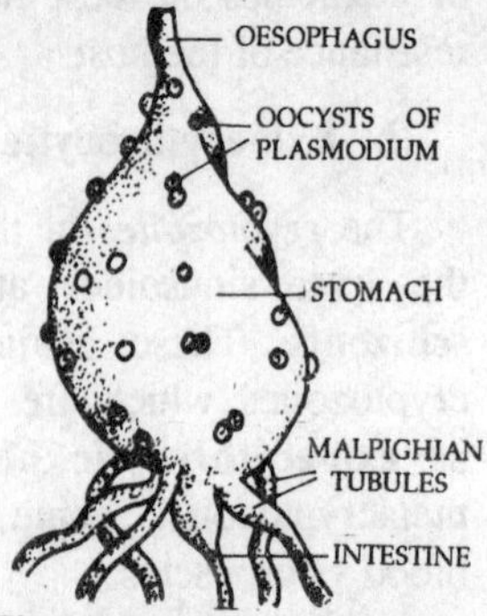

Fig. 7. 2. Stomach of an infected female *Anopheles* mosquito with oocvsts of *Plasmodium*.

The *sexual or Exogenous* phase takes place in female Anophels. It is divided into two stages :

(a) **Gamogony.**
(b) **Sporogony.**

(a) ***Gamogony***: After many sexual cycles some merozoites increase in size within the red blood corpuscles and form gametocytes. Some of these are many and known as **microgametocytes** while others are large and called **macrogametocytes**. Further development of these gametocytes is not possible in man because of the high body temperature.

Females or **macrogametocytes** are round and their cytoplasm is laden with food. The nucleus is eccentric i.e., placed on one side. **Male** or **microgametocytes** have clear cytoplasm with a central nucleus.

If a female Anopheles mosquito bites a man having this stage of plasmodium, then along with merozoites some gametocytes are also sucked up with blood and reach the stomach of mosquito, where their development takes place. The nucleus of microgametocytes divides into 6 to 8 small nuclei around each of which a little cytoplasm collects forming long flagellated structures known as **microgametes**. This process is called **exflagellation**.

Macrogametocyte undergoes little changes. It increases in size and its nuclues divides into two. One of these nuclei moves out along with some cytoplasm and form the polar body. In the remaining larger part a small conical structure is formed which is known as reception zone. Thus a macrogamete is *formed from* only one macrogametocyte.

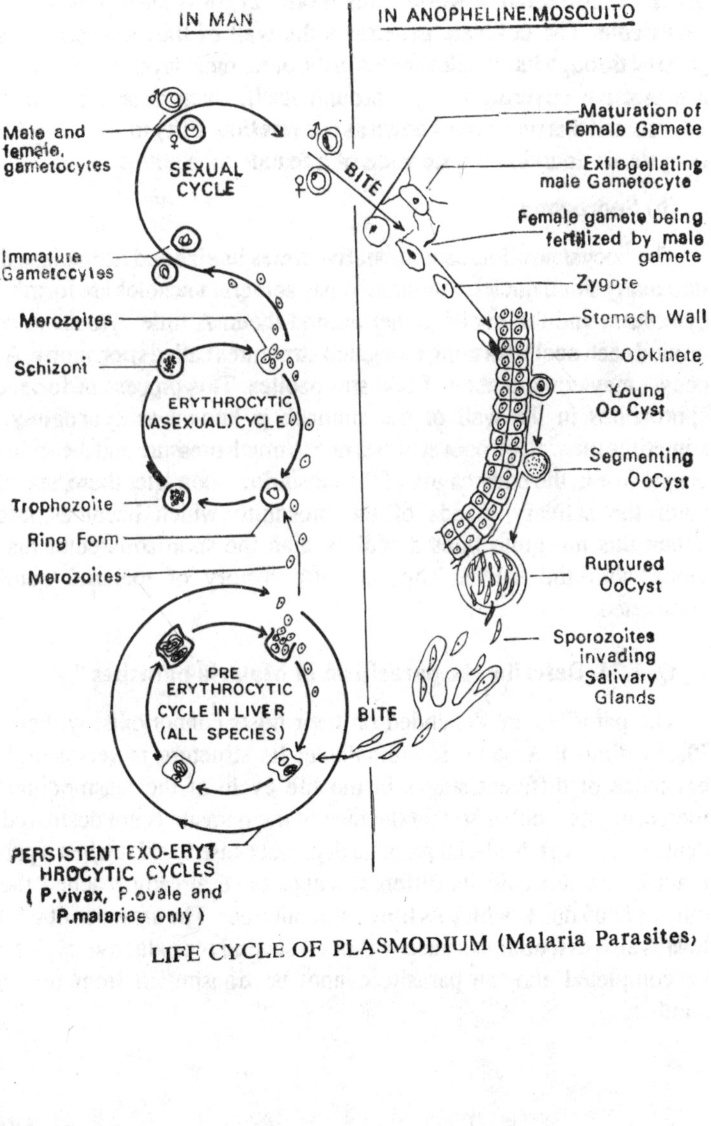

LIFE CYCLE OF PLASMODIUM (Malaria Parasites)

Fertilization :

Microgamete is attracted towards the macrogametes and enters the later in its reception zone. The nucleus and cytoplasm of both the gametes fuse and forms a zygote. This process is known as *fertilization.*

The zygot remains inactive for sometime after which it lengthens and beocmes motile like a worm. This motile zygot is known as **ookinete** or **vermicule.** The ookinete penetrates the wall of the stomach and after passing through its muscles settles in the outer most layer where it forms a protective covering or cyst around itself. Such structures are called oocysts and this process is known as **oocystation.** Fifty to five hundred oocysts are found in the stomach of a female mosquito.

(b) Sporogony :

The oocyst now increase about five times its size and its nucleus divides into many small nuclei. Simultaneously serveral vacuoles are formed in the cytoplasm and the nuclei gather around them. A little cytoplasm collects around each nuclei forming elongated structures called **sporogony.** A single occyst may contain about 1,000 sporozoites. This process of formation of sporozoites in the wall of the stomach is known as **sporogony.** After sometime the wall of oocyst bursts due to much pressure and the sporozoites are set free in the body cavity of the mosquito. Soon after these, sporozoites enter the salivary glands of the mosquito which becomes infective. When this mosquito bites a healthy man the sporozoits enter his blood along with the saliva. Thus the life history of malarial parasite is completed.

Q. 1.24. Describe the parasitism of Malaria parasites ?

The parasites are depended on their hosts cannot exist without them. Plasmodium is a parasitic animalcule. Its structure is very simple. The existence of different stages in the life cycle of the plasmodium is for increasing its number so that the race of the parasite is not destroyed at the death of the host. Malarial parasite does not cease to exist when a patient of malaria dies because its different stages have already reached the mosquito's body due to which its life cycle continues. The presence of secondary host is also essential, because without it several reproductive cycles cannot be completed and the parasite cannot be transmitted from one man to another.

PLATE IV

LIFE CYCLE OF MALARIA PARASITE (*Plasmodium vivax*) IN MAN AND MOSQUITO

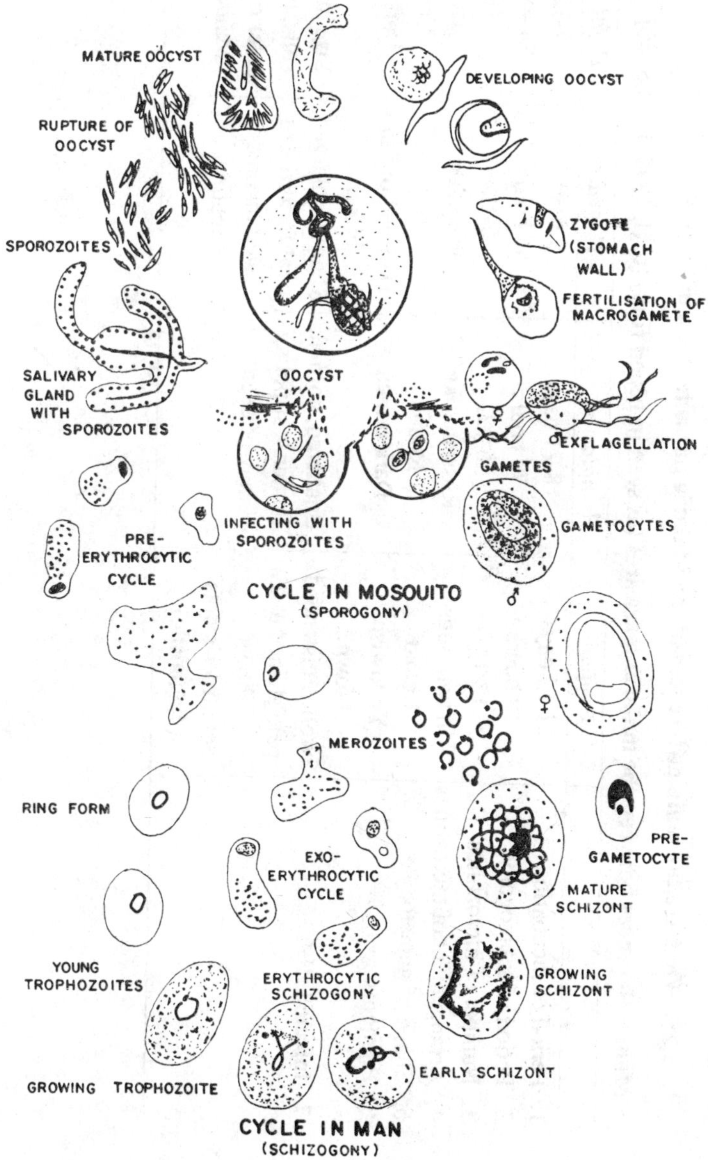

Q. 1.25. What are the main differences of the Malaria parasites seen in blood film ?

Main differences between the malarial parasites (as seen in Blood film) [C.U. 1979, D.M.S. 80]

	P. vivax	*P. malariae*	*P. ovale*	*P. falciparum*
1. Period of incubation	11-14 days	18-21 days	9 days	9-12 days
2. Period of schizogony	48 hours	72 hours	48 hours	24-48 hours
3. Number of merozoites	12-14	6-12	6-12	18-24
4. Arrangement of merozoites	In two rings	Rossette like.	Irregular	Irregular
5. Shape of gametocyle	Round	Round	Oval	Crescent
6. Pigments	Yellowish brown.	Dark brown.	Dark-yellowish brown.	Dark brown
7. Infected RBC.	Swollen,distended pale stained and shows Schuffner's dots (diagnostic).	Unaltered, normal, Zeiman's stippling may be seen.	Slightly enlarged oval frimbriated well marked stippling.	Size not altered, cells, containing older rings. Show Maurer's dots.

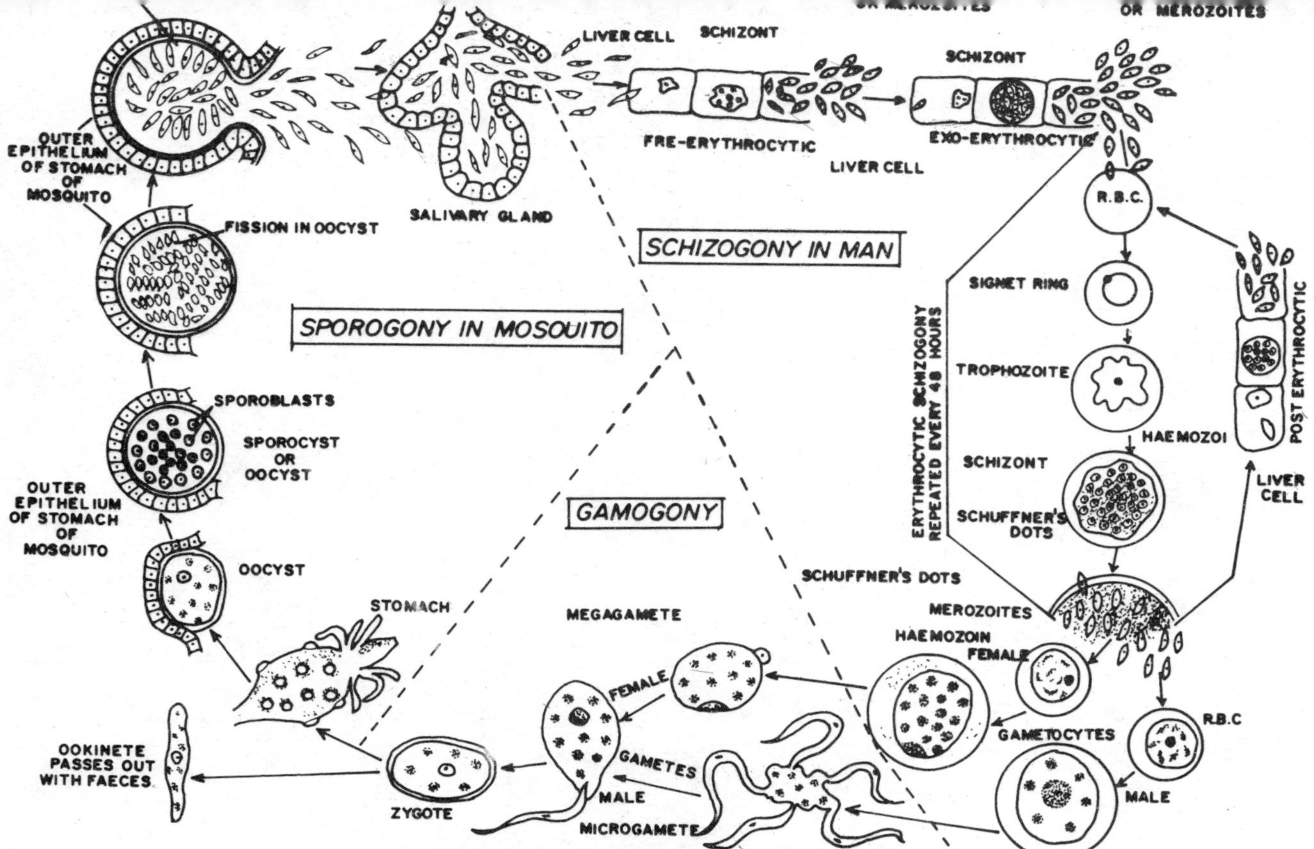

LIFE CYCLE OF PLASMODIUM VIVAX

Q. 1.26. What are the causative organism of the disease?
[C.U. 1979, D.M.S. 1980, 82, 84]

The causative organism of the disease malaria are :

(1) *Plasmodium vivax* (B.T)

(2) *P. malriae* (Q.T.)

(3) *P. falciparum* (M.T.)

(4) *P. ovale.* (O.T.)

Generally they cause *Benign tertian* (B.T), *Quartan* (Q.T), *Malignant* (M.T) and *Ovale tertian* fever respectively. In Benign tertian outbreak of fever occurs every other day, in quartan fever the outbreak sets in every day, while malignant malaria is irregular occurring almost daily and is often fatal.

COMPARASION BETWEEN P. VIVAX AND P. FALCIPARUM IN BLOOD FILM [D.M.S. 1976, 80]

Q. 1.27. Compare between P. Vivax and P. Falciparum as seen in Blood film :

P. VIVAX	P. FALCIPARUM
I. TROPHOZOITE (ringform)	
Ring usually large (3μ), 1/3 RBC: round or oval.	Small, 1/5 RBC, Slender accoleform characteristic.
(a) **Growing** : Highly amoeboid, vivacious, hence the name.	Multiple infection often with two Chromatin dots.
(b) **Pigment** : Fine, granular or delicate rods evenly distributed scattered with little tendency to coalesce.	Dark black in compact masses. Early collection of pigment seen in pre-schizont stage.
(c) **Infected RBC** Swollen, distended, Pale stained and shows Schuffner's dots (diagnostic).	Size not altered, cells containing older rings show Maurer's dots.
II. SCHIZONT	
Chromatin divided, Pigment brownish black as fine grains or tiny rods.	Not seen in peripheral blood, except in moribund cases.

(a)	**Sporulating Schizont** Almost fill the distended RBC, 9-10μ.	Fills 2/3 RBC, 6.5-7μ.
(b)	**Merozoites-8-24, usually 12-18.**	8-26, usually 8-18.
III.	**GAMETOCYTE** Round, almost fill the RBC; Host cell enlarged.	Cresent shaped RBC, hardly recognisable.
(a)	**Male** (Microganmetocyte) Cytoplasm greenish blue; Chromatin and pigment scattered.	Short and stout cytoplasm purplish blue; Chronatin and pigment scattered.
(b)	**Female** (Macrogametocyte) Larger than male; Cytoplasm deep blue, pigment coarse, con - densed; chromatin stains deeply.	Longer and thinner than male; cytoplasm deep blue pigment condensed chromatin stains deeply in centre.
IV.	**SCHIZOGONY** 48 hours	36-48 hours
(a)	**Forms in peripheral blood:** All stages of Schizogony and gametocytes seen.	Rings and ametocytes usually seen.
(b)	**Development period in mosquito:** 16-17 days; at 20°C; 10 days at 25°C.	22-23 day at 20°C
(c)	**Usual incubation period :** 18-31 days; Average 14 days	17-27 days; Average 21 days.
(d)	**Appearance of gametocyte** *after parasite potency 3-5 days.*	7-12 days.

Q. 1.28. What are the Parasites seen in peripheral blood ?

Parasites in Peripheral blood are of 2 types :

1. *Intra-cellular.*
2. *Extra-cellular.*

1. Intra-cellular:

(a) Within R.B.C.— Malarial parasites:

P. vivax
P. falciparum
P. malaria
P. ovale

(b) Within the W.B.C.'s— L.D. body (Leishmanoid form present within Monocyte — rare in peripheral blood)

2. Extra-cellular-i.e. in the plasma.

(a) Microfilaria.
(b) Trypanosomes.
(c) Larva of Trichinella spiralis (rare).

Q. 1.29. What are the Parasites seen in Urine?

1. **Microfilaria—** In case of chyluria resulting from filarial infection.
2. **Ova of Schistosoma haematobium —** Commonly associated with haematuria and the condition is called Bilhar Ziasis.

*Associated with Trophozoite form, hence if a blood film shows both ring and trophozoites forms we consider B.T. parasite.

Q. 1.30. What are the forms of Malarial Parasites seen in blood?

All forms (the ring form, the growing trophozoites, Schizont and the gametocyte) of Plasmodium vivax and P. malaria.

In case of P. falciparum causing M.T. malaria — We get only the ring form and gametocyte form. Other forms of this parasite are not seen because the schizogony occurs in the capillaries of internal organs.

The gametocyte form of M.T. parasite is known as 'cresent' and it is called falciparum because of the sickle shaped character of the gametocyte.

Q. 1.31. What are the differences between B.T. Ring and M.T. Ring ?

B.T. Ring	M.T. Ring
1. **Change in infacted RBC:** Affected RBC is enlarged, pale irregular outline and may show fine stippling (eonsinophilics, stipplings known as *Schuffner's dot*).	1. Affected RBC is normal in size and shape — There may be few granules present known as *Maurer's dot*.

2. **Apperance of ring:** Large ring — (1/3 of diameter of RBC). The chromatin dot stained purple is always solitary and the bluish cytoplasmic outline of the ring is very thick and vary.

2. It is a small rign (1/6 of diameter of RBC), the outline of the ring is thin and clear cut. M.T. ring may show some special features : they are: (a) within a single RBC there may be more than one ring (called multiple infection). (b) The ring may be in the periphery of RBC so that a part of the ring coincides within margin of RBC. (This is known as accole form). (c) There may be more than one chromatin dot in a single ring.

Q. 1.32. What is meant by Trophozoite and Schizont ?

So long as the chromatin mass is solitary but the cytoplasmic outline of the parasite is irregular due to psecudopodia we call it a *trophozites*. When the chromatin starts dividing into fragments it becomes as Schizont (Immature and Mature).

Q. 1.33. How to differentiate Tropozoites and Schizonts, of all types of Malaria parasites ?

Differntiation is made by the number of young merozoites present within the schizont in case of B.T. This varies from 16-24, in M.T. it is 24-32, in P. malariae it varies between 0.8.

Trophozoites	Schizont
1. **Ring form (early):** Vacuole present, size small.	1. **Early**—shape round, *size* : Larger than RBC. Haemozoin pigment scattered in cytoplasm.
2. **Growing trophozoite:** Irregular size, vacuole present.	2. **Late shape rounds,** ***size*** : large than RBC. No vacuole, chromatin divided called merozoites and masses of Haemozoin pigment aggregated in centre.

Mature schizont in P. vivax contains 16-24 merozoites, arranged around Haemozoin pigment, P. falciparum : 24-32.

MALARIA PARASITES OF MAN (*Erythrocytic Phase*)

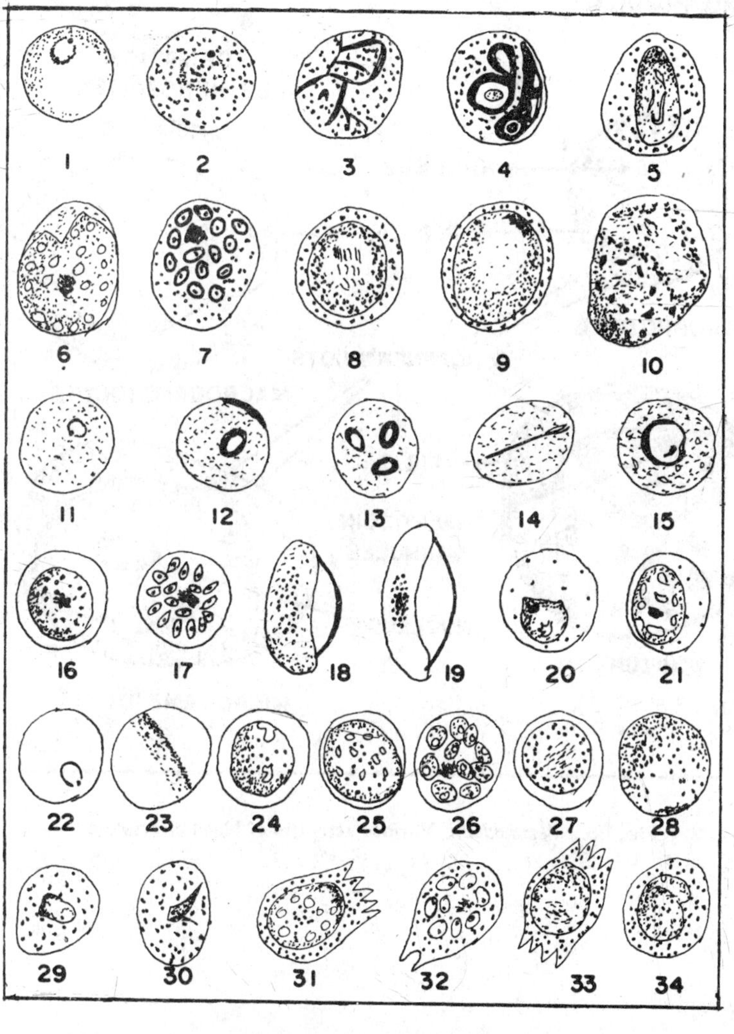

Malaria parasites of man (*Erythrocytic Phase*)

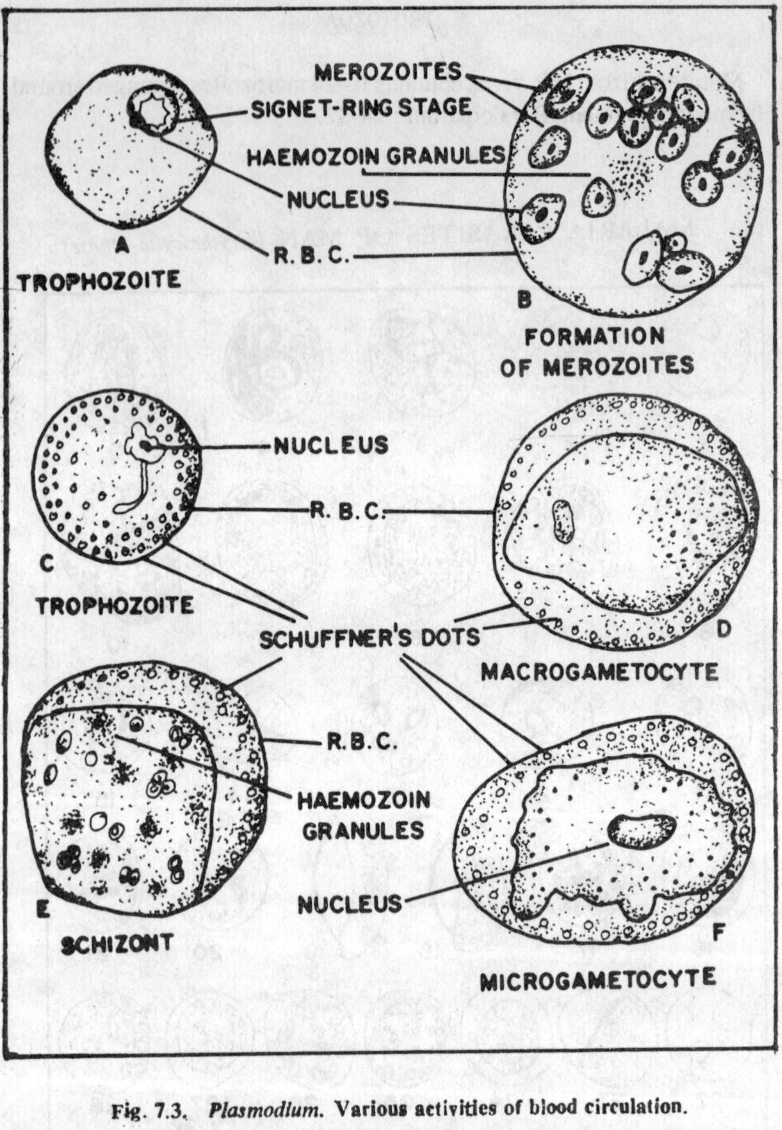

Fig. 7.3. *Plasmodium*. Various activities of blood circulation.

CHAPTER 2

HELMINTHES

[DISCUSSION FOR LEARNING]

1. PLATYHELMINTHES

(A) Cestodes:

1. *Taenia solium, T. sagginata.*
2. *Taenia echinococcus.*

(B) Trematoda:

II. NEMATHELMINTHES

(C) Nematodes :

1. *Ascaris lumbricoides.*
2. *Enterobius vermicularis.*
3. *Ancylostoma duodenale.*
4. *Wuchereria bancrofti.*
5. *Trichinella Spiralis.*
6. *Strongyloides Stercoralis.*
7. *Trichuris Trichiura.*

Q. 2.1. What is meant by Helminthes ?

Helminthes are worms, multicellular and metazoal animals arising from more than one embryonic layers. Their tissues are differentiated into : (i) alimentary, (ii) excretory, (iii) reproductive, and (iv) nervous system developed partially or completely. They are free-living but some are endo-parasites of man and animals. In man they may produce disease by depriving the host of his food and/or by liberation of toxic substances.

They are divided into two phyla :

(a) **Pltyhelminths** (flat worms).

(b) **Nemathelminths** (round worms).

HELMINTHES
(Metazoa)

Platyhelminthes — classes:
- **Cestoideae** (Tape worm)
- **Trematoda** (Flukes—leaf like)

Nemathelminthes:
- **Nematoda** (Round worm)

Characteristics:

Cestoideae	Trematoda	Nematoda
Body : Tapelike, segmented.	*Body* : Leaf like unsegmented.	*Body* : Cylindrical and unsegmented.
Sex: Hermaphrodite.	*Sex:* Usually hermaphrodite.	*Sex:* Male and female
Head: Often with hook and suckers.	*Head*: without hooks but with suckers.	*Head:* Hooks and suckers absent.
Alimentary canal: Absent.	*Alimentary canal* : Incomplete.	*Alimentary canal* : Complete with Anus.
Body cavity : Absent.	*Body cavity* : Absent.	*Body cavity* : Present.

I. PLATYHELMINTHES

Q. 2.2. What are the main characteristics of the Phylum-Platyhelminthes ? [C.U. 1982]

This phylum comprises worms which are dorse — ventrally flattened. They are mainly parasites, and have solid bodies without a body cavity. They have no respiratory or blood vascular system, but have an elaborate, bilaterally symmetrical excretory system. They are usually hermaphrodites, but in some cases the sexes are separate.

The phylum contains three classes, two of which are of medical importance.

These are :

(1) **Turbellaria or Eddy worms** : They are mainly fire-living, and are covered with cilia. None are parasitic in man.

(2) **Cestoideae or Tapeworms** : (a) Worms of this class are endoparasitic, and the adults are found exclusively in the intestine, (b) A tapeworm consists of a head which bears sucking organs and sometimes hooks in additon, and a long chain of segment, (c) There is no intestinal canal, (d) They are all hermaphroditic.

(3) **Trematoda or Flukes** : (a) Worms of this class are also endoparasitic, and are usually leaf -like in shape (as in Fasciola), but some are cylindrical (as are female Schistosomes).

(b) A fluke has no distinct head, its body is not segmented, and it has two suckers for attachment. The intestine is usually shaped, the two limbs terminating blindly at the posterior ends; there is no anus.

(c) They are hermaphroditic, except for the Schistosomes in which the sexes are separate.

Q. 2.3. What are the main characterisitcs of Cestoidea or Tapeworms and Trematoda or Flukes ? [C.U. 1979]

For Answer see Q. 2.2.

A. CESTODES

1. TAENIA SOLIUM

Q. 2.4. What is meant by tapeworms ?

All *flatworms belonging to class—Cestoda, Phylum — platyhelminths are known as tapeworms.* They generally live as endoparasites in the intestine of vetebrates. They do not possess any cilia but possess cuticular body and the body is divided into many Proglottides. For anchorage to the intestinal walls they possess hooks, suckers and other organs. They are hermaphrodite and involve more than one host in their life cycle, which shows hexacanth embryo during development.

Gyrocotyle, Echinobothrium, Tetrashynchus etc. are tapeworms of fishes, and *Taenia solium, Echinococcus, Hymenolepis* etc. are tapeworms of mammals and birds. *Taenia solium* and *Taenia saginata* are typical intestinal tapeworm of human beings.

Q. 2.5. What is the systematic position of Taenia solium ?

Systematic position (According to Hyman, 1951)

Phylum	Platyhelminthes
Class	Cestoda
Sub-class	Encestoda
Order	Taenodea
Genus	Taenia
Species	Solium

Q. 2.6. Where Taenia Solium is found ?

Or

Where they live in ?

(a) Taenia solium lives as an endoparasite in the intestine of man and is found specially in European countries where eating of pork without thorough cooking is a regular practice. But now it is comparatively rare. *Taenia solium* adheres to the mucous membrane of the intestine and injures it. It also causes mechanical injury by obstructing the alimentary canal. It causes abdominal pains, loss of weight and loss of appetite.

(b) Eggs passed in human faeces, usually in the gravid proglottid; infection to both pig and man.

(c) Larvae usually in the musculature and other organs of the pig, and also accidentaly, in the subcutaneous tissue, brain, orbit and musculature of man.

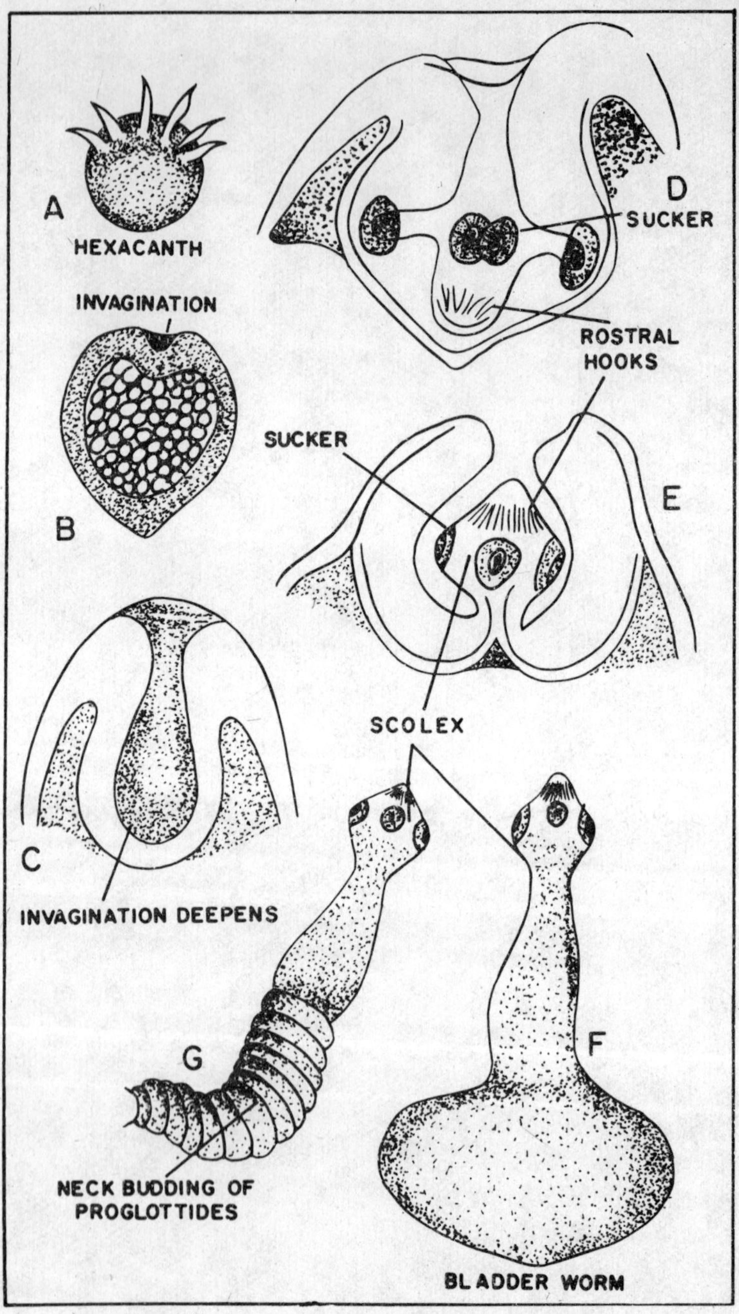
A
HEXACANTH
INVAGINATION
B
C
INVAGINATION DEEPENS
D
SUCKER
ROSTRAL
HOOKS
SUCKER
E
SCOLEX
G
NECK BUDDING OF
PROGLOTTIDES
F
BLADDER WORM

[MORPHOLOGY]

Q. 2.7. Describe the Morphology of T. solium.

The body of *T. solium* is long dorsoventrally flattened, narrow, ribbon-like, reaching a length of about ten feet. The colour of the body is opaque white. The body is divided into 3 regions : **(a) Head or Scolex, (b) Neck, (c) Strobila or body segment, (d) Proglottides.**

(a) Scolex: The anterior end of the Taenia has a knob - like scolex which is just like the head of a pin. This pinhead scolex has a diameter of 1 mm and 4 cuplike suckers having radial muscles. The anterior round prominences at the tip of the scolex is known as **rostellum**. It has 22 — 32 hooks in two circles. The inner circle has larger hooks while the outer one has smaller hooks. With the help of hooks had suckered scolex Taenia adhers to the intestinal mucous membrane of human beings.

(b) Neck : Behind the scolex is a thin, narrow unsegmented portion, which proliferates proglottides by transverse fission or asexual budding. This portion is known as *neck*.

(c) Strobila : The part next to the scolex is a segment which is the body of the worm, known as *strobila*.

(d) Proglottides : They are the remaining segments, and are produced by the strobilia. The body of a mature tape worm has 800-900 proglottides the *youngest proglottides* are nearest to the strobilia, they are broader than long and devoid of sex organs. The middle region has Squarish proglottides and in them first the male organs develop, then both male and female organs are found. These called **matured proglottides.** The oldest proglottides are towards the end of the body. They are filled with eggs and are called **gravid proglottides.** The proglottides alternately bear a genital papilla and pore alternately on the left or right side. **This animal has no mouth, alimentary canal and anus.** They absorb digested food as liquids from the mucous membrane of the host. They store reserve food as glycogen and lipid.

Q. 2.8.(a) Where Taenia solium is found and its life cycle is of what type ? Give an account of the life history of Taenia solium. [D.M.S. 1974]

For First part see Q. 2.6.

The life history of Taenia is complicated and is completed through two hosts, therefore, it is called a **digenetic life cycle**. Its primary host is **man** and secondary or intermediate host is **pig**.

1. Fertilization: Self fertilization takes place in Taenia, in which the cirrus of a reproductive proglottid enters the vagina of the same proglottid. Fertilization takes place in the ovi duct. The fertilized eggs are covered by the yolk secreted by vitelline glands. After fertilization the uterus increases in size and gives off 7 to 12 branches, all of which are filled up by fertilized eggs. In this condition,. the proglottids are called gravid proglottids.

Fig. 11.

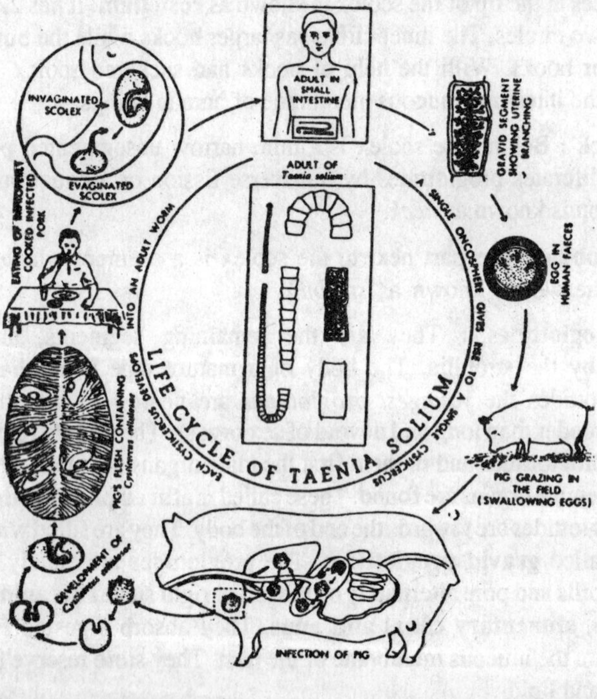

2. Cleavage: The eggs start developing while they are in uterus. After first division the zygot divides into two cells of different size. The larger cell is called *vitelline cell* and the smaller cell is known as *embryonic cell.* Gradually the *yolk cells* disappear being used as food.

3. Morula: The *embryonic cell* divides immediately and large *macromeres* and *small micromeres* are formed. The viteline cell decreases in size. A hard capsule is formed around the macromere and micromeres. The micromeres form the *morula*.

4. Onchophere : The micromeres of morula change into a small larva and three pairs of chitinous hooks are formed by the inner cells of the capsule. Thus a six hooked embryo is formed which is called ***hexacanth*** or ***onchosphere***.

Upto this stage the development takes place in the uterus of the gravid proglottid which now breaks off and comes out of the intestine of man with faeces. Thus onchospheres come out of the body of man in the gravid proglottids. When the faeces of man containing these proglottids is eaten by pig, the onchospheres reach its stomach. If onchopheres are unable to reach the stomach of pig then the further development of embryo does not take place.

CYSTCERCUS OR BLADDER WORM

The onchospheres are released from the gravid proglottids in the stomach of pig 24 to 72 hours after reaching there. The six hooks project on the outer side and the hexacanth embryos gradually reach the blood, lymph, heart muscles etc. of pig. Hexacanth now under-goes a change, its hooks disappear, its size increases and their central fluid filled cavity enlarges. It then becomes surrounded by a layer of cuticle and assumes a bladder-like form. A *proscolex* is formed, on the surface of which hooks and suckers are found. These structures are embedded towards the inner cavity. This state is called ***cysticercus*** **or** ***bladder worm*** and are disappeared in the flesh of pig. The further development of bladder worm takes place in the body of man.

When the half cooked meat of a infected pig is eaten by man, then these cysticercus reach the alimentary canal. The bladder is digested in the stomach and the proscolex is turned from inside to outside by which the rostellum and suckers come on the outer side. Soon a scolex and neck are formed and the scolex becomes attached to mucous membrane of the intestine. The neck forms new segments which change into a chain of proglottids. In this way they gradually develop into adult Taenia. This process takes about 2 or 3 months.

Q. 2.8.(b) What is Cysticercus ?

These are the sack-like oval larvae of *T. Solium* or *T. Saginate* seen in the longitudinal areas of muscles. These are distended with clear or opalescent fluid and in their central part there is an opaque spot which represents the future scolex. They measure about 10 x 5 mm.

Larva of T. solium is called *cysticescus cellulosae* and that of T. saginate is known as *cysticercus bovis.*

Q. 2.9. Why T. Solium is more dangerous than other Taenia ?

T. solium is more dangerous because it can be both definite and intermediate hosts in human beings.

Q. 2.10. What are the adaptation seen in tape worms due to their parasitic mode of life ?

Adaptation of Taenia due to Parasitic Life

As the Taenia lives as endoparasite within body of human being it shows both morphological and physiological adaptation.

(I) Morphological adaptations :

These are as follows :

1. Due to an economy of space within the intestine of the host of the body of Taenia has become just like a tape.
2. As locomotion is not required, the locomotary organs (cilia) have disappeared.
3. For the protection of the body from the succus entericus of the host, the body of Taenia has been covered with cuticle.
4. For perfect anchorage to the intestinal wall of the host suckers and hooks have developed in Taenia.
5. As the food is directly absorbed from the body of the host, so mouth and diagestive system have not at all developed and there is no sense organ in the body of Taenia.
6. Nervous system is ill developed and there is no sense organ in the body of Taenia.
7. Reproductive system is well developed and even each proglottid contains the reproductive system. Eggs are in very large number and these are encapsulated so that these are not destroyed during transmission.

(II) Physiological modifications :

1. In order to get rid of the difficulties in osmo-regulation the parasite is more or less equal.
2. They perform anaerobic respiration and glycogen is the source of energy.
3. Taenia excites the cells of the intestinal wall of the host which secrete mucous that acts as a covering over the body of the parasite.
4. They secrete antienzyme to neutralize the gastric juice.

So it is seen that parasitims does not always bad to degeniracy of organs but it is a special mode of life that leads to specialization of organs due to differential livings.

Q. 2.11. What are the differences between T. saginata and Taenia solium.

Like *Taenia solium, Taenia saginata* is also found in large number in the intestine of human beings. Apparently it appears that there is no difference between the two but scientific analysis distinguishes them as follows :

	T. Solium	T. Saginata
1. Length	2-3 metres	5-10 metres
2. Head	Large square, rostellum and hooks present.	Small and round, no rostellum, no hooks.
3. Proglottides	Below 1000	Ranging from 1000-2000.
4. Mode of expulsion.	5-6 proglottides at a time.	One proglottid at a time.
5. Uterus	Lateral branches 3-10	Lateral branches 15-30.
6. Ovary	Bilobed one extra lobe.	Bilobed, no extra lobe.
7. Testis	150-500 follicles	300-400 follicles.

8. Intermediate host. Pig. Bovine.

** Besides the above differences their life cycles, physiology, creation of disease etc. are identical.

Fig. 12

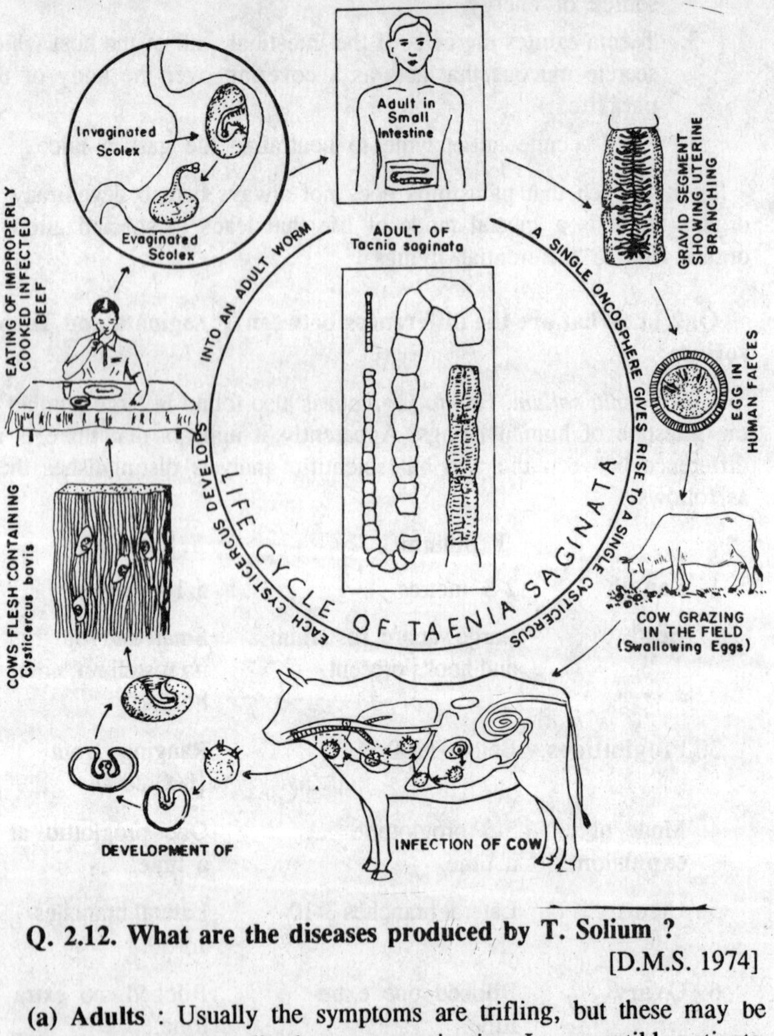

Q. 2.12. What are the diseases produced by T. Solium ?

[D.M.S. 1974]

(a) Adults : Usually the symptoms are trifling, but these may be indigestion with either diarrhoea or constipation. In susceptible patients, vomiting, loss of appetite and anaemia

(b) Cysticercus cellulosae : This larva has been recorded from partically every part of the human body, most commonly from the subcutaneous tissues, the brain, orbit and muscles. It is a dangerous parasite when it occurs in the brain, eye or other vital organs; calcification of older cysts takes place. It is the commonest identifiable cause of epilepsy in African and may be an important cause of mental disorder.

Q. 2.13. How can we diagnosis a case of T. Solium and T. Saginate infected person ?

Diagnosis :

Adults : In making a diagnosis of human infection with a species of *Taenia* the following points should be noted :

1. The worm can be diagnosed by the form of the uterus in the gravid segments which are passed in chains or singly, in the faeces of persons infected. In T. saginata the uterus bears 11 to 30 compound branches on each side, and in T. solium from 8 to 10 branches, they are counted where they arise from the main stem. This may be done by the naked eye but more easily with a hand lens, if the segments, after boiling them to kill the eggs, are pressed between two slides, and held up to the light. In these circumstances the uterine branches appear milky-white.

2. Single segments of both *T. solium* and *T. saginate* are frequently passed in faeces, and can be seen moving. They are apt to be mistaken by the untrained observer for trematodes, but the taller are only very rarely found in faeces and are never white. Trematodes all possess suckers and an intestine, and none has a pore on the lateral margin. They, thus, differ from the segments of Taenia which do not possess suckers or an intestine but do have a genital pore on the lateral margin.

3. The eggs of *T. solium* and *T. saginate* cannot be distinguished from each other, so that when Taenia eggs are found in faeces one cannot say to which species they belong.

4. The head of *T. solium* measuring about 1 mm. in diameter is armed with hooks whilst that of *T. saginata,* measuring upto 2 mm. in diameter, is unarmed. A diagnosis can, therefore, be made easily, if

the head is available, as it may be following successful treatment; it is however, difficult to obtain the head.

5. The larval stage of *T. saginata* does not occur in man. *But cysticercus cellulkosae in man are seen in T. solium* infection. If the cysts are superficial they can excised for examination, otherwise diagnosis depends on X-ray examination which will reveal the cysts when calcified.

1. ECHINOCOCCUS GRANULOSUS

Synonym—Taenia granulosa, T. echinococcus.

Q. 2.14. What are the main differences of T. echinococcus from other speices of Taenia ?

Adult worms of this species differ from Taenia species—in their small size, limited number of segments and in the absence of lateral branches from the gravid uterus which is sacculated.

Q. 2.15. Where do they live in ?

Habitat

(a) Adult: *Not in man*, but in dogs, jackals and wolves. The worms lie attached to the mucous membrane of the small intestine of the host, and post mortem appear as small white specks on the reddish mucous membrane.

(b) Eggs: in faeces of hosts of the adult are infective to man, and to herbivorous domestic and wild animals hosts.

(c) The larval form: is a hydatid cyst which is common in many species of herbivourous animals, but particularly in sheep, cattle and horses. It has been recorded from every organs in the body but is most commonly found in the liver and lungs. Multiple infection, especially of the liver of cattle is common, and when extensive, the cysts tend to the both small and sterile, i.e., they contain no infective scoleces (hydatid sand). Infection also occurs in man.

Q. 2.16. What are the Morphological characteristics of T. echinococcus ?

Morphology

(a) Adult :

The worm is very small, ranging from 2 to 9 mm in length and its maximum breath is 500μ. It is composed of a head and usually 3 segments, the last one being somewhat longer than the rest of the worm. The first segment contains no genital organs, the second is mature, and the third is gravid. The uterus in the mature segment becomes sacculated laterally and these vaginations become filled with eggs.

The head bears from 28 to 40 hooks in a double crown, the large hooks measuring about 37μ in length and the small one up to 28μ.

(b) Larval form (hydatid cyst) :

The cysts grow slowly to a diameter of 1 cm. in five months and may eventually attain the size of a child's head. They are vesicular bodies full of fluid; when the fluid is drained into a container, a sediment often referred to as "**hydatid sand**" settles to the bottom. This contains an enormous number of heads, each one of which, when swallowed by the dog, may become an adult worm, in that animal.

(c) Eggs : The ova are generally passed in the dog's faeces. The individual egg is spherical, containing thick brown radially striated embryophore, surrounding a hexacanth embryo. It is 30-37μ in diameter.

LIFE CYCLE

Q. 2.17. Describe the life cycle of Echinococcus ganulosus.

Host :

Definitive host : Dog, wolf, jackal etc.

Intermediate host : Sheep, cattle, pigs, rodent, horse and **man.** [Different stain is adopted to different host e.g. Horse is the common host in England.]

Transmission to Intermediate Host :

1. Eggs :

(i) Large number of eggs are discharged along with faeces which are swallowed by intermediate host while grazing in the field.

(ii) Man may be infected along in the food and drinks contaminated with

infested canine faeces or by handling infected dogs (accidental swallowing).

2. HYDATID ÇYST FORMATION

[How Hydatid cysts are formed ?] [C.U. 1979]

(a) **Hatching of hexacanth** : Swallwed eggs pass down the oesophagus into stomach, where shell wall is lost and active hexacanth embryo hatch out in duodenum is called Onchosphere.

(b) **Onchosphere** : (i) Unhatched hexacanth is covered by a shell and thin onchosphere membrane which are lost at the time of hatching.

(ii) About 8 hours after ingestion the onchospheres bore their way through the intestinal wall, entre the portalvein and are to the liver. Some embryo is left in sinusoidal capillaires. (Liver acts as first filter).

(iii) Rest embryo pass through the hepatic capillaries and enter the pulmonary circulation. Lung filter some embryo (2nd filter).

(iv) Few embryo enter the general blood stream and may infect : kidney, spleen, brain, genital organ, bones, muscles, cardiac muscles etc.

(v) Where the embryo settles, it forms *hydatid cyst*-with a hollow bladder. By 30 days the hydatid cyst becomes 1 mm in diameter.

[Onchosphere remain unaffected by pepsin in stomach but is acted by trypsin (pancreatic enzyme). This result is the liberation of the embryo (Reed 1971). Onchosphere are also actived by bile.)

3. HYDATID CYST

(I) Cellular reaction of the host with the embryo forms an fibrous layer (pericyst) around the cyst wall of the parasites.

(II) Cyst wall of the embryo compose of 2 layers :

1. **Ectocyst** : thick laminated, non-cellular layer.
2. **Endocyst** or germinal layer: celluler with nuclei embedded in protoplasmic mass.

(iii) Endocyst gives rise to broad capsule or multiple daughter cysts and lateral scolices or protoscolices.

(iv) Brood capsule secretes (endocyst) : hydatid fluid which act as buffer and serve nutrition to developing scolices.

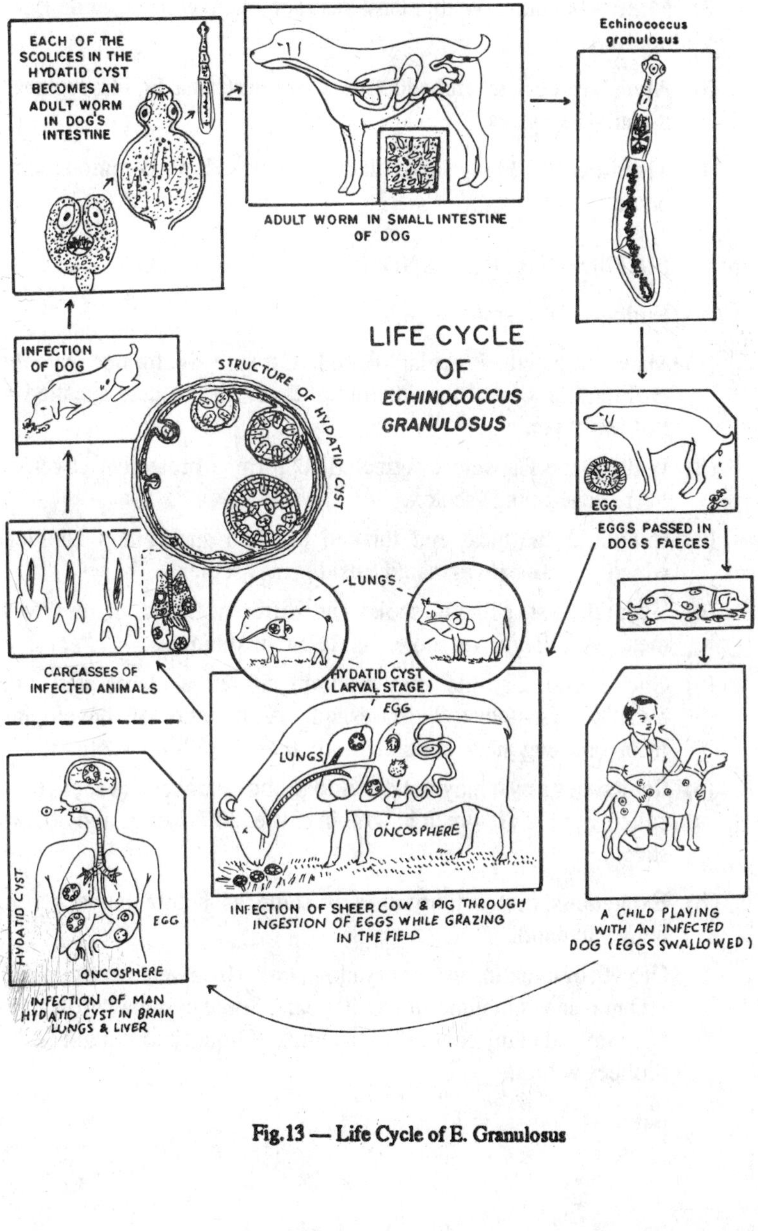

Fig.13 — Life Cycle of E. Granulosus

**TYPES OF HYDATID CYST

Cyst vary in different species. (Reed 1962)

1. **Unilocular**: With one bladder.
2. **Multi-vesicular**: With many bladder each with separate connection.
3. **Alveolar:** Vesicles embedded in common strama. Fluid is replaced by jelly-like mass.
4. **Multilocular:** Many small bladder, enclosed in a common membrane.

4. PROTOSCOLICES AND BROOD CAPSULE

(A) Endogenous Cyst :

(1) Many rounded vesicular Brood Capsule is formed by the proliferation of cell from germinal layer, the process is called—**Polyembryony**.

(2) Wall of the Capsule evaginated to form a protective covering over developing scolex.

(3) Cuticle at the head end thicked to form sucker and hooklets which remain invaginated inside the scolex.

(4) Hydatid cyst contain scolex at different stage of development. A full grown scolex is 160μ in diameter.

(5) One Brood Capsule may contain 5—20 scoleces and one hydatid cyst—several thousand. A hydatid of developing from one egg may contain more than 2 million scolices.

(6) Sometimes a cyst may not develop brood chamber and scolices—called sterile cyst which is 40% in cattle, 20% in pigs and 80% in sheep.

(B) Exogenous cyst : Formation is same as before but occur in bony hydatid.

Growth of hydatid cyst is very slow, take 10-12 years to attain 50-100 mm and sometimes up to 50 years. Some cyst may grow upto 500 mm and many contain 12-18 litres of liquid and contain 12-18 scolices within.

5. TRANSMISSION TO DEFINITIVE HOST

Dogs and other carnivores become infected by eating raw meat of the affected sheep, cattle or pig which contains scolices inside the hydatid cyst.

6. DEVELOPMENT OF ADULT WORM IN DEFINITIVE HOST. Or FATE OF HYDATID CYST.

(1) The brood capsules are lost and protoscolices are liberated by the action of pepsin in the stomach of carnivores.

(2) The evagination of protoscolex is activated by bile salt — Taurcoholate and attachment to gut wall "trigger" development.

(3) The protoscolices established in the small intestine with the rostellum buried in the crypt of Lieberkhum and remain dormant for 4-5 days.

(4) Scolex grows, at 14th day first segment appear, 2nd segment appear at 18th day and fully formed embryo.

Life Cycle of E. granulossa (T. echinococcus)

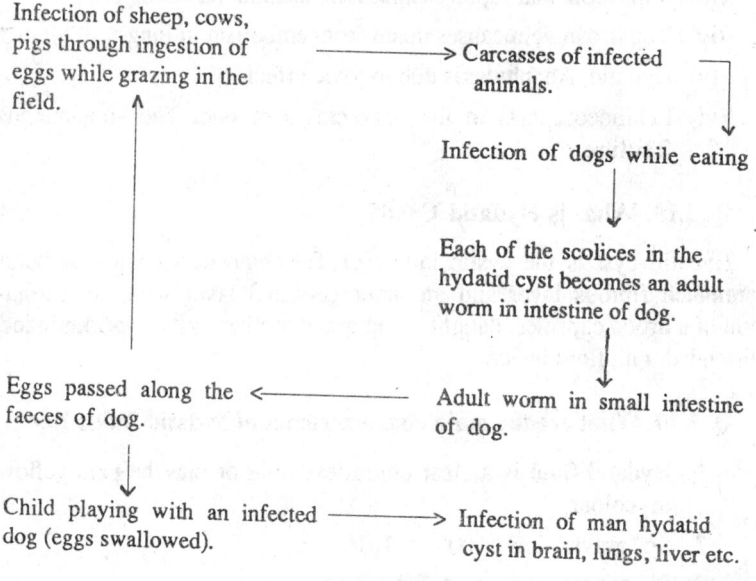

Infection of sheep, cows, pigs through ingestion of eggs while grazing in the field. → Carcasses of infected animals.

↓

Infection of dogs while eating

↓

Each of the scolices in the hydatid cyst becomes an adult worm in intestine of dog.

↓

Adult worm in small intestine of dog. → Eggs passed along the faeces of dog. (↑ back to infection of sheep, cows, pigs)

↓

Child playing with an infected dog (eggs swallowed). → Infection of man hydatid cyst in brain, lungs, liver etc.

Q. 2.18. What are the pathogenic effect of T. echinococcus on man ?

1. *Larval stages causes Echinococcus or hydatid diseases*. The % of the cyst in different organs are as follows :

	Produce tumour	5%	Brain
	Cyst	12%	Heart
	Malignent growth	70%	Liver
HYDATID	Cyst	12%	Lungs
CYST	Hydronephrosis	7%	Kidney
	Same as liver	27%	Spleen
	Crast at bone and spontaneous fracture	1%	Bone
	Cyst	5%	Ovary
	Cyst	2%	Genital organ

2. Other effects due to toxin released by cyst are :

(i) Intra -biliary rupture causes obstructive jaundice.

(ii) Ureter rupture produces renal colic, haematuria.

(iii) Intra-bronchial rupture causes suffocation haemoptysis.

(iv) Rupture in vein causes death from embolism in lung.

(v) Hydatid, Anaphylaxis due to toxic effect.

(vi) Echinococcus is in the bone-crases of bone and spontaneous fracture.

Q. 2.19. What is Hydatid Cyst ?

Hydatid cyst is the cystic larvae of T. echinococcus with an outer laminated fibrous layer and an inner germinal layer with the formation of a brood capsules, daughter and grand mother cyst of various sizes, distended with fluid inside.

Q. 2.20. What are the main characteristics of hydatid fluids ?

1. Hydatid fluid is a clear colourless fluid or may be pale yellow in colour.
2. Sp. gravity low, 1005 to 1010.
3. Reaction slightly acid, PH 6.7.
4. Contains NaCl, Na_2SO_4, Na_2PO_4 and Sodium and Calcium

salts of succinic acid.

5. Hydatid sand — A granular deposit found to settle at the bottom. It consists of liberated brood capsules, free scolices and loose hooklets.
6. It is highly toxic, when absorbed gives rise to anaplylactic symptoms.
7. It is an antegenic fluid and used for immunological tests.

Q. 2.21. What are the functions of the hydatid fluid ?

1. It acts as a buffer i.e. it protects the developing larvae from trauma inflicted from outside.
2. It supplies nutrition to the developing larvae.
3. This fluid is antigenic in nature and can be utilised as a diagnostic agent.

Q. 2.22. What is hydatid sand ?

It is the granular deposits collected at the bottom of the cyst. It consists of detached brood capsules, scolices and hooklets liberated from disintegrated scolices.

Q. 2.23. How can we diagnosis Echinoccous infection ? For diagnosis test is done : [C.U. 1979]

Casoni's intradermal test :

In this test 0.2 ml of sterile hydatid fluid is used as an antigen together with negative control. **Wheal upto 5 mm. within 20 minutes is diagnostic.**

II. NEMATOHELMINTHES

C. NEMATODES

Q. 2.24. What are the main characteristics of class—Namatoda ?
[C.U. 1980, 82, D.M.S. 78,79,80,82,84]

1. Nematodes are elongated, unsegmented, cylindrical or filiform worms having a body cavity with organs bilaternally symmetrical, and pointed towards the anterior and posterior ends.

2. The size varies greatly, the smallest being less than 1 inch (*T. spiralis and Strogyloid stercoralis*) and the largest measuring upto 10 inches (e.g. femal *Dracunculus medinensis*).
3. The body is covered with a tough cuticle of 2 layers : Cuticle and Subcuticle.
4. The alimentary canal is complete with a mouth and anus at the opposite ends.
5. The body wall consists of longitudinal muscle fibres and the body cavity is an unlined pseudocele.
6. It has no circulatory or respiratory organ and the excretory organ is simple.
7. The worm is sexually differentiated into male and female. The caudal end of the male is coiled ventrally and tapering in the female :
   (a) The male genital system consists of a single long coiled or convoluted tube differentiated into testes, vas deferens, seminal vesicle and ejaculatory duct which opens with the anus into a common cloaca. The compulatory apparatus consists of one or two unsheathed spicules with or without a gubernaculums.
   (b) The female genital system consists of a single tube (as in *Trichuris*) or a bifurcate tube as in *Enterobius*, *Ancylostoma* differentiated into ovijector, vagina and vulva, opening on the ventral aspect of the worm near the middle of the body or near the mouth (as in *Trichinella* and *Wuchereria*).
8. The nematode may, however, be :
   (i) **Oviparous** e.g., *Ascaris, Oxyuris* etc. and the egg consists to a fertilised cell and numerous yolk granules.
   (ii) **Viviparous** in *Dracunculus medinensis* and *Trichinlla spiralls*.
   (iii) **Ove-viviparous** in *Strogyloids* in which the eggs containing larvae hatch out immediately.

Q. 2.25. What are the common Nematodes seen in nature which are parasitic to man. [D.M.S. 1978]

I. INTESTINAL NEMATODES

(A) Small Intestine only

Ascaris lumbricodies : Common round worm.
Ancylostoma duodenale :The old world hook worm ?
Necator americanus : American hook worm.
Strongyloides stercoralis :
Trichinella spiralis :Trichina worm.
Capillaria philippinensis.

(B) Caecum and Vermform Appendix

Enterobius vermicularis : Thread worm or pin worm.
Trichuris Trichiura : Whip worm.

II. TISSUE OR SOMATIC NEMATODES

1. Lymphatic system
Wuchereria bancrofti : Filaria.
Brugia malayi.

2. Subcutaneous tissues
Loa loa : African eye worm.
Onchocerca volvulus.
Dracunculus medinensis : Guinea worm.

3. Lungs : *Strongyloides stercoralis.*

4. Mesentery :
Dipetalonema perstans.
Mansonella ozzarid.

5. Conjunctiva : *Loa loa.*

Q.2.26. How are they transmitted?

Modes of Transmission

Ingestion of embryonated eggs.	*Inhalation* of infected dust or with embryonated eggs.	Penetration of skin mucous membrane filariform larvae	Ingestion of mature larvae	By the bite of blood sucking insects
e.g. *Ascaris lumbricoides* *Trichuris trichura* *Enterobius vermicularis.*	*e.g.* *A. lumbricoides* *E. vermicularis.*	*e.g.* *Ancylostoma duedenale* *Necator americanus* *Strongyloides stercoralis* .	*e.g.* *Trichinella spiralis* *(in port meal)* *Dracunculus medinensis.* *(in infected cyclops).*	*e.g.* *Wuchereria bancrofti* *Dipetalonoma perstans* *Mansonella ozzardi* *Loa loa* *Onchocerca* volvulus.

Q.2.27. How can we diagnosis intestinal Nematodes seeing their eggs ?

Intestinal Nematodes

Larvae in stool	Eggs in stool		Eggs on perianal skin
S. stercoralis	Coloured (Bile-stained) 1. *A. lumbricoides* 2. *T. trichura* .	Colourless (Not bile stained) 1. Hook worms *A duodenale* *N. americanus.* 2. *E. vermicularis.* (Rarely)	Colourless (Not bile : stained) *E. vermicularis.*

III. ASCARIS LUMBRICOIDES

Q. 2.28. Where they live in ?

(a) Adult : In the intestine of man and pigs. The normal habitat is in the small intestine, but owing to the fact that they wander about within the body they often found in other sites.

(b) Eggs : In human faeces are not infective to man when passed.

(c) Infective larvae : Present inside the eggs which are found in soil, water, or on green vegetables.

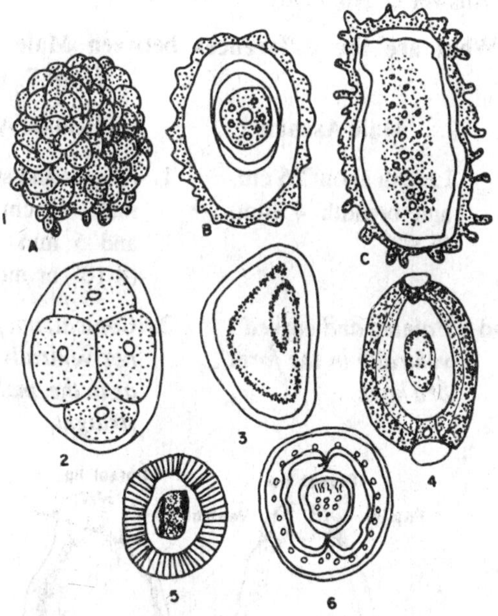

Fig.—9 Helminthic eggs in stool of Man

1. Fertilised eggs of A.Lumbricoides
   A. Surface focus
   B. Medium focus
1. C.Unfertilised eggs of A. lumbricoides
2. A. duodenale
3. E. vermicularis
4. T. trichiura
5. T solum or T.Saginata
6. H.nana

Q. 2.29. What are their morphological characters ?

[D.M.S. 1978, 79, 80, 82, 84]

The worm is the largest of the human intestinal nematodes, and in shape and size it resemblems, somewhat, the ordinary earthworms; it is brownish-yellow in colour. The three lips lie, one dorsal, and the other two subventral, and they are finely toothed. The digestive and reproductive organs float inside the body cavity containing an irritating fluid—*ascaron* or *ascarase*, which is probably of the nature of primary albumoses (proteose).

*[Also see Answer Q. No. 2.30]

Q. 2.30. What are the differences between Male and Female Ascaris ?

[D.M.S. 1978, 79, 80]

	Male Ascaris	Female Ascaris
1. Size :	Length about 25 cm. and breadth 4 mm. (6-8").	1. Longer and stouter than male, 40 cm. in lenght and 5 mm. breadth. (8-10" or more).
2. Tail end :	*Pointed and curved ventrally in the form of a hook.*	2. *Conical; not pointed nor ventrally curved, as in the male; but straight.*

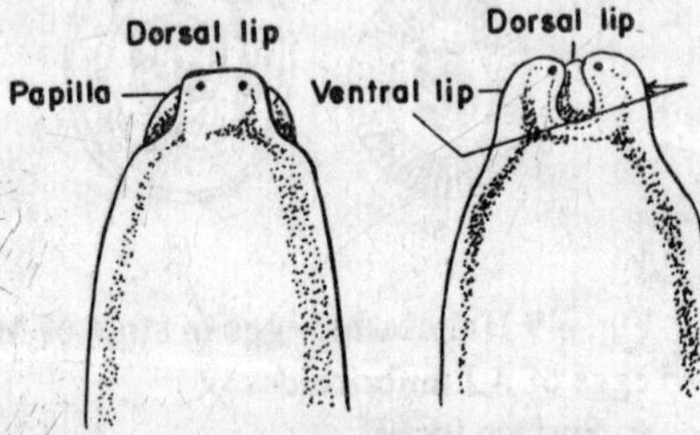

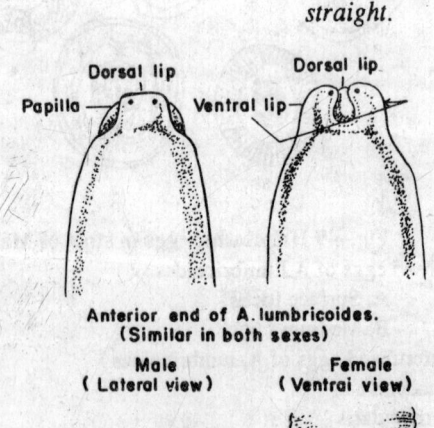

Anterior end of A. lumbricoides.
(Similar in both sexes)

Male (Lateral view) Female (Ventral view)

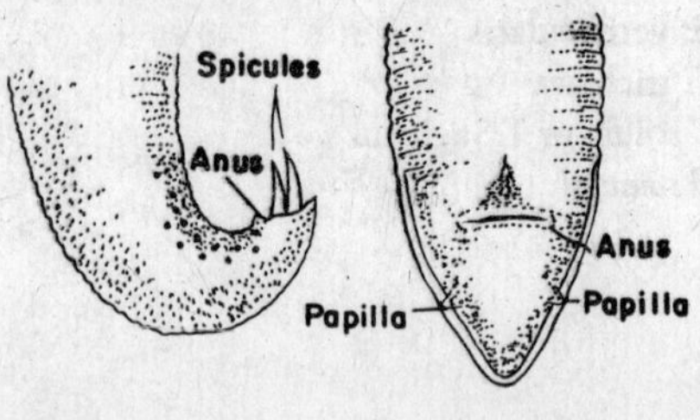

3. **Genital pore :**	Genital pore opens into the cloaca. Two sicules (copulatory bursa) each measuring 2 mm. in length can often be seen protruding from the orifice of the cloaca, around which there are large numbers of minute papillae.	3. **Vulve**: The vulva is very minute and situated ventrally, at the junction of the anterior and middle thirds of the body and becomes narrower i.e. **vulvar waist**. The vulva leads into a stout duct, the vagina, which divides into two branches; these tubes lie coiled antero-posteriorly within the worm. That portion of each duct close to the common vagina functions as a uterus. The middle part is the oviduct and the distal part the ovary.
4. **Anus :**	Anus opens with the ejaculatory duct into the cloaca.	4. **Anus** : Anus opens on the ventral surface as a transverse slit.

Q. 2.31. What are the differences between Fertilized and unfertilized eggs of Ascaris ?

	Fertilised Eggs	**Unfertilised Eggs**
1. **Size and shape :**	Round or oval in shape, 60 to 75μm. in length and 40 to 50μm. in breadth.	1. Narrower, long (80-μm. in length and 55-μm. in breadth), and more elliptical.
2. **Colour :**	Brownish or golden brown in colour i.e. always in bile stainned.	2. Brownish in colour.
3. **Eggs :**	(a) *Shell* —Thick, smooth and colour-	3. (a) Has thinner shell with an irregular coa-

	less (translucent) ; and with an outer albuminous coat which is thrown into rugosities or mammillations; it stains brown after absorbing bile pigments in the faeces.	ting of albumin.
	(b) **Vitalline layer :** within the egg shell there is a very delicate vitalline envelop which is even more resistant than the egg shell; as a result eggs can remain viable for about a year.	
	(c) **Ovum**: The egg contains a very large, conspicuous, fertilized unsegmented ovum, which is contracted away from the vitelline membrane at the poles.	(c) The egg contains a small atrophied ovum with a mass of disorganised highly refractile granules of various sizes.
4. Salt flotation:	Floats in saturated solution of common salt.	Does not float in salt solution.

N.B. (i) **Both fertilized and unfertilized eggs** may be found in a sample of stool but if specimen shows only the unfertilized eggs, it signifies that the host is harbouring the females Ascaris or mating between males and females has not occurred.

(ii) Occasionly, in human faeces, the protein coat of fertilized eggs is lost, and the eggs are the somewhat difficult to recognise. The presence of a large ovum within the egg is, however, sufficient to identify them.

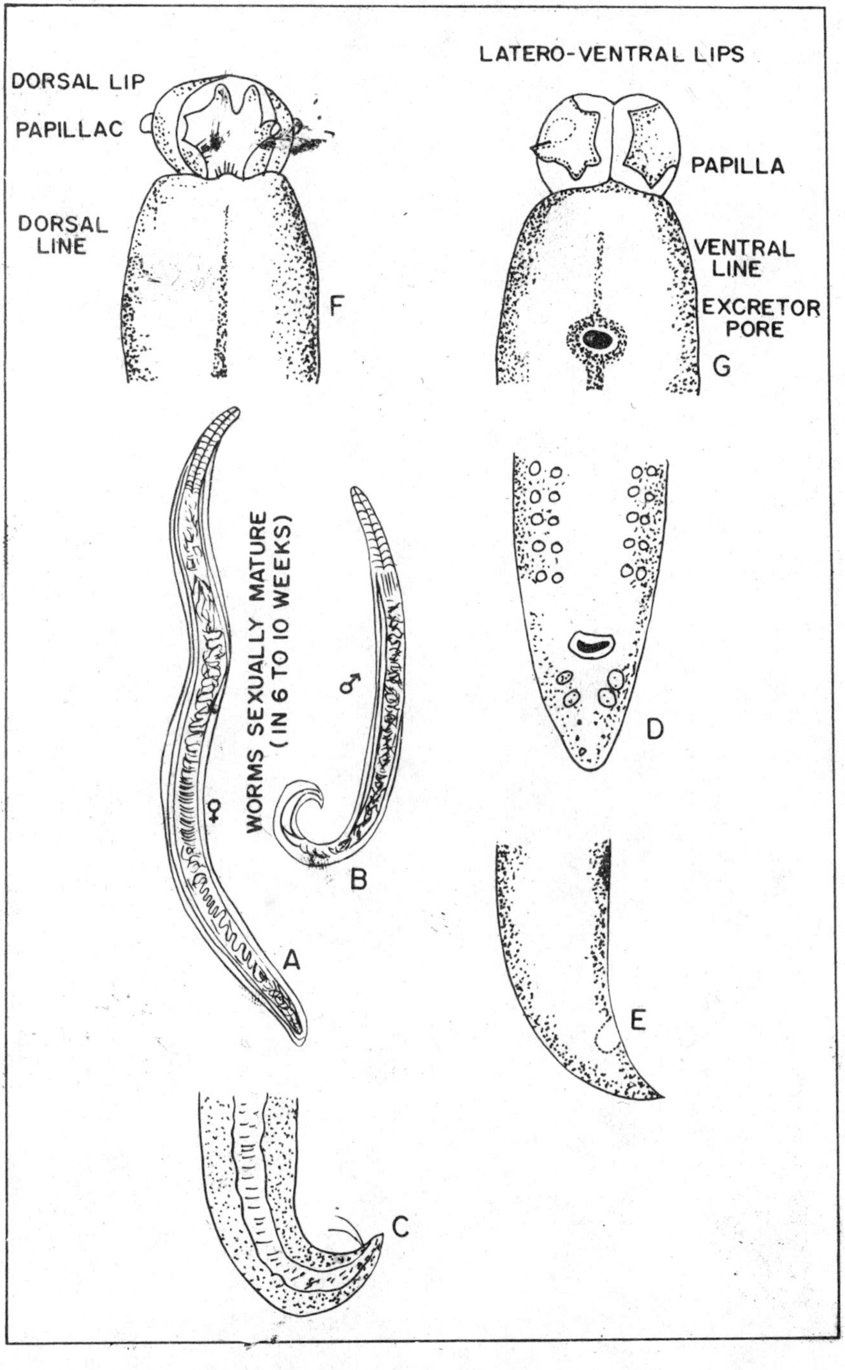

DORSAL LIP
PAPILLAC
DORSAL LINE
F
LATERO-VENTRAL LIPS
PAPILLA
VENTRAL LINE
EXCRETOR PORE
G
WORMS SEXUALLY MATURE (IN 6 TO 10 WEEKS)
♀
A
♂
B
C
D
E

Q. 2.32. Give an account of the life history of Ascaris.
[C.U. 1980, 82, 84]

Ascaris is a parasite found in the alimentary canal of man. Its life **history** is completed in one host (man) only.

1. Copulation and Fertilization : Copulation between male and female *Ascaris* takes place in the intestine of man. During copulation, a male and female Ascaris come close to each other in such a way that the cloacal aperture of male attaches with the genital pore (vulva) of the female. Penial setae open the vulva and spermatozoa are transferred into female by repeated contractions of the ejaculatory duct. The spermatozoa reach the uterus through vagina. The fertilization takes place in uteri or distal ends of oviducts. After fertilization, the eggs move downwards and during their course they are covered by an albuminous coat and a thick, very resistant chitinous shell.

2. Eggs : The eggs are elongated, oval or spherical in shape. There is a thick, transparent, chitinous, egg shell around the eggs. Below the egg shell is an albuminous layer. The egg shell is uneffected by chemicals and atmospheric changes. Under unfavourable conditions they can remain in dorment condition for years.

3. Segmentation or Cleavage :

How fertilization takes place in Ascaris ?

The segmentation in fertilized egg takes place outside the body of the host when they come out along with the faeces. The segmentation is of **determinate type.**

The first division is transverse as a result of which a dorsal cell (AB) and a ventral cell (P_1) formed. The dorsal cell divides vertically to form an anterior cell (A) and a posterior cell (B). Simultaneously, the ventral cell (P_1) divides transversely into an upper cell (EMST) and a lower cell (P_2). The four-celled embryo is now T shaped. P_2 cell moves upward to come on the right side of EMST. A and B cells divide together and form a right and a left cell. These cells divide again to form ectoderm of the embryo. EMST and P2 cells divide to form EMST, P3 and C cells. E cells divide to form endoderm and MST cell forms mesoderm and part of ectoderm, P_3 cells divide to form P_4 and D cells. C and D cells form ectoderm. P_4 cells divide into G_1 and G_2 cells which form primordial germ cells. In this way a blastula is formed. By invagination the blustula turns into a gastrula which grows into a mobile juvenile representing **rhabditoid stage.

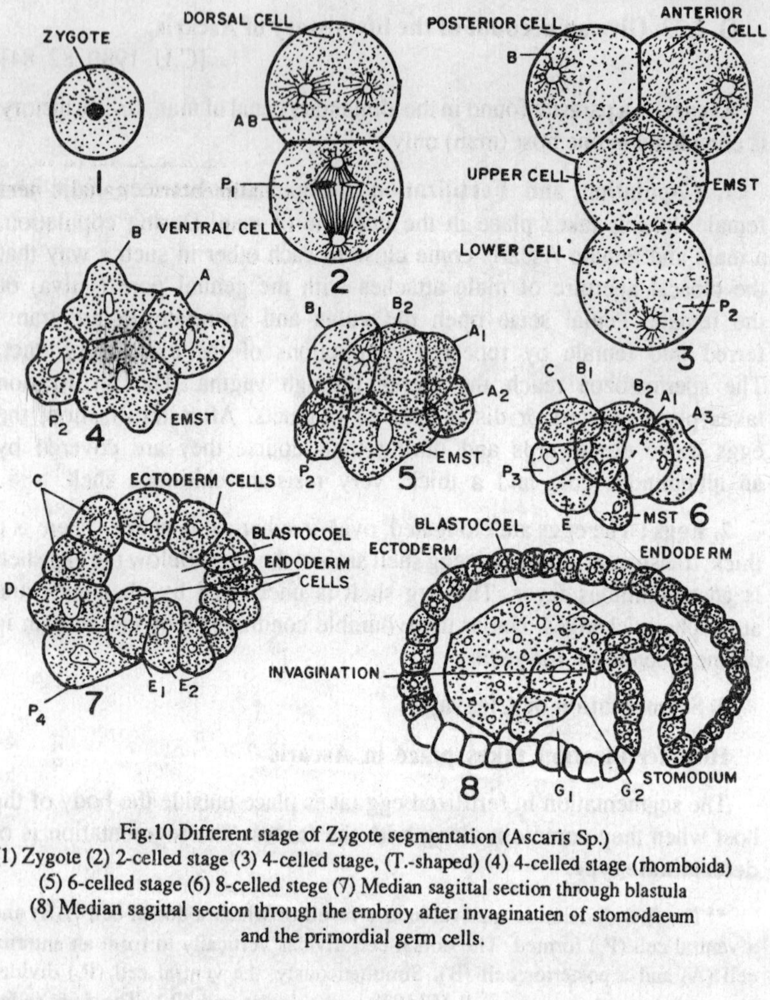

Fig.10 Different stage of Zygote segmentation (Ascaris Sp.)
(1) Zygote (2) 2-celled stage (3) 4-celled stage, (T.-shaped) (4) 4-celled stage (rhomboida) (5) 6-celled stage (6) 8-celled stege (7) Median sagittal section through blastula (8) Median sagittal section through the embroy after invaginatien of stomodaeum and the primordial germ cells.

Under favourable conditions of temperature and moisture, the fist larva (juvenile) from egg is formed in 10-12 days. *First moulting* of larva takes place within the egg shell. In about a week's time the larva reaches the second larval stage and comes out of the egg shell.

4. Egg laying : The eggs are laid in the intestine of the host and come out of its body along with faeces. A female Ascaris lays about

27,000,000 eggs in its life time and about 200,000 eggs in a day. After coming outside the body of host, the eggs develop into infective stage. If these are swallowed by the host then they develop into new worms in its intestine. There is no intermediate host in the life cycle of Ascaris. Further development of larva is possible only if the eggs reach the intestine of man otherwise they die.

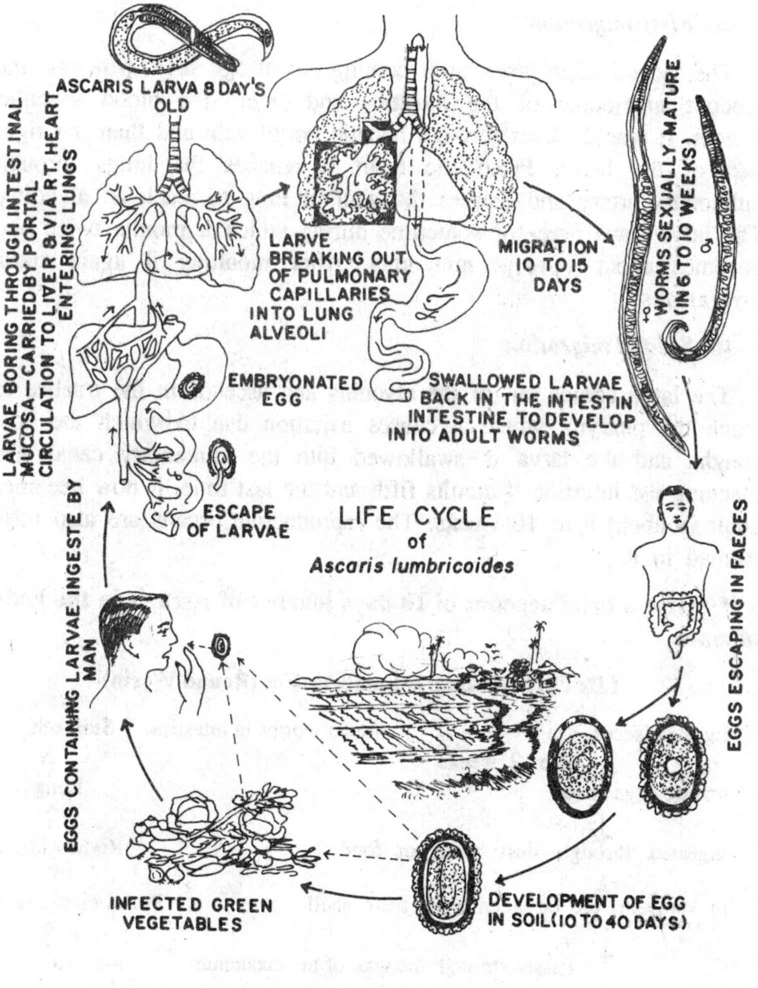

5. Infection : The eggs reach the alimentary canal of host with contaminated water and raw vegetables. In deuodenum the egg shells are dissolved and second stage **rhabditoid larva** come out.

Rabditoid larva is about 0.2 to 0.3 mm long. It has fully developed alimentary canal, nervous system and excretory system. Before starting life in intestine they lead a ten days migratory life in the body of the host. During this period it moults twice and becomes adults.

(a) ***First migration*** :

The second stage larva, after coming out of egg shell, penctrats the mucous membrane of the intestine and enters the blood vascular system. It reaches liver through hepatic portal vein and then the right part of the heart. From the heart it reaches the lungs through pulmonary artery and pierces the wall of lung to reach an alveolus. The larva stays here for sometime during which it moults twice and becomes about 1 to 2 mm long. After moulting it again starts migrations.

(b) ***Second migration***:

The larva comes out of the alveolus and ascends in the trachea to reach the pharynx where it causes irritation due to which the host coughs and the larva is swallowed into the alimentary canal. On reaching the intestine it moults fifth and the last time. It now becomes adult in about 8 to 10 weeks. The reproductive organs are also fully formed in it.

**** Give a brief account of 10 days journey of Ascaris in the body of man.**

Life Cycle of Ascaris Lumbricoides (Round Worm)

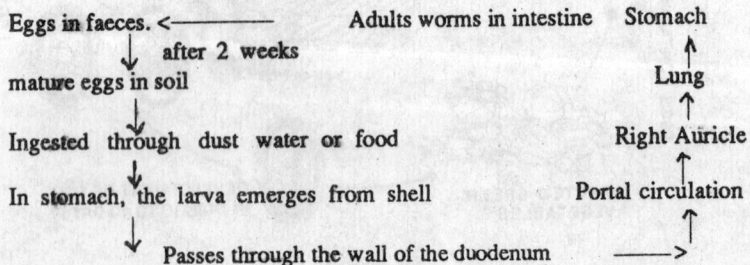

Eggs in faeces. <———— Adults worms in intestine **Stomach**

↓ **after 2 weeks** ↑

mature eggs in soil **Lung**

↓ ↑

Ingested through dust water or food **Right Auricle**

↓ ↑

In stomach, the larva emerges from shell **Portal circulation**

↓ ↑

Passes through the wall of the duodenum ————>

Q. 2.33. What are parasitic effects of a Ascaris on man ?

[C.U. 1980]

Pathogenic effects of Ascaris are due to *adult parasites* or by the larve and due to certain chemical substance produce by then.

(a) Due to larvae :

In the *early stages* of a heavy infection the migration of the lungs gives rise to numerous minute haemorrhages and to oedema and exudation; in *severe infections* they may produce symptoms resembling lobar pnumonia and may cause death in young children.

(b) Due to adult parasite :

1. Allergic manifestations may result from the presence of these parasites.
2. The worms frequently migrate, and may be obstructed the lumen of the intestine.
3. Single worms may enter the bile or pancreatic ducts, or the appendix, and they may even penetrate the intestinal wall causing peritonitis.
4. Sometimes, 500 to 5,000 adult Ascaris are found in a single host.
5. Due to large number of Ascaris in the intestine, irritations and colic start.

(c) Toxic product :

Generally they form certain chemical substances which destroy trypsin and hinder digestion of proteins. Its infection also causes *vomiting, delirium, convulsions. general nervousness, diarrhoea* etc. Sometimes mental and physical development is retarded in children.

Q. 2.34. How can we diagnosis a case of Ascariasis ?

Diagnosis is generally based on the identification of *worms passed* or on *finding eggs in faeces. Fertilized eggs* are more commonly found, but presence of unfertilized egg indicates presence of female parasites only. When the infection limited to male worms, diagnosis is impossible unless a worm is obtained. In Ascaris pneumonia of infants the faeces of the mother should be examined for evidences of infection locally; she may be infecting here child with ova on her fingers. The infant's sputum may be examined for larval Ascaris.

****Fertilized eggs** : They are more commonly found, but presence of unfertilized egg indicates presence of female parasite only.

IV ENTEROBIUS VERMICULARIS

(Synonym : Oxyuris vermicularis)

Common name : Thread worm, Pin worm.

Q. 2.35. Describe the habitat, Morphological characteristics and life history of a Thread-worm.

Habitat

(a) **Adult** : The worm is a common parasite of man, especially of children. The young and mature forms occur in the terminal ileum but the gravid females lives in the colon, especially in the rectum.

(b) **Eggs** : Deposited on the perianal skin.

(c) **Infective larvae** : They are found in eggs on the buttocks a few hours after being passed.

Morphological Characters

Enterobius vermicularis : It is a small nematode parasite of the caecum and large intestine of man.

(a) **Adults** : The male worm measures about 4 mm. in length and has a miximum diameter of about 150μ. The posterior extremity is curved and sharply truncated ; there is a single brown, hook-like spicule, measuring 70 μ in length.

The female is much larger than the male; it measures about 1 cm. in length and has a diameter of about 400 μ. The tail is long, tapering, straight and pointed.

(b) **Eggs** : The eggs are plano convex in shape, with an albuminouscoat, colourless and symmetrical, one side being a little flattened within it coiled up tadepole larvae, and they measure about 55 μ by 25 μ.

N.B. : It is to be noted that this worm is peculiar in that, it does not lay eggs in the intestine, but on the perianal skin. When deposited, they contain a tadpole-like larva, which becomes infective to man in about six hours, as a coiled up young worm in the egg. The larva remain viable for several days.

Life History

When the infective eggs are swallowed by man, the larvae escape in the upper intestine. After moulting twice they become adult in the lower ileum. The life cycle from egg to adult takes two to four weeks.

Fig-15

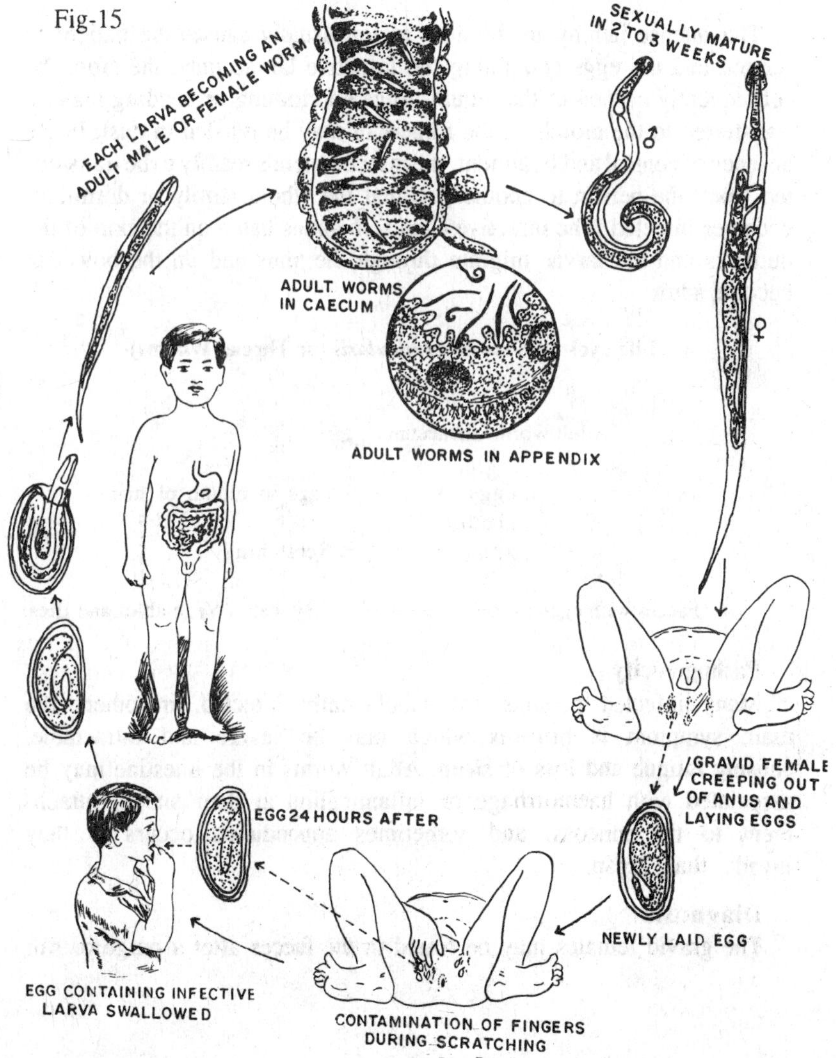

As the worms become mature in the small intestine, the male fertilizes the female ; the male worm is rarely seen except after a purge. The female, when gravid, migrates to the rectum and, during the night, passes out of the anus, deposits its eggs on the perianal skin and dies. As a result of the itching caused by moving over the skin, the female worms may be crushed by the patient scratching the affected part and, occasionally, masses of eggs are to be found on the buttocks.

The intense itching in the anal region usually causes the patient to scratch and the eggs containing the infective larvae may, therefore, be subsequently carried to the mouth. Eggs on clothing or bedding may be transferred to the mouth on the fingers or may be inhaled in dust. In the absence of control and treatment, the infection tends readily to be transmitted from one person to another, so that the whole family or dormitory becomes infected. The infective eggs sometimes hatch on the skin of the buttocks and the larvae migrate through the anus and up the bowel to become adult.

Life cycle of *Oxuris vermicularis* (or Thread Worms)

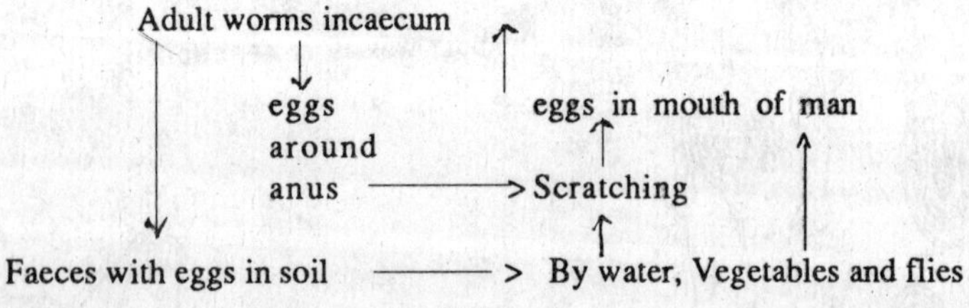

Pathogenicity

Many infected persons are subclinically infected, in others the main symptom is pruritus which may be severe and intractable, causing fatigue and loss of sleep. Adult worms in the intestine may be associated with haemorrhage or inflammation at their site of attachment to the mucosa, and sometimes appendicitis occurs if they invade that organ.

Diagnosis

The gravid females may be found in the faeces after a purge or salt enema, or they may be seen if the buttocks are examined at night during sleep. Occasionally the characteristic eggs are found in the faeces. The best diagnostic method is to examine the skin of the buttocks for eggs by means of the swab (either the NIH swab or adhesive cellulose tape).

(3) ANCYLOSTOMA DUODENALE (Hook Worm)

Q. 2.36. What is Ancylostoma duodenale ?

Ancylostoma duodenale is a blood feeding Nematode of human and commonly known as, the '*old world Hook-worm*' as they are hook like in structure.

Q. 2.37. What are the various species of Ancylostoma and where they live in or what is their habit or habitat ?

Various species of Ancylostoma are :

1. **Necator americanus**: mainly seen in South India.
2. **Ancylostoma** duodenale : in North India.
3. **A. Ceylanicum** : recently reported from Calcutta.

(Saxena and Prasad 1971)

Habit and Habitat :

1. Adult lives in the jejunum and less often in the duodenum of man.
2. Eggs passed in human faeces.
3. Infective larvae free in soil and water.

They suck tissue fluid, blood at a rate of 0.67 cc./ day (Faust 1940). Oesophagacal gland secretes a ferment which prevent blood cloting.

Q. 2.38. What are the morphological characteristics of A. duodenale or Hook worm ? [D.M.S. 19'81]

Morphological Structure :

(i) Cylindrical, greyish white with bent antetior end.

(ii) Buccal Capsule with 6 teeth 4 hooks on the ventral surface, and two dorsal knobs, two pharyngeal teeth.

Differences between Male and Female Hook Worm

	Male	Female
1. **Size :**	8-10 mm long and 0.4-0.5 mm in breadth.	1. Length : 10-13 mm. Breadth : 0.6 mm.
2. **Tail end :**	Tail end with umbrella like copulory bursa, with three lobes.	2. Pointed tail. No bursa
3. **Genital organ :**	It consists of tubular testes with deferences, Seminal vesicles, ejaculatory duct open in cloaca.	3. Genital organ consists of two coiled tubules of which the distal part form the *ovary*, middle part the *oviduct*, and terminal part the *uterus*. Two ducts united to form Vagina opening in Valva.
4. **Spicules :**	(2 mm long) used in copulation.	4. Absent.
5. **Genital : opening**	Posteriorly or opened in cloaca.	5. Genital opening posterly or by 2/3 from anterior end.

Eggs :

The eggs are oval and colourless, with broadly rounded extremities; there is a thin outer shell lined by a very fine vitelline layer. They measure about 60μ in length and 40μ in breadth and contain, when freshly passed, an *ovum* which has segmented into two to eight cells, there being a clear space between the egg shell and the segmented ovum.

Q. 2.39. Describe the life history of Hook worm. (A. duodenale)
[C.U.80 (Sup), D.M.S. 1976, 1977,81]

No intermediate host. Man is the definite host. After cross fertilization each female lays about 10,000-20,000 eggs/day within the host intestine. After eggs are passed by the infected persons in the field together with faeces, in sufficient moisture and at a temperature about 70-85°F, the 1st stage larvae which are known as **rhabaditiform larvae** from the eggs within 24 to 48 hours.

They are voracious eaters and feed for 2 to 3 days and moult to develop 2nd stage larvae which also feed and grow and within 5 to 10 days and they moult for the second time to become **filariform larvae.**

These **filariform** larvae cannot feed due to their closer of the mouths but they are infective form and can live for 2 months in the soil, if it is moist, shady and airy. The average and maximum longivity of filariform larva are 6 and 15 weeks respectively. They are found in upper inch of all soil. The upwards and larval movements of *filariform larvae* are 90 cm and 35 cm respectively.

Mode of infection :

The filariform larvae by active penetration enter the skin of a barefooted person and through circulation they pass their way to the right heart of the human host. From the right heart, the larvae pass through the lungs, alveoli, and they crawl up to trachea and then, pass through the oesophagus to the stomach, to settle in the small intestine, by this time, they undergo **third moulting**. In the intestin, they acquire provisional buccal capsules and after 3 weeks the worms undergo **fourth moulting** in order to develop permanent buccal capsules after which they become matured. After maturity fertilize the females and females start laying eggs.

Thus the various stages of the life cycle of hook worms take place following days :

Free living forms in soil	5 days
Skin to intestine	5 days
Third moulting	3 days
Fourth moulting	14 days
Maturity	15 days
Total	42 days or 6 weeks

The egg to egg cycle requires about 6 weeks to complete :

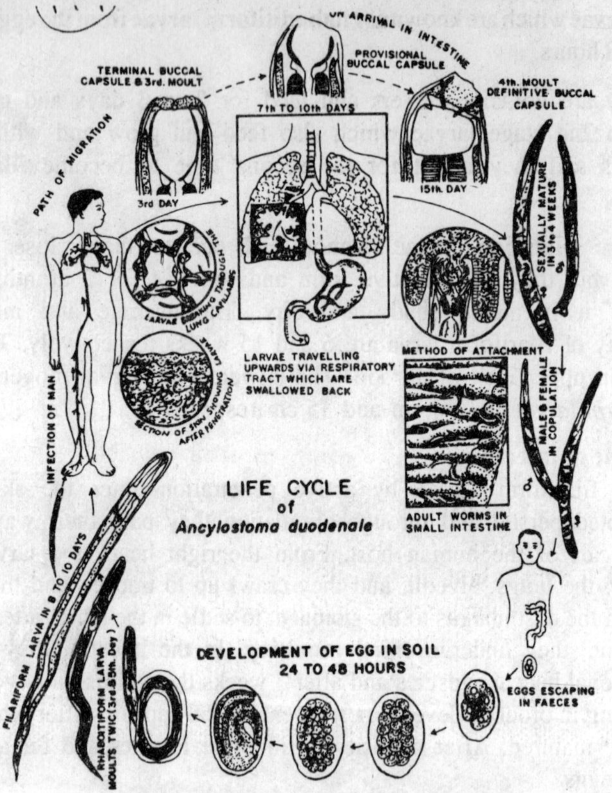

Fig.16—[*Morphology: After Looss and Brüimpt.*]

***(Life cycle of *Ancylostoma Deuodenale*)**

Adult worms are in duodenum : In stomach

Matures in a month — In lung

Eggs in stool

Rhabtidiform larve in soil — In blood vessels

Filariform larva in soil — In lymphatics

Remains on grass blade or moist earth for 2 months. — Larva pierces the skin through water or vegetables.

Q. 2.40. What happens, when a Hook worm infection occurs on man ? [D.M.S., 1976, 77]

1. Effects of Larva :

The penetration of the infective larvae causes a papular, urticarial erruption of the skin which may become pustular known as *ground itch.*

2. Effects of Adult Worm :

Symptoms are usually slight or absent when only a small number of worms is present, because each worm causes the loss of only about 0.1 ml of blood daily. The size of the worm load depends on the degree of exposure to infection and, possibly, to some extent on the resistance of the host to super infection, resulting from an existing infection. The level at which symptoms become evident is related to the number of worms present, possibly influenced by resistance acquired by the individual to the pathological effects of the worms, which enables him to limit or repair the damage done by them. This acquired resistance may be diminished or lost as a result of a variety of factors including maluntrition, intercurrent infection, heavy physical work or pregnancy.

Loss of over 6 ml of blood daily, indicated by 4,000 ova per gm of faeces, produces *slight anaemia,* and over 10,000 ova per g. is associated with *severe anaemia* resulting in lassitude, dyspnoea, *palpitation* of the *heart* and *oedema* of the *feet* and *ankles.*

N. B. [*Microcytic type of anaemia* is the usual feature. It has been found that A. duodenale removes about 0.5 ml of blood, per worm, per diem, against 0.2 to 0.5 ml each per diem that of N. americanus.]

Apart from these three may be creeping eruption, pneunonitis, watery diarrhoea, physical and mental retradation, etc.

Diagnosis: Based on finding the eggs in the faeces.

Q. 2.41. What are the differences between A. duodenale and N. americanus ?

	A. Duodenale	**N. Americanus**
Size :	Longer and thicker than *N. americanus.*	Shorter and thinners than *A. duodenale.*
Teeth :	2 pairs ventrally.	Absent but 2 cuting plates present.

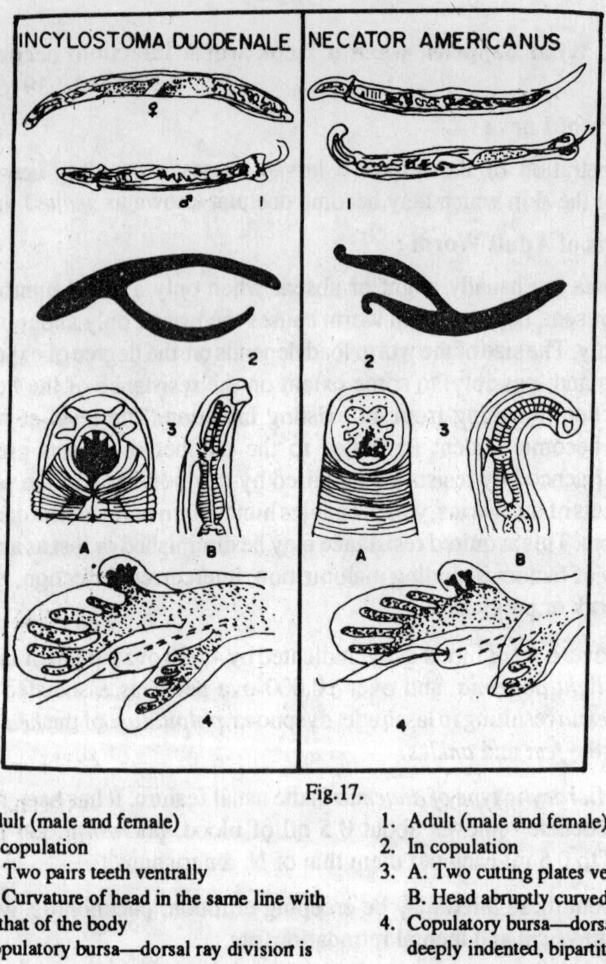

Fig.17.

1. Adult (male and female)
2. In copulation
3. A. Two pairs teeth ventrally
   B. Curvature of head in the same line with that of the body
4. Copulatory bursa—dorsal ray division is shallow, tripartite. Spicules-two, separate.

1. Adult (male and female)
2. In copulation
3. A. Two cutting plates ventrally
   B. Head abruptly curved, dorsiflexed
4. Copulatory bursa—dorsal ray is deeply indented, bipartite. Spicules-two, fused and hooklike at this tip.

Head :	'C' shaped, i.e. head is the same line with its body.	'S' shaped, i.e. head is in opposite curve with its body.
Males :	8-11 mm x 0.4 mm *Copulatory bursa* : Total no. of rays 13, Dorsal ray is triprtitie *Spicule* :2 long and slender.	7-9 mm x 0.3 mm Total no. of rays 14, Dorsal ray is deeply indented; each division bipartite. *Spicule* : long,slender, united and terminate in a barbed end.

Females :	10-13 mm x 0.6 mm. Posterior tip spined. Vulva-situated behind the middle of the body (posterior half).	9-11 mm x 0.6 mm. No. spine situated in the front of the middle (anterior half) of the body.
Life Span :	6-8 years.	4-5 years.

Q. 2.42. (a) What are the differences between the 2 types of larva of Hookworm.

Two types of larva develop within the soil : Humid warm (27 °C) and free oxygenation and dilute faeces is favourable for larval development).

Rhabditiform Larva	Filariform Larva
i) 250μ long with rhabiditics oesophagus (3 segments).	i) Do not grow any more size 500-600μ, long elongated, cylincrical oesophagus.
ii) Varacious feeder of organic matter in faeces or soil.	ii) Do not feed.
iii) Larva grows rapidly and moults twice in one week-1st at 3rd day and 2nd at 5th day, and form 2nd larval stage (filariform larva) at 8-10 days.	iii) It cast off sheath and enters into the new host through skin.

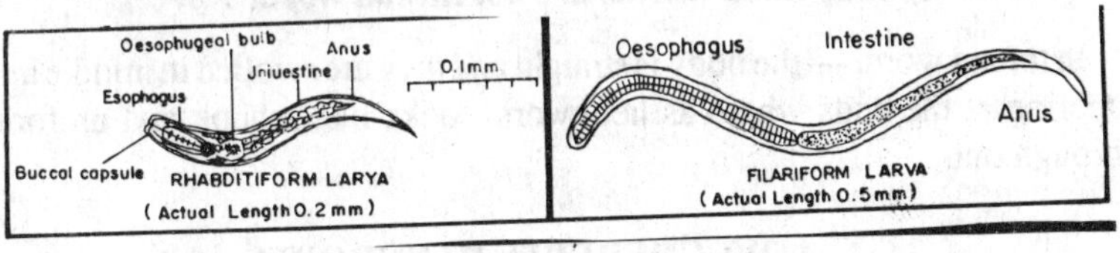

Fig.18—Larvae of an intestinal nematode (Hook Worm)

Q. 2.42. (b) What are the causes and type of Anaemia seen in Hook worm disease ?

It is due to chronic blood loss due to :

1. The adult parasite utilise about 0.6 — 0.7 cc of blood per day as their meal.
2. There is punctiform haemorrhage in the intestinal mucosa at the site of lodgement during its blood meal.
3. There is show oozing from these spots as the parasites secretes an anticoagulant during its blood meal.

Type :

Commonest type is microcytic, hypochromic due to chronic blood loss. Sometimes we may have dimorphic (macrocytic hypo chromic) anaemia.

Q. 2.42. (c) How to assess severity of infection in hookworm disease ?

1. By the degree of anaemia — noted from blood picture.
2. By ova count of stool — on average if 40 ova is present in 1 gm of foecal materials it indicates the presence of *1 adult* parasites in the intestine. Thus from the ova count we can know how many adult parasite are present in the intestine.

The infection is said to be severe if the number of adults be above 1000. It is said to be heavy if the number be between 500 —1000 and said to be moderate if it is between 100 — 500.

Q.2.42. (d) How do you explain such large number of parasites?

It means so many larva have penetrated through the skin and the parasites does not multiply in the system.

Q. 2.42. (e) Why hook worms are not thread worm ?

In thread worm — the body is straight and they are swollen in middle and tapering at the ends where as hookworm looks like a hook and uniform through out.

4. WUCHERERIA BANCROFTI

Q. 2.43. What is filariasis ?

The term **filariasis** is often used to indicate various morbid conditions produced by different nematods, or filariae constituting super family : **Filariodiea** of the sub-order — **Spirurata.**

Q. 2.44. Where do they live in ? Or Where do we get the adult parasite ?

(a) Adult worms :

These are found in extricably coiled in lymphatic glands, or lying in lymphatic vessels, in superficial abscesser, or wandering in retroperitoneal tissue and other sites.

(b) Microfilariae :

The microfilariae occur in lymph vessels, and in the peripheral blood *normally at night* (10 P.M. to 2 P.M.). During the day microfilariae are absent from the peripheral blood or are found only rarely, and are present mainly in the lungs and in other organs.

(c) Infective larvae :

Developmental forms are found in the gut and muscles of certain species of mosquitoes which taken up infected blood, later, infective larvae are present in their mouth parts.

Q. 2.45. (a) What form of the parasite cause lesion ?

It is the adult parasite responsible for lesion.

Q. 2.46. Describe the morphology of Wuchereria bancrofti in adult and Embryos forms. (Microfilaria)

Morphology of the Adult Worms :

These are long hair like transparent namatodes (often creamy white in colour). They are *filiform* in shape and both ends are tapering, the head end terminating in a slightly rounded swelling.

Male :The male measures 2.5 to 4 cm in length by 0.1 mm in thickness. Its *tail-end* is curved ventrally and contains two spicules of unequal length.

Female : The female measures 8 to 10 cm in length by 0.2 to 0.3 mm in thickness. Its *tail-end* is narrow and abruptly pointed. The females, though liberating active embryos, are really *ovoviviparous* (laying eggs with well developed embryos).

Male and female remain coiled together and can only be separated with difficulty (female are usually more or numerous than males and the latter are difficult to find).

The life span of the adult worms is long, probably several years (5 to 10 years).

MICROFILARIA

*** [What are the morphological characteristics of Microfilaria ?]**

Generally *Microfilaria* live in circulating blood of the lymphatic channels and they are very active in their habits as they can move both with and against the blood stream.

(a) When Unstained :

When unstained microfilariae appear as colourless and transparent bodies with blunt heads and rather pointed tails. The embryo measures about 290 m m in length by 6 to 7 m m in breadth.

(b) When Stained :

When stained with Romanowsky's stains they become dead and shows the following *morphological peculiaritis* :

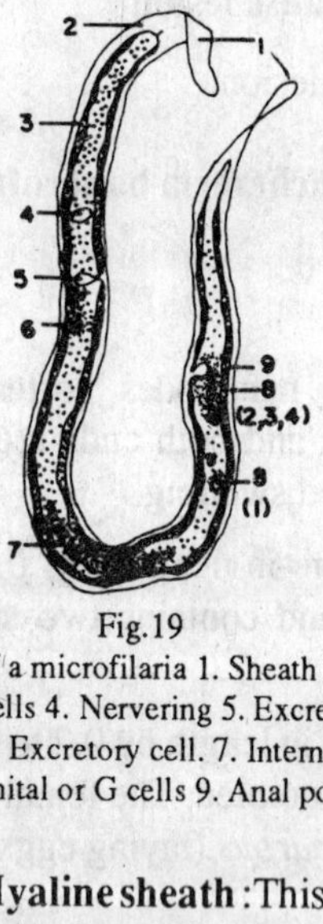

Fig.19
Structure of a microfilaria 1. Sheath 2. Stylet 3. Somatic cells 4. Nervering 5. Excretory pore (V Spot) 6. Excretory cell. 7. Internal body 8. Genital or G cells 9. Anal pore

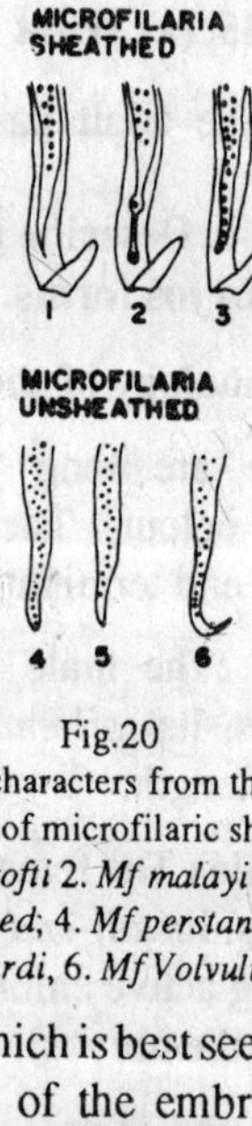

Fig.20
Diagnestic characters from the postrior extremity of microfilaric sheathed: 1. *Mf bancrofti* 2. *Mf malayi* 3. *Mf toa unsheathed*; 4. *Mf perstans* 5. *Mf Ozzardi*, 6. *Mf Volvulus*.

(i) **Hyaline sheath** :This is a structureless sac which is best seen where it projects slightly beyond the extremities of the embryo. The sheath is much longer (359 m m) than the larval body so that the larva can move forwards and backwards within it. The sheath represents the chorionic envelope of the egg; it remains as an investing membrane round the larva.

(ii) **Citicula** : is lined by subcuticular cells and is seen only with vital stains.

(iii) **Somatic cells or Nuclei** : Those appear as granules in the central axis of the body and extended from the head to the tail-end. The granules do not extend up to the tip of the tail (terminal 5 per cent) and serve as a distinguishing feature of *Mf. bancrofti.* At the anterior end there is a space, also devoid of granules, called the *cephalic space* which is as long as it is broad. With vital stains the presence of a *stylet* is seen.

(iv) **The granules** : are broken at definite places serving as the land-marks for identification of the speices. They include the following:

(a) **Nerve ring** : an oblique space.

(b) **Anterior V-spot**, represents the rudimentary excretory system.

(c) **Posterior V-spot** or tail spot, represents the terminal part of the alimentary canal (anus or cloaca)

(v) A few G-cells (the so-called ''genital cells) posteriorly; while G-cells 2, 3 and 4 are just infront of the anal pore, G-cell 1 is situated further infront.

(vi) Innenkorper of Fullebron or Central (Internal) Body of Manson extends from the anterior V-spot to the G-cell 1. It represents the rudimentary alimentary canal.

Q. 2.47. Describe the life history of W. bancrofti.

[C.U. 1981, D.M.S. 1977, 81]

Wuchereria bancrofti passes its life cycle in 2 hosts : *man* and *mosquito*. Man is the definite host and *Culex pipiens fatigans* (Culex fatigans) is the intermediate host.

1. Development of Microfilaria in the Mosquito :

When female *Culex pipines fatigans* takes a blood meal from a human carrier containing microfilariae the further developmental changes of the microfilariae take place in the gut of the mosquito in the following ways :

(i) Sheathed microfilariae ingested by the mosquito during its blood-meal collect round the anterior end of the stomach. They cast off their sheathed quickly, penetrate the gut wall within an hour or two and migrate to the thoracic muscles. Hence they rest and begin to grow.

(ii) In the next 2 days the slender, snake-like organism changes to a thick, short, sausage-shaped form with a short spiky tail, measuring 124 to 250 mm in length by 10 to 17 mm in breadth (the first stage larva). It possesses a rudimentary digestive tract.

(iii) In 3 to 7 days time the larva grows rapidly, moults (sheds cuticle) once or twice and the end of this stage measures 225 to 355 μm in length by 15 to 30 μm in breadth (the second stage larva).

(iv) *On the 10th or 11th day the metarmosphosis becomes complete :*

The tail atrophies to a mere stump and the digestive system, body cavity and genital organs are now fully developed. This is the *third stage larva* which measures 1,500 to 2,000 μm in length by 18 to 23 μm in breadth and has 3 subterminal caudal papillae (B. malayi has 2). At this stage it is infective to man and enters the proboscis sheath of the mosquito on or about the 14th days. It should be noted that one microfilaria gives rise to one infective larva in the proboscis sheath. There may be several larvae remaining coiled up, waiting for an opportunity to infect man while the mosquito is having its blood-meal.

The time taken for the complete development of microfilaria in the mosquito varies from 10 to 20 days or more, depending, however, on the automspheric temperature, humidity and also to a certain extent on the species of the mosquito. The mean temperature and humidity required for development of microfilaria in a mosquito are 80°F and 63 percent respectively.

2. Entrance into Man and development into Adult worm :

When the infected mosquito bites a human being, the thrid stage larvae are not directly infected into the blood stream like malarial parasites but are deposited on skin near the site of puncture. Later, attracted by the warmth of the skin, the larvae either enter through the puncture wound or penetrate through the skin in their own.

The *third stage larvae* (infective larvae), having penetrated the skin, reach the lymphatic channels, settle down at some spot (inguinal, scrotal or abdominal lymphatics) and begin to grow into adult forms. In course of time, probable after a period of 5 to 18 months they become sexually mature. The male fertilises the female and the gravid females give birth to larvae.

A new generation of microfilaria is emitted which passes either through the thoracic duct or the right lymphatic duct, to the venous system and pulmonary capillaries and then to the peripheral (capillaries of the systemic circulation), thus completing th cycle.

The time requires from the entry of infective larvae to the appearence of microfilariae in the blood of a new host is about one year.

The *life span* of adult worms is about 4 to 5 years.

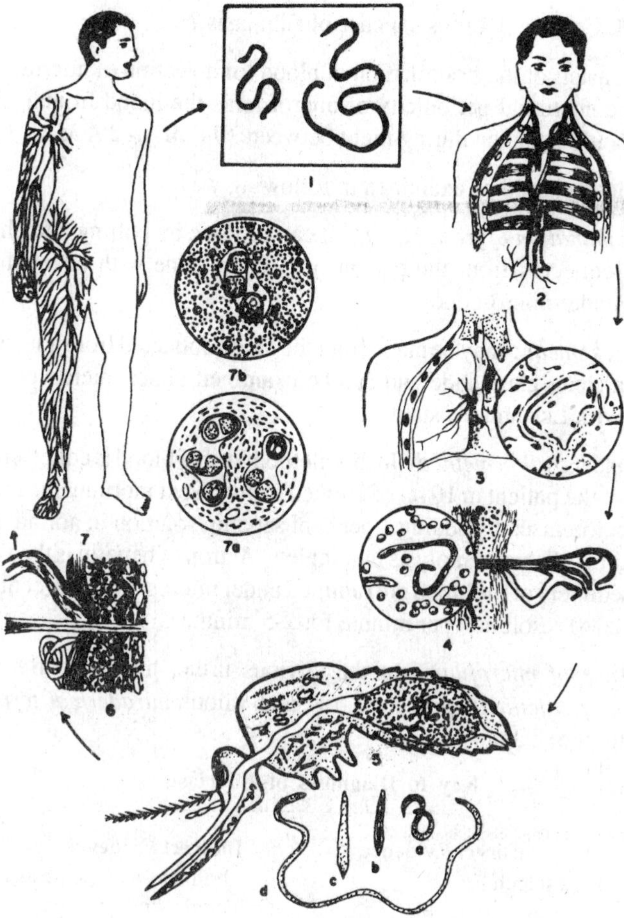

Life Cycle of Wuchereria Bancrofti (Filiaria)

In a year adult male and female in lymph gland ← mature microfilaria in skins lymphatic Culex bites man.

↑ ↑

Immature microfilaria ← mature microfilaria in 14 days.

↑ ↑

Lymphatic circulation ← sucked up by Culex

↑ ↑

Pulmonary circulation

↑

Systemic circulation ← In capillaries of skin at night.

Q.2.48. Can we diagnosis a case of filariasis ?

This consists of the examination of blood for detection of microfilariae. Due to the nocturnal periodicity of microfilarae the blood from a filarial patient should be taken during night between *10 P.M. to 2 A.M.*

The blood should be examined in following ways :

(a) *Examination of fresh blood :* It can be done by putting a fresh drop of blood collected from the patient on a clean slide with coverslip and examine under microscope.

(b) *Thick smear* : may be made from the blood collected from a suspected case on a clean glass slide and can be examined under microscope after staing it with Leishman's stain.

(c) *Concentration method*: In this method 5 ml of blood is collected from the vein of the patient in 10 ml of citrated saline. Next morning the blood is dehaemoglobinised by adding 1 per cent saponin solution in normal saline drop by drop till the haemolysis is complete. A drop of heparin is then added and the sediment of the blood is examined under microscope after centrifuging it at 2000 resolution per minute for 2-5 minutes.

Presence of microfilaria in the chylous urine, hydrocele fluid. *The detection of calcified worm* by X-ray and vaious *intradermal tests* may also help the diagnosis.

Key to Diagnosis of Filariasis

Direct Evidence This includes a search for :		**Indirect Evidence** Immuno-allergic Tests :	
Microfilariae (A sheathed microfilaria having tail tip free from nuclei.) (i) In the peripheral blood. (ii) In the chylous urine. (iii) In the exudate of lymph varix.	*Adult worms* (i) In the biopsied lympt node. (ii) Calcified worm by x-ray.	Allergic tests (i) Blood examination Eosinophilia (5 to 15%) (ii) Intradermal test. An immediate hypersensitivity reaction.	Immunological test and complement fixation test.

(iv) In the dydro-
cele fluid.

Q. 2.49. What are the effects of W. bancrofti on man ?

[D.M.S. 1977]

Pathogenicity :

The worm causes, or is closely associated with, the disease **filariasis**. This is characterized by attacks of irregular fever, lymphangitis, enlargement of lymphatic glands, hydrocele, thickening of the skin, elephantiasis of the legs, scrotum, and vulva, and less commonly of the arms and breast. Lymph varices due to stoppage of lymph flow by adult worms in the lymphatic glands, often occur. If the pre-aortic glands are blocked, the condition of true chyluria may arise, the urine containing chyle. More frequently a condition indistinguishable from chyluria arise, when the lymphatics of the kidneys ureter, or bladders are blocked; this is due, not to true chyle, but possible to cellular degeneration in the walls of the lymphatics.

Q. 2.50. (a) What is the essential pathological change in filarial infection ?

The basic pathological change in lymphatic obstraction caused by :

(1) Mechanical obstraction by adult parasite either living or calcified clumps of parasites may behave as emboli.

(2) There is endothelial proliferation of the lymphatic trunk and also fibrous thickening of the wall : a process known as obliterative endolymphangitis.

(3) The draining lymph glands may undergo focal necrosis and healing by fibrosis.

(4) Super added bacterial infection specially by haemolytic streptococci may add to lymphatic obstruction. According to many this bacterial lymphangitis which is often recurrent precipeitates complete obstruction.

Q. 2.51. Notes on :

Microfilaria :

The eggs of the *W. bancrofti at the time of eviposition contain uncoiled embryos which are delicate, snake-like minute, larvae called microfilariae.*

Its size varies from 100 to 300μ, *Mf. bancrofti, Mf. malayi* and *Mf. loa* are sheathed and others are unsheathed. Its anterior end is pounded off has a stylet. Certain clear spots are seem is embryo which are :

(i) Nerve ring, (ii) Anterior V spot rudimentary excretory pore, (iii) Posterior V spot is anal pore. There are four genital spots and an internal body. The number of cells as distributed throughout the body represent rudimentary intestine run from head to pointed tail.

The diagnosis of the species of *microfilaria* is actually made by the study of the larvae form.

*Tail uncleii not up to the end : W. bancrofti.

**Tail nucleii up to the end : L. Loa.

***Terminal nucleii : W. malai.

Q. 2.52. (a) What is Elephantiasis ? [D.M.S. 1977]

The affected skin (by microfilariae) becomes markedly thickened due to a process of hyperplasia and hypertrophy which is caused by a irritant action of high protein content of the tissue fluid. Due to the inflammatory process the tissue fluid canot drained out due to lymphatic obstruction and known as elephantiasis.

Q. 2.53. What are parasites enter through the skin ?

Parasites entering through the skin are :

1. Those penetrating directly through skin :
   - (a) Larva of hook worm (filariform).
   - (b) Blood flukes or Schistosoma.
   - (c) Microfilaria.

2. Parasites introduced into skin by other agents :
   - (a) Malarial parasites.
   - (b) L.D. Body.
   - (c) Trypanosomes.

Q. 2.54. What are the parasites present in body tissue ?

1. Hydatid cyst.
2. L.D. Bodies : Leishmanoid form within the endothelial cells of bone marrow.

Q. 2.55. What are the parasites seen in brain ?

1. Ring form of plasmodium falciparum with RBC's in capillaries of brain.
2. Trypanosomes may be demonstrated even in C.S.F.
3. Larva of Taenia solium (cysticereus cellulosae) these may remain calcified within the brain tissues giving rise to convulsions.
4. Hydatid cyst.

Q. 2.56. What are the parasites causes microcytic anaemia ?

1. *Dibothriocephalous latus.* The adult parasite utilises the haematinic principle in the intestine.
2. Rarely in *hookworm* infection there may be Macrocytic anaemia which is probably due to lack of absorption of haematinic principle as a result of diarrhoea.
3. Rarely chronic *kala-azar.* This is also true in diarrhoea and dysentery which are common complication in *kala-azar.*

Q. 2.57. What are the parasites causes skin lesion ?

1. Protozoa :

(a) *L.D. Body* : Causing dermal leishmaniasis. This is a manifestation of post kala-azar skin lesion but the peculiarity is that the serological tests for kala-azar like AT, CT, CFT etc. become negative. The only way to diagnosis the condition is to demonstrate leishmanoid form of L.D. body in the scraping materials from the local skin lesion.

(b) *Leishmania tropica* : Causing oriental sore.

(c) *Leishmania brazilenses* : Causing a chronic granulomatous lesion in the skin and mucus membrane of mouth and upper respiratory tract and this condition is called **Espunida.**

(d) Entamoeba histolytica causes amoebiasis, out of it the skin lesion is due to mechanical implantation of the trophozoite form of E. histolytica on the adjacent area of skin, affected sites are perianal skin, skin adjoining liver drainage would in case of amoebic liver abscess.

2. Heminths :

(a) *Ground itch or Collie's itch* : caused by penetration of the skin of the foot by the filariform larve of hook worm. The affected area shows oedema, redness and papulovesicular eruptions. With the onset of secondary bacterial infection pustules are formed.

(b) *Creeping eruption* : caused by *Ancylostoma brasiliensis* and A. canilum (very rare).

(c) *Dracunculus medinesis* : causing ulcer near about the ankle through which the gravid female parasite comes out.

(d) Lesion caused by filaria. Elephantiasis of skin.

(e) Affection of peripheral skin by the irritation caused by the ova of thread worms this is an important cause of pruritus.

Q. 2.58. What are the parsites found in the liver ?

(A) Protozoa :

1. Malaria parasite found within the liver cells in the pre and exoerythrocytic phase. Erythrocytic forms are present within the RBC's in the sinusoids of the liver.
2. Entamoeba histolytica : trophozoites forms of the parasites.
3. Leishmanoid form of L.D. body : within the kupffer's cells of the liver.
4. Trypanosomes, in the stage, if systematic disemination of the parasite.

(B) Helminths :

1. Hydatid cyst.
2. Larva of Taenia solium.
3. The Liver flukes.
4. Blood flukes.
5. Migrating larva of *Ascaris lumbricoides.*

5. TRICHINELLA SPIRALIS

5.1. General characters :

The genus *Trichincilla* is a smooth worm; the male-1.5 mm x 44-60 μ, has no spicule or copulatory sheath; the female, 3-4 mm x 60 μ is viviparous,

with vulva close to the anterior end. The male dies shortly after fertilizing the female. It is a parasite of rats and pigs transmitted to man by eating uncooked or inadequately cooked infected pork.

5.2. Habitat : Adult worm lives in small intestine; larvae gain entrance to circulation by boring through its wall and pass through liver to the capillaries of lungs and from there to the striped muscles of the body where they become encysted. Although one host serves as the definitive host and intermediate host the live cycle is completed in two hosts. Each adult female liberates about 1500 larvae of the size 500μ x 250μ. *Cysts* are also small-800μx 300μ and remain infective for long periods (10-30 years).

5.3. Life cycle : The whole life cycle is passed in one animal-the *pig, rat* or *man*. A transference of host is required for the preservation of the species. Two hosts are required to complete the cycle. When man consumes raw or undercooked flesh infected with the cysts of *T. spiralis* the cyst gets digested out of the flesh, in the stomach by the gastric juices. The cyst passes to the duodenum where excystment takes place and the larva invades the duodenal/jejunal mucosa and undergoes development into male or female adults. After fertilisation the females being to deposit larvae. Some of these may escape into the lumen of the intestine but the great majority get into the intestinal lymphatics or the mescenteric venules and are distributed throughout the body. They finally settle in the striated muscles where they encyst.

The cyst is formed by a tightly coiled larva encapsulated by host tissues. The long axis of the cyst is parallel to that of the muscle fibres.

The cycle thus ends in the host. Continuation requires transference of host. The pig is the natural host of the parasite. *Disease in man has not been reported in India. Prophylaxis* consists in the proper inspection of meat and avoiding the consumption of raw or undercooked meat.

6. STRONGYLOIDES STERCORALIS

6.1. General characters :

There are two kinds of adult worms (a) *parasitic form* and (b) *free-living form.* The latter is the basic life cycle of the parasite. The parasitic males are seldom seen and are found in the lungs rather in the intestine. The parasitic females are colourless, transparent, slender and filiform 2.2 mm x 0.3-0.75 mm., with a finely striated cuticle and pointed posterior end. In the female the cylindrical oesophagus extend through the anterior one-thrid and open into the midgut. The anus opens near the posterior end. The vulve opens ventrally at the junction of middle and posterior thrid from this a pair of uteri extend anteriorly and posteriorly to continue as oviducts which join the clindrical ovaries. Eggs are oval, thin-shelled and transparent and measure 50 x 30μ. They are segmented at oviposition in the intestine of the host and hatch out in a few hours to form rhabdititi form larvae before passing out in faces.

6.2. Life cycle : The worms pass their life cycle in *man*. No intermediate host is required. When man walks barefoot on faecally contaminated soil, the filariform larvae penetrate his skin. They invade the tissue enter the venous circulation and are carried by the bloodstream to the right side of the heart and thence to the lungs. From the pulmonary capillaries they enter the lung alveoli where they develop through post-filariform and preadolescent stages to adolescent worm. If both males and females are present, fertilisation of the adolescent female may occur in the bronchi and trachea or later after the worms have reached the intestine.

The fertilisation of the female has to take place before the female penetrates the mucosa of the intestine since the males are not tissue parasites and after a brief stay in the gut, get voided. Probably *S. Stercorales* females usually developed parthenogenetically. The adolescent larva which have reached the pulmonary alveoli climb up the pulmonary tree and get swallowed and reach the intestine. The females migrate into the mucosa mature and begin to deposit eggs in the tissues. The rhabdiform larvae hatch out immediately and enter the lumen of the bowel and passing down with the food and faeces, get excreted in the stools. These then undergo development in the soil and go through other a *direct* or *indirect* cycle.

In the direct cycle the rhabditiform larva directly develops in 3-4 days into a filariform larva infective to man in the indirect cycle the rhabditiform larvae develop into free living sexual forms. Fertilise, lay eggs and develop into rhabditiform larvae when conditions become unfavourable the indirect cycle ceases and the rhabditiform larvae develop into filariform larvae; the infective stage. Thus the cycle continues.

Some of the rhabditiform larvae while still in the intestine may develop into filariform larvae, penetrate the intestinal epithelium and constitute a *reinfection*.

They get into the circulation and follow the normal cycle. Some of these larvae in their transit along with the faeces may penetrate the perianal and penrieal skin without leaving the host and may cause autoinfection.

6.3. Clinical manifestations : Urticarial rash at the site of entry and erythematous urticarial wheals around the anus, caused by migrating filariform larva are seen. Haemorrhages in the lung alveoli and bronchopneumonia during the migration of larvae through the lungs occur. Intractable diarrhoea or dysentery may result.

**Diagnosis*: Rhabditiform larvae are seen in freshly passed stools.

**Prophylaxis* : This is achieved by personal hygiene, the proper disposal of faeces and the use of footwear.

7. TRICHURIS TRICHURA

7.1. General character :

The adult worm is 30-50 mm long (Females 40-50 mm). Its anterior 3/5th is thin and resemble the lash of a whip and hence the name. The posterior 2/5th are thicker than the anterior part. The mouth at the anterior end is simple and opens into a long minute chanelled oesophagus having a single column of secretory cells. The anus is terminal. The male has a long sacculate tubular testes and a single lanceolate spicule, 2-5 mm long protruding through the retractile penile sheath. The female has a sacculate tubular ovary over hall the thick part of the body. The evid'ict runs posteriorly and open into the uterus, which in its turn run forwards to open into the vulva through a short vagina situated on the ventral surface of the anterior end of the thick part of the body.

7.2. Habitat : There is no intermediate host but change of host is necessary to continue the new life cycle. Eggs containing larvie are infective to man. From the eggs in the faeces the infective larvae develop in moist soil without hatching. When these are ingested by the human host with food and water the shell is digested and the larva is liberated through one on pole and attach itself to the small intestine where they attain maturity in about three months.

Prevalence-all over world :

7.3. Life cycle : The worm passes its life cycle *in man*. A change of host is necessary for the continuance of the species. The eggs which are voided in the faeces develop in water or damp earth and inside the egg a rhabditiform larva develops in 3-4 weeks. Such an egg is infective to man. Man gets infected by taking in contaminated food or water. The egg shell is dissolved by digestive enzymes and the larva is liberated. It passes down to the caccum where it grows into the adult worm and gets embedded in the mucosa. When sexually mature fertilisation of the female takes place and the fertilised female lays eggs which are voided in the faeces. The cycle is repeated.

7.4. Clinical manifestation : It does not usually produce any disease. In heavy infestations abdominal pain, mucus diarrhoea - often blood-stained- and loss of weight occur occasionally appendicitis and prolapse of the rectum may occur.

******Diagnosis :* The eggs can be easily demonstrated in the faeces. Occasionally adult worms may also be present.

**Prophylaxis :* This is possible by preventing the consumption of uncooked vegetables and fruits grown in contaminated fields and by the proper disposal of faeces.

PART — III

GENERAL PATHOLOGY
AND
SPECIAL PATHOLOGY

GENERAL & SPECIAL PATHOLOGY

DISCUSSION FOR LEARNING

1. *Inflammation*
2. *Necrosis*
3. *Gangrene*
4. *Oedema*
5. *Thrombosis*
6. *Embolism*
7. *Infarction*
8. *Degeneration*
9. *Tumour*
10. *Jaundice*
11. *Anaemia*
12. *Immunity*
13. *Aids*
14. *Peptic Ulcer*
15. *Corcinoma of Stomach*
16. *Carcinoma of Liver*
17. *Lobar Pneumonia*
18. *Broncho Pneumonia*
19. *Pulmonary Tuberculosis*
20. *Adult Type of Tuberculosis*
21. *Bronchogenic Carcinoma*
22. *Glomerulunephritis*
23. *Nephrosis*

"History of Medical Science is the history of pathology". This proverb is dealt with by many since the early days of our research. It has been proclaimed from the **hoary**—of old age that inflammation is the basic process by dint of which human body can be capable of protecting itself. So **Celsus** in the first century A.D. described the cardinal signs of inflammation in clinical practice. **Conheim** (1879) described the important role played by blood vessels in the process of inflammation by his study of vessels in frogs intestine. After that **Metchnikoff** and **Virchow** postulated different pathological phenomenons in order to consolidate Medical Science. Now here we are dealing with some pathological processes in lucid expressions so that we can comprehend this phenomenon in proper way.

As we know that inflammation gives us the basic concept of pathological process, so we are giving a glimpse of inflammation in brief.

1. INFLAMMATION

It is derived from the Greek word, "*Phalogos*", suffix meaning "*fire*".

Its suffix is added to denote inflammation e.g. *Bronchitis*, *conjunctivitis* etc. but *Pneumonia* is exception.

Q. 1.1. What is meant by Inflammation ?

Literally it means *flaming* or *fireing* or *burning*; *Pathologically* : by the term inflammation we mean a set of pathological changes associated with local vascular reaction and cellular response of the living tissue to an injury insufficient to kill the tissue. The effect of inflammation is of two fold, i.e.:

(a) To destroy or to remove the causative organism.
(b) To repair the damaged tissues.
For the first one, wandering cells or mesodermal cells of blood or tissue come to the picture, but for the second one fixed cells or giant cells of the tissue take part.

Q. 1.2. Define Inflammation. Or, What is Inflammation?

[C.U. 1979,80 (Sup.), D.M.S. 74,77,79,81,82,84]

Inflammation is a complex reaction of organisms—(series of pathological changes) *against the action of noxious agents that render the thiamine pyrophosphate* (T.P.P.) *inactive; to stimulate further phosphorllisation in Mitochondria and associated with local vascular reaction and cellular response of the living tissue, provided noxious agents are not sufficient to kill the tissue.*

[Here it is noteworthy to mention that in R.N.A's (Ribo Nucleic Acid) are quickly synthesised to cope out the demand of this situation, and different cellular enzymes are stimulated to secrete. In this time, smooth endoplasmic reticulum are prominant and Lysozome becomes enormous in size. A.T.P's are rapidly broken down into

A.D.P.+Pi. So whole process of inflammation lies in the intricate Bio-chemical processes.]

Or

It is a complex phenomenon due to some noxious agents manifested by some structural and functional changes of the living tissues and blood vessels which are produced in diseased conditions.

Or

Inflammation means series of changes that take place in living tissues when it is injured by various noxious agents or irritants provided, the injury is insufficient to cause immediate death of the tissue.

Q. 1.3. What are the causes of Inflammation ? [C.U. 1980 (Sup.)]

(Aetiology of Inflammation).

Causes of Inflammation

- **Predisposing causes**
  e.g., allergic conditions, diabetes mellitus, alcoholism etc.
- **Exciting causes**
  - LIVING (Animate)
  - NON-LIVING (Inanimate)

LIVING (Animate):

Bacteria	**Animal parasites**	**Fungus**	**Virus**	**Rickettsiae**
e.g., Streptococcus, Staphylococcus, My. tuberculosis, C. diphtheriae etc.	e.g. E. histolytica, A. duodenale, W. bancrofti- etc.	e.g. Nocardia.	Echo, Polio, Hepatitis A, S.H., virus. Hepatitis B. Australian virus etc.	R. peowazekii.

NON-LIVING (Inanimate):

Mechanical	**Physical**	**Chemical**
Any type of *Trauma*, *Foreign body* like silk worm, gut or any metallic agents, *Dead tissue*—sequestrum.	Extreme heat or cold, X-ray, Radium, electricity, Atomic radiations, rays etc.	Strong acids or alkali, poisons like $CHCl_2$, Cl_4 etc.

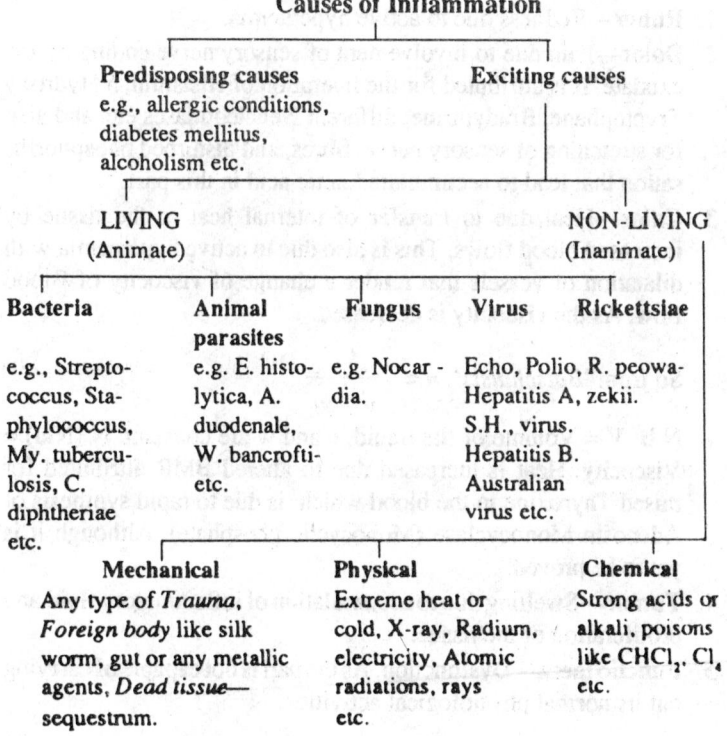

Q. 1.4. What are the Cardinal Signs of Inflammation ?

Or, What are its (inflammation) Classical Signs? Mention their underlaying causes? [D.M.S. 1974, 77, 79, 81, 82, 84]

Cardinal Signs of Inflammation

(Classical Signs of Inflammation)

1. **Rubor**—Redness
2. **Dolor**—Pain
3. **Calor**—Heat
4. **Tumor**—Swelling
5. **Functio laesa or Functio lessae**
(propounded by Galen)—Loss of function.

Underlaying causes :

1. **Rubor**—Redness due to active hyperaemia.
2. **Dolor**—Pain due to involvement of sensory nerve ending by the exudate. It is attributed for the liberation of Histamin, 5 Hydroxy Tryptophane, Bradypirine, different Neucleotidases etc. and also for stretching of sensory nerve fibres, and disturbed phosphorilisation that lead to accumulate Lactic acid in this part.
3. **Calor**—Heat due to transfer of internal heat to the tissue by increased blood flows. This is also due to active hyperaemia with dilatation of vessels that render a change of viscocity of Blood flow. As the viscocity is decreased.

   So from '*Batschinski*'. $n = \dfrac{c}{v - w}$

   N.B: V = Volume of the liquid, c and w are constant. N (Niu) = Viscocity. Heat is increased due to altered BMR attributed for raised Thyroxine in the blood which is due to rapid synthesis of Adenosin Monocyclase (Monocyclic phosphate). Although it is yet to be proved.
4. **Tumor**—Swelling due to accumulation of inflammatory fluid and proliferation of the tissue.
5. **Functio laesa**—Dysfunction. As the part is not capable of carrying out its normal physiological activities.

These signs are very much characteristis for the invading organisms and manifestations are also often correlated with these. But besides these, it has got some general *symptoms* :

(i) *Mallaise.*
(ii) *Bodyache.*
(iii) *Fever*, due to liberation of pyrexial substances by the causative organisms.
(iv) *Leucocytosis.*

1. **Bodyache** (a) *Due to the production of lactic acid.* [From disturbed Glycolysis as already been said that Thiamine Pyrophosphate can not act properly.

[CH_3 COCOOH——>CH_3 CHOHCOOH]
Pyruvic Acid Lactic Acid

(b) *Liberation of Leucotoxin, Histamin 5 H.T. etc.*

2. **Leucocytosis** : Due to the invasion of Bacteria or exposure to Aetiological agents *opsonin index* is raised (more than 1), so Leucocytes are increased to cope out the demand of this situation resulting Leucocytosis.

Besides the above mentioned signs and symptoms, Viraemia, Bacteriaemia and pyaemia are found during inflammation, provided the inflammation is caused due to Virus and Bacteria.

Q. 1.5. What are the differences between Exudate and Transudate?
[D.M.S. 1974, 79]

	Exudate	**Transudate**
1. Def./Origin	It is an inflammatory fluid, partly derived from the blood and partly from the tissue as in cases of acute inflammation such as acute tonsillitis, acute appendicitis etc.	It is a non-inflammatory fluid due to passive venous congestion as in cases of cardiae and renal failure.
2. Mechanism:	It is due to increased permeability.	It is due to passive venous congestion.
3. Specific : gravity	High above 1020.	Low : below 1010.
4. Physical : appearance	High coloured, may contain fibrin flakes. Turbid due to leucocytes or	Pale yellow in colour, mostly transparent in nature.

	Exudate	Transudate
	haemorrhagic due to presence of blood. (In Tuberculosis or Malignant diseases.)	
5. Chemicals :	Protein 3 to 4 gms%. seromucin present.	0.25 to 6 gm% absent.
6. Cytological :	RBC and pus cells must be present (in profuse number).	Endothelial cells are present (scanty in number).
7. Organisms :	Bacteria present.	Absent
8. Total : Leucocytes	Leucocytosis	Leucopinea
	(a) In acute inflammation polymorphonuclear leucocytes as in T.B. (b) In chronic inflammation lymphocytosis.	
9. Coagulability	Spontaneous coagulation due to presence of fibrinogen.	No coagulation.

Q. 1.6. What are the various types of Inflammation ?
Or, Classify Inflammation.

I. Pathologically inflammation is divided into three groups:

(1) *Alternative*
(2) *Exudative*
(3) *Proliferative.*

(1) Alternative

It is characterised by the degeneration of the parechymal cells with exudation and repairvative process. This condition starts during the injury and continous until the irritant ceases off. This type of inflammation is due to physical or chemical agents and endotoxins or extoxins of Bacteria.

(2) Exudative

It is characterised by the different process of exudation like serous exudate, fibrinous exudate, haemorrhagic exudate, serofibrinous exudate and putrifactive exudate.

(3) Proliferative

It is mainly found in chronic type of inflammation where fixed cell or giant cell take part for repairation of the damage tissue e.g. in chronic tuberculosis and chronic syphilis.

II. Clinically inflammation is divided into four groups :

(1) *According to mode of onset duration and severity* ; e.g. Acute, Subacute, Chronic.

(2) *According to causative organisms*; e.g. Tiubercular, Syphilitic, Streptococcal, Staphylococcal etc.

(3) *According to predominate of exudate*; e.g. Serous, Fibrinous, Serofibrinous, Haemorrhagic etc.

(4) *According to tissues or organ involved*; e.g. Peritonitis, Appendicitis etc.

Q. 1.7. What are the differences between acute, subacute and chronic inflammation ?

	Acute	**Subacute**	**Chronic**
1. Clinically :	Signs of inflammation must be present with constitutional symptoms.	Less marked	Absent
2. Durations :	Few days to weeks.	Few weeks	Months to years.
3. Vascular phenomena :	Present	Less marked	Absent
4. Exudation of plasma	Present	Less marked	Absent
5. Cellular response :	Polymorphonuclear leucocytes, Fibroblasts and Lymphocytes are present.	Lymphocytes, Platelets, Histocytes and Fibroblast present.	Luymphocytes, Giant cells. Macrophages are present.

6. Types :	Exudative	Both-exudative and Prolifera-tive.	Only Prolifera-tive.
7. Repair :	Preparation sets on after the removal of debris.	Follows on along with vascular and cellular proliferation.	Follows on side, by side vascular and cellular. Proliferation.

Q. 1.8. What are the various types of Acute Inflammation ? Describe them in short.

Types of Acute Inflammation :

1. Catarrhal
2. Suppurative
3. Haemorrhagic
4. Gangrenous
5. Serofibrinous
6. Fibrinous
7. Phlegmonous
8. Pseudomembranous.

1. Catarrhal Inflammation:

It is mainly characterised by erosion of superficial part of mucous membrane causing excessive secretion of mucin from the goblet cells including dead endothelial cells and other debris. This inflammation generally takes place in case of upper respiratory tract and urogenital tract infection, e.g. common cold and cough.

2. Suppurative Inflammation :

It is mainly characterised by accumulation of pus caused by pygenic organisms e.g. streptococus, staphylococcus, penumococcus, Gonococcus etc.

****Pus**-The pus is composed of dead tissue debris, dead and living W.B.C. and Bacteria.

This type of inflammation is mainly found in the superficial parts as well as internal parts inlcuding epithelial and connective tissue.

3. Haemorrhagic Inflammation :

It is mainly characterised by liberation of R.B.C. from the damage blood vessels causing Haemorrhagic Inflammation.

It is mainly found in case of glomerular nephritis (Inflammation of glomerulonephron).

4. Gangrenous Inflammation :

This type of inflammation is found in gangrenous condition of the patient where massive death of the tissues takes place in the rapid way, where resistant power of the patient is lower than the causative organism.

5. Serofibrinous Inflammation :

It is mainly characterised by the composed of serous and the fibrin, which are liberating from damage tissue cell and are mainly found in the suberficial mucous membrane of endothelial layer e.g. pericarditis and peritonitis.

6. Fibrinous Inflammation :

It is generally affect the subcutaneous tissues liberating plasma protein which is mainly composed of fibrinogen and other dead endothelial cells.

This type of inflammation is mainly found in case of pleurisy and pericarditis and lobes of the lungs.

7. Phlegmonous Inflammation .

It is mainly found in poor resistant body persons.

This type of Inflammation is mainly found in diabetic patient where causative organisms take the upper hand; in regard to host for repairation. As a result the inflammation more causes detoriation of the patient ultimately causes death.

8. Allergic Inflammation :

Allergic Inflammation is mainly found in superficial part of the body liberating toxin which is known as *histamin* – Causes death of the tissue by their toxic effect and ultimately infected by secondary pyogenic organism result inflammatory condition of that particular part.

As in case of Asthma, Autoimmune disorders like — S.L.E. (Systemic Lupus Erythromatosus).

9. Pseudomembranous :

It is characterised by the formation of false membrane, of fibrious material as seen in case of Diphtheria, Bacillary dysentery and Ulcerative coilitis.

Q. 1.9. What are the various types of Chronic Inflammation ?

Chronic Inflammation

1. **Diffuse**
2. **Suppurative**
3. **Granulomatous**
4. **Fibrinoid.**

1. Diffuse Inflammation :

It is mainly characterised by infiltration of leucocytes or by the perivascular part with fibrosis or inflliltrationof lymphocyte to pervivascular part without fibrosis.

In case of *chronic gastritis*—infiltration of lymphocyte—*lesser in amount*. But in case of *cholecystitis infiltration of lymphocyte* greater amount ultimately leads to fibrosis.

2. Suppurative Chronic Inflammation :

Suppurative Chronic Inflammation is characterised by the formation of pus as seen in case of Chronic suppurative Osteomyelitis.

3. Granulomatous Inflammation :

It is mainly characterised by granules in inflmmatory part e.g. Syphilitic, Tubercular and Leprotic Inflammation.

4. Fibrinoid chronic inflammation (accumulation of fibrin in the inflammatory parts).

It is mainly characterised by deposition of fibrin in the synovial membrane leading to a lump formation which is known as Fibrinoid Chronic Inflammation.

This type of Inflammation is found in case of Rheumatoid arthritis and Rheumatic fever.

Q. 1.10. Describe the Pathology of Inflammation ?
[C.U. 1979,80 (Sup.), D.M.S. 76,77,82,84]

Pathology of Inflammation can be categorically divided into three parts:

1. Vascular Phenomenon.
2. Cellular Response.
3. Repair or Healing.

These three are also divided into various parts which are as follows:

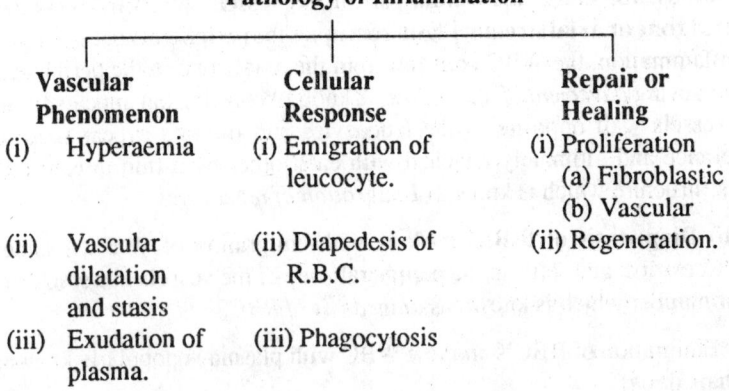

Pathology of Inflammation

Vascular Phenomenon	**Cellular Response**	**Repair or Healing**
(i) Hyperaemia	(i) Emigration of leucocyte.	(i) Proliferation (a) Fibroblastic (b) Vascular
(ii) Vascular dilatation and stasis	(ii) Diapedesis of R.B.C.	(ii) Regeneration.
(iii) Exudation of plasma.	(iii) Phagocytosis	

(1) VASCULAR PHENOMENON

Q. 1.11. Discuss the vascular response in acute inflammation.

It follows the following sequence of events:

1. Vasodilatation preceded by vaso-constriction.
2. Increase blood flow to the arteries, arterioles, capillaries vein and venules (which is known as *hyperaemia*).
3. Capillary dilatations, slowing of blood flow and ultimately *stasis*.
4. Packing of RBC in the capillaries.
5. Pavement of leucocytes.
6. Exudation of fluid without pouncing of polymorphos cells and other cells to the inflammatory part.

In case of **local injury** at first constriction of the vessels take place causing local anaemia of that particular part leading to hyparemia with dilatation of arterioles and venules; capillaries in a lesser quantity. This stage lasts for one hour or few hours. After few hours vascular changes take place, blood stream gradually slow in nature and stasis of form elements take place inside the vessels.

(2) CELLULAR RESPONSE

(a) Emigration of leucocytes: When blood moves in the blood vessels the corpuscles occupy the central part of the vessels which is known as **central zone or axial stream**. Plasma occupies the peripheral zones. In case of inflammation, the WBC cells fall from the axial zone to the peripheral zone causing *pavement of leucocytes*. A knob like projection appears from the vessels wall opposite to the leucocytes and roduces a pear shaped apperance and ultimately attached with each other by a thin thread like tissue structure which is know as *Emigration of leucocytes.*

(b) Diapedasis of R.B.C : Along with emigration of W.B.C., some R.B.C. escape and settle at the peripheral zone of the vessels in a single or a fair number which is known as *diapedasis of RBC*.

[*Emigration of RBC's and few WBC with plasma is popularly known as Diapedasis]

(c)Phagocytosis: It is a process by which dead tissues, bacteria and other debris are engulf by the Microphages and Macrophages cells i.e. by *Neutrophil and giant cells.*

(3) REPAIR OR HEALING

Q. 1.12. What is Repair or Healing ? How does healing occur in case of open wound ? [C.U. 1982]

Repair-*It is a process by which damaged or dead tissues are preplaced by new and healthy cells (parenchymal or stromal).*

Repair is of 2 types i.e. by **: 1. Proliferation** and **2. Regeneration**.

It generally occurs under following heads :

I. *Proliferation by connective tissue as in fibroblast.*

II. *By the proliferation of the parenchymal cells.*

I. Parenchymal proliferation :

(a) In case of nerve and muscle tissues injury.
(b) In case of lymphoid tissue injury.
(c) In case of Epithelial tissue.

II. Repair by connective tissue :

In this type proliferation involves in following 2 types of pathological process :

1. Vascular proliferation.

2. Fibroblastic proliferation.

1. Vascular proliferation: The endothelial cells of the injured blood vessels become hypertrophoid swollen and marked mitotic cell division occur. That swelling part of the cell turns into solid buds and that solid buds ultimately turn into a canalised blood vessels which helps for circulation and regeneration of that injured blood vessels. Generally that canalisation takes place with in three days from the date of injury of the blood vessels.

Lymph vessels also undergo similar proliferation of that particular injured part.

2. Fibroblalstic proliferation: It is characterised by proliferation of fibroblast in which oval and round cells and enough cytoplasm play most important role in fibroblastic proliferation.

From the swelling part of the cell some watery substances are secreted, which deposited outside the cell membrane and is known as *pre-collagenic* soluble. That pre-collagen ultimately form collagen which is solid in nature. That collagen ultimately turn into fibroblast and it is a connective tissue proliferation.

(2) REGENERATION

Regeneration denotes multiplication of the functioning cells.

It is a new growth of the tissue stimulated by injury or destruction of the tissue resulting with complete or partial restoration

It may be (a) **Physiological** or (b) **Pathological.**

(a) **Physiological** means replacement of lost tissue as a physiological process or it is the restoration of tissue elements destroyed under normal condition e.g. regeneration of the glandular cells, regeneration of Erythrocytes etc.

(b) **Pathological** regeneration means replacements of the lost tissue during trauma or infections. In place of lost tissue new tissue beings to grow from the retain tissue elements, capable of proliferation leads to elimination of defects.

Q. 1.11. What are the factors influence the healing wounds?

Healing depends on :

1. Close approximation of the divided segments.
2. Rest to the part.
3. Absence of foreign bodies.
4. Absence of infective organisms.
5. Absence of any other complication, like diabetes.

Q. 1.12. Describe the healing non-infected, incised, sutured wound. [C.U. 1982]

This type of healing occurs by **First intention**-i.e. when the incised wound contains blood and lymph due to the injury, the divided surfaces of the wound are brought together and fixed in opposition by the thin layer of fibrin coagulum formed out of the blood and lymph in the wound. A few leucocytes migrate to the spot and remove if there is any becteria present. The fibroblasts and endothelial cells, present in the connective tissues, proliferate and fillup the gap. The fibroblasts absorb the fibrin from the coagulum. New capillaries are formed and restore the blood supply to the part. (This type of healing also occurs in case of operated wounds).

Q. 1.13. Describe the healing of cut wound where the divide surfaces are separated in a long gap due to excessive tissue damage.

Healing occurs in this type by formation of granulation tissue from the bottom of the wound. The granulation tissue consists of W.B.C.s, endothetial cells, fibroblests and newly formed blood vessels. W.B.C.s remove the bacteria by phagocytosis, gap of the wound is filled by the granulation tissue and the blood supply to the part is restored. The epithelial cells start growing on the surface of the wound. Then the scar formation

As this wound is wide and the opposition surfaces do not come together, the gap is filled with excessive amount of fibrin clot. A large number of fibroblasts and endothelial cells cover the wound leading to the formation of a dense fibrous layer which is of white colour. This is brown or black according to the colour of the skin. If excessive scar formation occurs it leads to keloid formation.

Q. 1.14. What are the causes of Vascular changes ?

According to **Menkin** and **Lewis** the vascular causes are of the following types :

1. Chemical.

2. Neural (Axon reflex).

1. Chemical causes

(a) Chemical factors :

(i) H. substances
(ii) Leucotoxin
(iii) Anoxia
(iv) Increased Co_2 tension
(v) Proteolytic enzymes.

(b) Permeability factors :

(i) Polypetides : Kinins (Brady kinin).
(ii) Amines like 5 Hydroxy tryptamine.
(iii) Nucleic acids and tissue breakdown products.
(iv) Including toxins of Gas-gangrene. Cl. oedematines may directly act upon blood vessels and increase their permeability.

2. Neural causes (Axon reflex)

It is recognised that a sensory fibre has a vasodilator branch to an arteriole, supplying the part. When receptor organ is stimulated the nerve impulse, as it reaches the branch and causes dilatation of the arteriole, that is to say the blood vessels.

Q. 1.15. What is Chemotaxis ?

It is a chemical action by which leucocytes come at the sites of Inflammation, outside the blood vessels through inter-tissues spaces.

They are of 2 types :

(1) Positive Chemotaxis.

(2) Negative Chemotaxis.

(1) **Positive** : By which leucocytes attracts or draw (Polymorpho-nutrophils) at the site of the Inflammation through inter tissues spaces outside the blood vessels. It is only occur in a acute inflammation and the emigration of leucocytes occur by the positive chemotaxis action.

(2) **Negative** : When Lymphocytes and Monocytes migrate the vessel wall by a process of amoeboid movement aided by a chemical stimulus to the site of injury hence it is negative chemotaxis.

Generally bacterial products and injured tissues act as chemotactic agents.

Q. 1.16. What is Phagocytosis ?

It is a process by which dead tissues, bacteria, and the other debris engulf by the phagocytes.

Q. 1.17. What is Phagocytes ?

These are microphages and macrophages cells which are responsible for phagocytic action.

Microphages : Which are responsible for bacteria engulfication e.g. polymophonuclear nutrophils. It is seen in Chronic inflammation.

Macrophages : Which are responsible for engulfing bacteria, (Lympho, Monocytes) as in case of Tuberculosis. It is seen in acute inflammation.

Q. 1.18. What are the various types of cells involved in Inflammation ?

Different cells which are involved in inflammation are :

1. *Leucocytes.*
2. *R.E. Cells.*
3. *Giant Cells etc.*

1. Leucocytes : Among the Leucocytes-Polymorphos, Lymphocytes and Monocytes part in inflammation.

(a) Polymorphos : They engulf foreign bodies, in acute inflammation large number of phagocytes are killed, as a result new batches of cells from

the bone marrow appear in the circulation in excess which we can determined by total leucocytes count.

(b) Lymphocytes and Monocytes : Act as Macrophages and antibody forming cells in chronic inflammation like Tuberculosis.

2. R.E. Cells : They are usually of 2 types : *Fixed* and *Wandering* types. There are found in Liver, Spleen, Bone marrow etc. They are seen in chronic inflammation.

3. Plasma Cells : Cart wheel like appearance are believed to be prepared from R.E. Cells and Lymphocytes, they are responsible to prepare globulin, found in Myeloma, Plasmacytoma etc.

4. Giant Cells :
(a) Foreign body giant cells.
(b) Osteoblastic giant cells.
(c) Tumour giant cells.

(a) Foreign Body Giant Cells

(i) **Langhan's type of Giant cell** : found in Tuberculosis, Leprosy, syphilis etc.

(ii) **Aschoff Giant cell** : found in Rheumatic fever.

(iii) **Sternberg : Reed cells**- found in Hodgkins disease.

(b) **Osteoclastic Giant cells** : found in osteoclastoma, osteitis fibrosa cystica etc.

(c) **Tumour Giant cells** : found in Osteogenic Sarcoma and other different tumours — Glioblastoma Multiforme.

[**N.B** : These cells are seen in Chronic inflammation, containing a large number of Nuclei as much as 50 to 100.]

(d) **Fibrocytes** : These are highly differentiated cells and from connective tissue fibres, reticulin and collagen.

Q. 1.19. What is Chronic infective granuloma ? Mention some important varities ?

Granuloma is a condition of swelling, caused by granulation tissue due to chronic inflammatory changes, characterised by vascular proliferation and cellular response as a protective or separative process.

*The characteristic feature of this kind of Chronic inflammation is the collection of cells followed by destructive changes in the inflamed tissues

The collection of cells, consisting of epithelial cells, plasma cells, lymphocytes and giant cells, from a noduble called "*Infective Granuloma*".

**This type of Ch. inflammation reaction can be distinguished from acute inflammatory reaction by the absence of vascular changes. The infective granuloma has no blood supply, hence necrosis and caseation and ulceration follow the nodule formation. Cavities formed in Pulmonary Tuberculosis is the sequele of infective granuloma.

TYPES OF INFECTIVE GRANULOMA

1. Bacteria:	Tuberculosis.
	Leprosy.
	Rhinoscleroma.
	Glanders.
	Granuloma inguinale.
2. Spirochettal :	Syphilis.
3. Viral :	Lymphogranuloma.
4. Mycotic :	Actinomycosis.
5. Protozoal :	Amoeboma; Dermal Leishmanoid
6. Idiopathic :	Sarcoidosis.

2. NECROSIS

Q. 2.1. What is meant by Necrosis ? [C.U. 1979, 81]

It means cellular death of the living body in a localised area due to some bacteria, toxin or by chemical and mechanical injury with severe irreversible characteristic changes of the cells.

Q. 2.2. What is meant by Necrobiosis?

It signifies the physiological death of the cells, such as RBC and cells of epidermis due to infiltration of abnormal constituents or degeneration of the contents of the cells. Cells die when the vital functions cease.

[The term "**Necrobiosis**" means a gradual process when the cells are passing through various stages of degeneration and is on the way to necrosis. These changes in Necrobiosis are reversible, If favourable condition is restored later on, affected cells may come back to their normal state.]

Q. 2.3. What are the causes of Necrosis ?

The causes of Necrosis are of following types :

1. *Loss of blood supply to the particular part.*
2. *Bacterial or allied causes.*
3. *Physical and chemical agents.*

1. Loss of blood supply to the particular part :

1. Loss of blood supply leading to Ischaemic condition of that particular part—that leads to failure of nutrition and ultimately necrosis develop.

Loss of blood supply to the particular part is due to:

(a) *Thrombosis of the arterioles.*
(b) *Lodgement of the embolus inside the vessels.*
(c) *Pressure of the small arterioles.*

2. Bacterial or other organisms :

Bacteria, Virus, Protozoa and their toxins and enzymes causing obstruction of the artery with the formation of thrombus leading to necrosis.

3. Physical causes :

Sun-rays, X-Ray, extreme cold, extreme heat causes cellular death of the living body (i.e. necrosis).

4. Chemical agents : Strong acids, strong alkali, Arsenic, Phosphorus etc. cause cellular death of the body.

Q. 2.4. What are the Pathological changes occur in Necrosis? [C.U. 1979]

Pathology: 1. *Macroscopical appearance.*
2. *Microscopical appearance.*
(a) *cytoplasmic changes.*
(b) *nuclear changes.*

1. Macroscopical

Normally skin is glazy i.e. transulent. But the necrosed part of the living body looses its normal appearance turn into white opaque whitish and yellowish in colour.

2. Microscopical

(a) **Cytoplasmic changes**: Cytoplasm turn into opaque haemogeneous in character and looses its granulation.

(b) **Nuclear changes**:

(i) *Pyknosis.*

(ii) *Karyorrhaxis.*

(iii) *Karyolysis or chromatolysis.*

(i) **Pyknosis**: Nucleus turn into opaque and small chromation looses its nuclear dilatation (shrink).

(ii) **Karyorrhaxis**: Nucleus chromation broken into small irregular fragments.

(iii) **Chromatolysis:** Destruction i. e. Nuclear chromatin undergoes gradual dissolution and losses its affinity.

Q. 2.5. What are the various types of Necrosis?

(A) Coagulated type of Necrosis.
(B) Casesous type of Necrosis.
(C) Coliquative type of Necrosis.
(D) Fatty type of Necrosis.
(E) Traumatic Type of Necrosis.
(F) Focal type of Necrosis.

(A) Coagulated type of Necrosis: It is characterised by Coagulation of Protein of the dead or dying cell by the intracellular enzyme liberated by autolysis, e.g. Infarct of the Spleen, Kidney or Tuberculosis.

Microscopically: The architecture of the tissue is preserved, cytoplasm is denser granular. Nucleus is Pyknotic or may show Karyorrhaxis followed by Karyolysis.

(B) Caseous Necrosis: This is classed under the coagulated type of Necrosis, but unlike the coagulated type, Caseous Necrosis renders total destruction of Cell wall. Here it forms a cheesy, granular mass that is found in Tuberculosis due to tubercular toxines. This substance does not attract Poly-Morphos. Very often Lesion is converted into cold abscess as the secondary infection invites Poly-Morphos to cause liquification of the Cheesy mass. Calcification is often noticed by the formation of insoluble Calcium soap as contains enormous quantity of fat particles.

Gummatous Lesion: is also one kind of Caseous Nercroses, found in Syphilis, where Ischaemia results endarteritis obliterans.

(C) Colliquative Necrosis: This is commonly seen in tissue containing excess of liquid, e.g. Brain due to Ischaemia, Brain tissue undergoes Softening. The fluid is partly absorbed but is often enclosed by the formation of a wall resulting in a cyst like space.

(D) Fat Necrosis: It is encountered in certain Pancreatic diseases, which allow release of Lipase, in the abdominal cavity. Splitting Neutral fats in the Lipid cells forming small, opaque, soft white areas in those parts giving a characterstics chalky-white appearance.

(E) Traumatic Fat Necrosis: Proliferation of connective tissue and presence of Macrophages and Foreign body type of giant cells are found following an injury to Breast or to the subcutanius tissue is known as Traumatic type of Necrosis provided the tissue contains splitting fat particles, that are chalky white appearance.

(F) Focal Necrosis: This indicates Necrosis of small areas of cells in certain organs in diseases like, Typhoid; Weils diseases as a result of endogenous Metabollc Toxin or Tomin of the organism. It is usually seen in the Liver, Spleen, Lymph Nodes.

Fate of Necrosis

(i) **Absorption,** (ii) **Abscess Formation,** (iii) **Fibrosis,** (iv) **Calification,** (v) **Encapsulation in case of tuberculosis of lungs.**

3. GANGRENE

Q. 3.1. What is meant by Gangrene ?

[C.U. 1980, 81, D.M.S. 76, 77, 81, 82, 84]

Gangrene *is a massive death of tissue; superadded by putrefaction due to action of proteolytic enzymes liberated by saprophytic organisms.*

So it has 2 processes:

1. **Massive death.**
2. Putrefaction due to proteolytic enzyme liberated by dead bacteria.

It is usually occurs when there is:

(a) Loss of blood supply.

(b) Bacterial infection, or
(c) Above two are combined to any aprt.

Q. 3.2. What are its Aetiology ? [D.M.S. 1976]

Aetiology

(a) Loss of Blood Supply—Causes anoxia of cell that renders neocrosis. It is modified due to obstruction of the blood flow e.g. *embolus or pressure that obliterates blood supply* e.g. strangulation, or *continous spasms of blood vessels* in case of Burger and Ragnaud disease or Thrombangitis obliterans, *sudden vesoconstriction*—frost bite etc. and *some chemical like strong acids and alkalies.*

(b) Bacterial Infections:

Inflammation of the part is often complicated by gangrene, specially when the vessels become thrombosed e.g. gangrene of an inflamed appendix.

Q. 3.3. What are the various types of Gangrene?
[C.U. 1980, D.M.S. 76, 81, 82, 84]

Essentially it is of 2 types:

1. Primary. 2. Secondary.

1. Primary: Death and putrefaction are carried out by bacteria, e.g. Gas gangrene by anaerobic bacteria (CL. welchii).

2. Secondary: Death of part due to some other causes like vascular obstruction and putrefaction due to bacteria.

Secondary gangrene is again divided into two:

(a) **Dry gangrene** : Obstruction is only arterials, so part is dry.

(b) **Moist gangrene** : Along with aterial obstruction there is superadded venous obstruction, so there is a lot of fluid inside.

Special types of gangrene are:
(i) Diabetic gangrene.
(ii) Senile gengrene.
(iii) Decubitus ulcer.
(iv) Norma pudentio (cervix).

**The conditions which determine the types of gangrene depends on : (a) Blood supply to the part.

(b) Fluid loss from the part by drainage or evaporation.

(c) Specific Bacterial injections.

Q. 3.4. What do you meant by Dry Gangrene and Moist Gangrene ? Describe their causes, signs and symptoms, and pathology.

Or, What are the differences between Dry Gangrene and Moist Gangrene ? [C.U. 1980, D.M.S. 74, 77, 80]

Dry Gangrene	Moist Gangrene
1. Definition	
It is an ischaemic massive death of the tissue of a particular part of body due to obstruction of vascular supply mainly arterial flow and the venous flow is intact, so that evaporation of water easily takes place. Secondary saprophytic organisms cause in putrifaction to the part.	It is a massive ischaemic death of tissue of a particular part of the organ due to obstruction of both arterial and venous flow, resulting in accumulation of fluid inside the dead tissues characterised by liberation of gasses due to proteolytic enzyme.
2. Causes/Aetiology	
(i) Gradual vascular (arterial obstruction as seen in thromboangitis obliterans.	(i) Blocking of arterial and venous blood flow.
(ii) Sudden vascular occlusion as in embolism, thrombosis etc.	(ii) Area that contains much fluid favours the growth of putrefying bacteria.
(iii) Extreme cold such as frost bite.	(iii) Burn.
(iv) Due to strong escharoties i.e. strong acid and alkali.	(iv) Bed sore.
	(v) Malnutrition.
	(vi) Strong Acid and Alkali.
	(vii) Long continue illness.
	(viii) Hypo-stasis from the feeble circulation.

	(ix) Diseases or injury of the spinal cord.

3. Seat of Lesion

Lower extremities fingers and nose and ears as in frost bite.	Mainly internal organs, such as strangulated Hernia, Intussasception Volvulus of intestine etc.

4. Clinical Findings

(a) **Onset** :	Gradual due to arterial flow obstruction but venous flow intact.	Sudden onset due to both arterial and venous flow blocked.
(b) **Skin : colour**	Dry, discoloured and mummified.	The part becomes dark with shades of blue, green or black due to the formation of Iron sulphate.
(c) **Line of : demarcation.**	Prominent	Not fully developed
(d) **Temperature: and pulsation.**	Cold and pulseless	Not found properly due to rapid Toxaemia
(e) **On Palpation:**	Egg shell crackling is absent or slightly present.	Emphysematous (Egg shell) crackling is present due to the present of gas.
(f) **Liberation: of gas**	Absent	Enormous quantity of gases are produced—**Indole and Skatole** due to the breakdown of N_2.
(g) **Toxaemia:**	Nil or less marked.	Rapid or more marked.
(h) **Odour :**	Foul smell less marked.	Offensive odour mostly marked.
(i) **Putrifaction:**	Less marked	More marked

5. Pathology

This is a term usually applied to Ischaemic infarction causing mummification of the part as a result of evaporation of water. Secondary saprophytic organisms are present in smaller number. The tissue becomes dried, shrivelled, greenish yellow and finally dark brown or black in colour. Haemolysis of the RBC's liberates Haemoglobin, the Iron of which combines with Hydrogen sulphide produced by Bacteria and forms Iron sulphide ($Fe + H_2S \rightarrow Fes$). This is why, is stained black. Inflammatory reaction in the adjacent living tissue causes a sharp "line of demarcation" of granulation tissue separating the healthy from the dead tissue, which acts as a mild irritant to the healthy tissue. The microscopic picture is one of Necrosis with disintegration of the tissue.

As the part contains sufficient fluid, it favours the growth of bacteria. Owing to abundant supply of moisture, there is rapid growth of putrefying bacteria invading the devitalised or dead tissue, with the production of indole and skatole and other products of Nitrogen breakdown. There is liquefaction of the tissue with the production of gas and these are responsible for the formation of blebs under skin, and for emphysematus or Egg shell crackling on palpation. The part becomes dark with shades of blue, green or black due to formation of Iron sulphide. For the presence of moisture local spread of infection is very rapid. The most important feature is great absorption of toxins and hence profound toxemia and death ensure. The disease spreads rapidly to the limbs and there is hardly any attempt for the formation of a line of demarcation.

Q. 3.5. What is meant by Gas gangrene ?
Describe the causes and pathogenesis of Gas gangrene.

Gas gangrene is an infective gangrene due to infection of anaerabic organisms, like Clostridium welchii, Cl. histolyticum, Cl. sprorogens etc.

Aetiology or Causes

1. Primary causative organisms:

(a) Pathogenic saccharolytic anaerobes.

(i) Cl. welchii.
(ii) Cl. oedematiens.

(b) Pathogenic proteolytic group of organisms.
(i) Cl. hystolyticum
(ii) Cl. sporogens.

2. Secondary causative organisms

For the infection, contaminations of secondary aerobic organisms are necessary e.g.

(i) *Staphylococcus.*
(ii) *Streptococcus.*
(iii) *Escheria coli* and *Proteus* group of organisms use up the oxygen of the tissue and help in maintaining the anaerobic constition.

3. Loss of circulation of the part: It may cause massive involvement and this often takes place by the process of thrombosis, which aggravates the condition.

4. There should be a **crush injury**, contaminated with SiO_2 and Ca^{++} and it requires a suitable pH for the growth of gas gangrene organisms. [pH (7.8—8)]

5. Haemorrhage and blood clot help in infection.

6. Inadequate supply of blood (circulation obstruction).

7. Foreign body.

8. Laceration.

9. Inadequate drainage of exudate or other debris.

10. Parts of splinters or fragments.

11. Dirty cloths etc.

PATHOGENESIS

The infection of traumatised tissue with *Streptococci, E. coli* and Proteus group of organisms etc. produces the primary anaerobic condition by using up or of the tissue and the anaerobes get an opportunity to multiply.

The saccharolytic group of organism grow on the sarcolemma e.g. *Cl. welchii* and breakdown the muscle glycogen into Carbon di- oxide, Hydrogen and Lactic acid.

Glycogen—>CO_2 + H_2 + CH_2 CHOH COOH
Lactic acid.

This lactic acid does not favour the growth of saecharolytic organisms as the pH is low. So protecolytic groups i.e. Cl. hystolyticum multiply with the liberation of proteinase and the formation of animo acids in the tissue. Amino acids are broken down into ammonia, when the acid produced by saccharolytic group is Neutralised.

$$R—NH_3—COOH \xrightarrow{\text{diamination}} NH_8$$

$$[NH_3 + CH_3\ CHOH\ COOH] \longrightarrow NH_4\ CH_3\ CHOH\text{-}COO.]$$

Amonium Lactate

Acidity is further nutralised by profuse exudation and calcium salts. There is liberation of toxin in blood associated with a fall of blood pressure. The toxin too damages the Myocardium and thus sudden Heart failure is explained.

Q. 3.6. Describe the pathology of Gas gangrene.

(I) Macroscopic or Gross Appearance

1. Degeneration of longitudinal muscle fibres.
2. Degeneration of circular muscle fibres and their sheaths.
3. Parts of gas inside tissues and the skin.
4. Muscles loses its elasticity and losses its normal colour.
5. Changes of skin—> yellow—> greenish—> black red—> Blackish due to production of Iron sulphide.
6. Muscles looked like cooked meat—due to liberation of sulphurated hydrogen (H_2S) from broken muscle Haemoglobin.
7. The exudate is sero-sanguinous.

(II) Microscopical Appearance

1. Present of a caustive organism inside the muscles fibres or muscular tisues.
2. Muscles sarcolemma lost.
3. Ultimately muscle nucleus disappears completely.
4. Present of gas and haemorrhagic spot inside the muscle fibres.

Q. 3.7. Why does Diabetes mellitus favour to cause Gangrene?

Diabetes mellitus causes gangrene in the following ways:

1. High Blood Sugar Level favours the growth of aerobic organisms, that can use up the oxygen in next turn.
2. Hypercholesterolaemia leads to atherosclerosis, which is due to diposition of cholesterol in the intimal layer of the artery.
3. Atheromatous plaques detached from the initimal layer as thrombus, and causes blocking the lumen of the artery and thereby it renders the circulation sluggish.
4. Lastly, Diabetic Neuropathy, causes Lower Motor Palsy, so the affected part is either hyperestics of anasthetics. So numbness leads the part insensible. This is why, any injury causes to the part, can lead to gangrene due to numbness.

Q.3.8. What do you meant by Senile gangrene?

This occurs in old age and due to arteriosclerosis. It is generally a **dry type of gangrene** characterised by change of colour and occurs in the extremities with a line of demarcation.

4. OEDEMA

Q.4.1. What is Oedema? [D.M.S. 1978, 81, 82, 84]

Oedema is an abnormal accumulation of fluid in the cell, intercellular tissue spaces or serous sac or cavities of the body due to disturb water metabolism.

This fluid is a transudate from the blood vessels which is different from haemorrhagic and inflammatory swelling.

Some Important terms related to Oedema or Varities of Oedema (D.M.S. 1981, 82, 84)

1. What is Effusion?

It is the escape of fluid from the blood vessels or lympthatics into the tissue or cavity. It is also referred to as the fluid effused.

2. What is Anasarca?

It is an accumulation of serum in sub-cutaneous connective tissue, e.g. Beriberi, Angio-neurotic oedema etc.

3. What is Hydrocele ?

It is an abnormal accumulation of fluid in sacs of tunica vaginalis of testis.

4. What is Dropsy ?

It is an abnormal accumulation of fluid inside the serous cavity i.e. known as dropsy.

5. What is meant by Hydrothorax. Hydrocaphalus and Hydro-pericardium ?

Hydrothorax : Collection of serous fluid in pleural space.

Hydrocephalus : Increased volume of cerebrospinal fluid inside the skull.

Hydropericardium : Accumulation of fluid inside the pericardium.

6. Ascitis : Abnormal accumulation of serous fluid into the peri-tonial cavity.

7. Myxoedema : It is solid oedema which does not pit on pressure. It is characteristic feature of hypothyroidism of adult.

Q. 4.2. What are sites of oedema ?

1. In case of loose connective tissue behind the eyeball and lower eyelids.
2. Sacs of serrous cavities as for examples: pleura, pericardium and peritonium etc.
3. Tissues of external genital area.
4. Subcutaneous tissues all over the body (generalised).
5. Dependent part of the body as in case of ankle or in the knee joint.

Q. 4.3. What are the various causes of oedema ? Mention their causes. [D.M.S. 1979]

Oedema of 2 types:

1.Local

2.General

(1) **Local :**
- (a) Inflammatory Oedema
- (b) Lymphoedema
- (c) Milory disease.

(2) **General :**
- (a) Cardiac
- (b) Hepatic
- (c) Nutritional
- (d) Oedema include Adenaline Hormone
- (e) Oedema of epidemic dropsy
- (f) Pulmonary Oedema.

(1) LOCAL

1. **Inflammatory Oedema:** It is due to the inflammatory condition of the tissues with accumulation of exudate. Accumulation of exudate occurs under following conditions :
   - (a) Increased permeability of the endothelial layer.
   - (b) Increased osmotic pressure.
   - (c) Increased capillary permeability.
   - (d) Stasis and Thrombosis of small vessels.
   - (e) Retardation of lymph flow.
2. **Lymph Oedema:** It is mainly characterised by elephantiasis of limbs due to obstruction of lymph flow. (Thoracic duct obstruction due to *W. bancrofti*).
3. **Miloray's disease:** It is a hereditary disease where oedema seen in successive generation and oedema is limited in one leg or both legs and never extents above the inguinal ligaments. It is due to obstruction of subcuteneous tissue circulation mainly lymphatic obstruction and this disease is symptom less without any pain or other constitutional disorder.

(2) GENERAL

1. **Cardiac oedema:** It is due to hydrostatic pressure or venous congestion, and anoxia of the tissue.
2. **Renal oedema :** (a) Increased permeability of the endothelial layer or injury by toxins damaging the endothelial layer.

   (b) It is marked due to chloride retention in case of Albuminuria.

(c) Renal oedema due to plasma retention (low plasma protein).

3. **Hepatic oedema** : (a) Increased permeability of the capillary wall due to increased pressure of portal vein.

   (b) Hepatic oedema due to retention of Sodium with increased plasma protein.

4. **Nutritional**-(a) It is due to low serum albumin caused by mal-nutrition.

   (b) Due to defective tissue regeneration caused by cardiac insufficiency.

5. **Adrenaline hormone**-Administration of Cortisone or of ACTH causing oedematous condition of subcutaneous tissue resulting oedema.

6. **Oedema of epidemic dropsy** : (a) It is a toxic origin and is due to damage of the endothelial wall of the capillaries, or

   (b) Due to enormous dilation of the capillaries, or

   (c) In sufficiency of Heart.

7. **Pulmonary oedema** : (a) It is due to peripheral vasoconstriction, or

   (b) Increased permeability of the vascular wall with increased protein fluid (serum albumin and globulin).

Q. 4.4. Describe the Pathology of Oedema. Or, How does Oedema occur ? [D.M.S. 1978, 79, 82, 84]

The pathogenesis of Oedema is based on a complex change or changes in the *inflow and outflow of tissue fluid or lymph.*

An important part in the mechanism of Oedema is played by increased transudation of fluid from vessels into tissues and retention of fluid by the tissue. The impeded outflow of the fluid through the lymphatic vessels is likewise conduction to development of oedema; although it plays a secondary role because there are many colateral lymph channels and the outflow of tissue fluid may also be affected through veins. hence oedema is caused by disorders of water interchange between the blood and tissues.

The water inter change between the blood and the tissue depends on 3 collodial systems :

1. The blood.
2. Connective tissue.
3. Cellular protoplasm.

DEVELOPMENT OF OEDEMA

Generally oedema develops as a result of changes in the*Hydro-dynamic factors or Increased Capillary hydro-static pressure.*

1. Increased capillary hydrostatic pressure:

This is the pressure exerted on the wall of capillaries by column of circulating blood and it is about 32 mm. Hg. at the arterial end of capillaries and 12 mm. Hg. at its venous end. As the hydrostatic pressure at the arterial end of capillary exceeds the colloidal Osmotic Pressure (25 mm. Hg.) the fluid is thrown outside into the tissue space which supplies nutrition to the tissue cells and is called tissue pressure (25 mm. Hg.). As the tissue pressure is more as compared to capillary hydrostatic pressure (12 mm. Hg.) of the venous end the fluid which was once thrown out of the vessel at the arterial end, is now readily reabsorbed. A minor fraction of tissue fluid is, of course carried to blood by way of lymphatics.

In a normal person this process of drainage of fluid from arterial end, and its subsequent reabsorption into the venous and capillary, goes on in such a perfect harmony that oedema fails to occur. In different diseases when this delicate balance is lost there is possibility of development of oedema. In congestive cardiac failure or in obstruction of vein draining a limb, there is marked rise of venous pressure causing in turn rise of capillary hydrostatic pressure. This higher hydrostatic pressure at the venous end reabsorption fails to take place and fluid is continuously driven out of the vessels into the tissue space causing progressive oedema. (This is the mechanism of oedema of cardiac failure).

Another very essential factors conductive to oedema are : **(a) Lowering of colloidal osmotic pressure and (b) Increased capillary permeability.**

(a) Lowering of colloidal osmotic pressure:

Plasma proteins of blood normally exert a binding or adhesive force, roughly equivalent to 25 mm Hg. which is known as **colloidal osmotic pressure.**

When blood protein level goes below 4 gm%, there is much lowering of colloidal pressure with the result that sufficient amount of fluid escapes out of the vessel into the tissue space. This mechanism works in the oedema of subacute nephritis, Nephrosis, Nutritional oedema and in cases of huge ascities.

(b) Increased capillary permeability:

Capillary wall normally behave as a semipermeable membrane allowing passage of water and electrolytes but proteins are held back. If due to any cause like anoxia, action of toxins etc. permeability of capillaries be increased, the plasma protein will diffuse out into the tissue space. Once the proteins start coming out of the vessel a vicious cycle is created as there is lowering of colloidal osmotic pressure of blood and rise of tissue osmotic pressure. Thus more and more fluid will escape out of the vessel. Protein molecule will also attract electrolytes along with water. This mechanism of increased permeability as cause of oedema works in acute anaemia, congestive cardiac failure and inflammatory oedema.

N.B. The *secondary factors* like *Tissue osmotic pressure, retention of NaCl, Endocrine or Nervous control factor*, etc. are never initiate oedema but once oedema is established these help to maintain the process.

Q. 4.5. What are the characteristic features of Oedema ?

1. It pits on pressure.
2. It is not red like inflammations.
3. It is not painful like inflammations.
4. When punctured, a thin water incoagulable fluid oozes from the wound.
5. It does not contain blood or pus or bacteria.
6. It contains small amount of proteins.

5. THROMBOSIS

Q. 5.1. What is Thrombosis ? [C.U. 1979, D.M.S. 77]

Thrombosis is a pathological process by which a solid mass or a thrombus form either intra-cardiac or intro-vascular; derived from formed elements of circulating blood during life time.

Q. 5.2. What is Thrombus ? [D.M.S. 1975, 77]

Thrombus is a solid mass derived from elements of blood i.e. composed of

WBC + RBC + Fibrin + Platelets. (Resulting thrombosis).

Q. 5.3. What are the differences between Thrombus and Blood clot ?

Thrombus	Blood Clot
1. It is a pathological phenomenon.	1. It is a physiological phenomenon.
2. Due to an active and a vital process in the living tissue.	2. Not so.
3. Composition : chiefly composed of platelets and pale in colour, other elements are RBC + WBC and + fibrin.	3. Composed of Fibrin and blood cells like RBC and WBC.
4. From either intra-vascular or intra-cardiac.	4. Extravascular.
5. Forms in a current of blood.	5. Forms in stagmant blood.
6. Adherent to the under lying tissue and when detached, a raw eroded surface is left.	6. Not adherent to the vessel wall and does not produce a raw surface.
7. Clot is retraced or organised with brownish colour, dry friable and variegated as serum has already extruded.	7. Colt is soft and red, currant jelly or yellow like chicken fat,. arranged in layers — RBC at the bottom and then plasma and Leucocytes.
8. Lines of zahn present .	8. Absent.

Q. 5.4. What is true Thrombosis ?

Where platelets formed thrombus and the R.B.C., W.B.C. and fibrin may be absent, this is a true thrombosis.

Q. 5.5. What are the conditions cause thrombosis ? Or, What do you meant by Virchow Triads ? [C.U. 1979, D.M.S. 77]

Generally the following factors are responsible for thrombosis and are known as Virchow Triads:

1. Injury to the vascular endothelium.

2. Slowing of blood flow.
3. Changes of the constituents of blood.

1. Injury to the Vascular Endothelium

Due to the following conditions:
(i) Trauma.
(ii) Infection.
(iii) Disorder of metabolism.
(iv) Presence of foreign bodies.
(v) Due to degenerative changes.

(i) Trauma: Due to ligature or sutering of blood vessels or injection by chemical substances.

(ii) Infection: In case of thrombosis it plays an important role, e.g. in case of phlebitis (acute inflammation of venous wall), and arteritis (inflammatory condition of the artery).

(iii) Disorder of Metabolism: In case of burn or in case of eclampsia.

(iv) Presence of Foreign Body : Presence of any foreign bodies causing injury to the inner vessels wall leading to thrombus formation.

(v) Due to Degenerative Changes : Atheroma of artery causing ruffness and destruction of inner wall leading to thrombus formation.

2. Slowing of Blood Flow :

(i) Aneurysm of aorta.
(ii) In case of dilated heart due to passive congestion.

3. Changes of the Constituents of Blood :

(i) After child birth or after surgical operation: Changes develop in blood.
(ii) Deficient supply of heparin helping formation of thrombus.
(iii) Excess supply of Vit. K. : Helping prothrombin formation leading to thrombus.
(iv) New formation of platelets: Precipitate on the wall of the blood vessels leading to thrombus formation.

N.B. The basic causes of thrombus formation are known as Virchow triads.

Q. 5.6. How does Thrombosis occur ? Describe the mechanism of Thrombosis.

Mechanism of Thrombosis :

Basic Process of Thrombogenesis depends upon three factors : (i) *A break in the wall of the vessel,* (ii) *Slowing of the blood flow,* (iii) *A change in the composition of the blood.*

All of these phenomenons are undergone a process of agglutination of Thrombocytes and deposition of the same, and formation of a clot.

The agglutination phase is the partial precipitation from the circulating blood of plasma proteins and then blood platelets which are deposited on the internal surface of the vascular wall. The agglutination and ppt. of platelets are due to decrease in their electric charge. The decrease in their charge is a result of disturbances in the proportions of protein fractions in the blood plasma increase in globulines and decrease in albumins. The decrease in the charge of platelets is also favoured by accumulation of CO_2 in the blood, which is due to slowing of the Blood Current at the given site and disturbance in the gas exchange between the blood and tissue. Furthermore CO_2 intensifies the fermentative process of glycolysis and accumulation of under oxidised products (for example Lactic acid) which hasten coagulation. In addition to the A.T.P. is broken down into A.D.P. and Pi — that gives sufficient amount of energy for agglutination.

During the coagulation phase the thrombokinase liberated from the platelets and Leucocytes causes coagulation of the blood flowing between white layers of platelets and lucocytes. The coagulated blood forms the red layers of the thrombus. The middle of the thrombus is of a mixed structure and consists of alternating red and white layers. The tail end of the thrombus consists of red coagulated blood. Such thrombus is called a **Stratified** or **Mixed thrombus.**

Primary platelet thrombus in which due to some intimal damage, platelets adhere to the wall of the vein to form an amorphous, pale thrombus, likened to snow drift during a snow storm. Normally, it would not produce any ill-effects but µ Stas occurs, coagulation factor accumulate locally with formation of fibrin, followed by formation of a **coraline thrombus.** This is due to formation of upstanding laminae going across the stream and are bent in the direction of blood flow by the force of the stream, arborise to form and intricate structure resembling Coral. Its complexity is ill understood but between the Laminae, there is a complete Stasis and fibrin is deposited in the meshes of which red cells and leucocytes are entangled. **On Section**, it is found to consist of fused Platelets and fibrin with blood cells. Refraction of Fibrin gives characteristic, **ribbed appearance** when the surface of the thrombus is viewed with hand lens. The elevated ridges are called lines of **Zahn.**

Coralling thrombus is transmitted from one vein to other through tributaries. Stages are as follows :

(i) **Occluding thrombus.**
(ii) **Consecutative clot.**
(iii) **Propagating thrombus.**

Q. 5.7. What are fates of a Thrombus ? [C.U. 1979, D.M.S. 75,81]

Fates of thrombus are: (i) Absorption, (ii) Organisation, (iii) Embolism, (iv) Calcification-Phlebolith.

(i) **Absorption**-When the thrombus is in the body, it is absorbed by phagocytosis.
(ii) **Organisation**-When thrombus present in the vessels, healing wound by proliferation of capillary and fibroblast with formation of fibrous, leading to the canalisation of blood flow.
(iii) **Calcification**-A thrombus may be calcified then it is called phelbolith.
(iv) **Embolism**-Most dangerous fate of the thrombus is its dislodgement from original site; causing embolism.

Q. 5.8. What are the various types of Thrombus ? Mention their formation. [D.M.S. 1975,81]

I. Varieties of Thrombus

Generally it is divided into seven groups :

(1) Pale thrombus or platelets thrombus.
(2) Red or coagulation thrombus.
(3) Erythrocyte coaglutination thrombus.
(4) Mixed thrombus.
(5) Ball thrombus.

(6) Aseptic thrombus.
(7) Septic thrombus.

II. Formation of Thrombus

(1) **Pale or Platelete thrombus** (Conglutination) : It is pure, composed almost entirely of blood platelets. e.g.-found in the vegetations of rheumatic endocarditis.

(2) **Red or Coagulation thrombus** : Composed largely of Fibrine that entangles R.B.C. and Leucocytes having initial basis of the platelets.

(3) **Erythrocyte Coagulation thrombus** : Arise from natural adhension of erythrocytes.

(4) **Mixed thrombus** : Large thrombi are of mixed types. They are composed partly of Platelets, partly of Fibrin mixed with R.B.C.s in alternate layers and Leucocytes.

(5) **Ball thrombus** : That forms in the auricle, is aseptic in nature.

(6) **Aseptic thrombus** : It is bland, does not contain any infective organism.

(7) **Septic thrombus** : It usually forms in the vein and contains pyogenic organism, when detached, it produces septic emboli and pyaemic abscesses.

Q. 5.9. Describe the various sites of Thrombosis ?

(I) In Heart :

(a) Azonal
(b) Ball thrombosis
(c) Appendages.

(II) In Artery.
(III) In Vein.

(I) Heart

1. **Azonal thrombosis** : It generally occurs in case of right heart failure and in some cases of pneumonia (shortly before death).
2. **Ball thrombosis** : This type of thrombosis occurs in case of mitral stenosis where thrombus looks like a red mass occuring generally at auricle.
3. **Appendages:** This type of thrombosis generally occurs in case of bacterial endocarditis (subacute).

(II) Artery

1. Anurysm.
2. Atheroma-coronary artery.
3. Thromboangitis — Cerebral artery.
4. Periarterium nodusa.

(III) Vein

1. **Thrombophlebitis** : *Inflammatory condition of the vein* with formation of thrombus, ultimately that thrombus is infected. This type of thrombosis is found in cavernocynus and transversecynus.
2. **Phlebothrombosis** : Thrombus form in the vein without any evidence of inflammation of vein, especially occurs in the independent part of the body (i.e. lower extremities). Generally it is found after perturition or after surgical operation.

Q. 5.10. What are the effects of thrombosis ? [D.M.S. 1981]

1. Embolism.
2. Infarction.
3. Gangrene.
4. Pyaemia.
5. Local oedema.

6. EMBOLISM

Q. 6.1. What is Embolism ? [D.M.S. 1981]

Embolism is a process by which an undisolved material is impacted in the blood vessels which is carried by the blood stream from its point of origin and ultimately lodged into the distal part of the body, causing obstruction to the lumen ofbloodvesselsmore or less completelyorpartially.

Q. 6.2. What are the various types of Emboli ?

Emboli are classfied under following heads :

1. ***Aseptic embolus.***
2. ***Septic embolus.***
3. ***Miscellaneous embolus.***
4. ***Tumour embolus.***

1. **Aseptic embolus** : It is originated from detached aseptie part of the thrombus.

2. **Septic embolus** : It is originated from detached thrombus, containing bacteria e.g., in case of bacterial endocarditis.

3. **Miscellaneous** :
   (a) *Air embolus* — Produced by the inter venous injection.
   (b) *Parasitic embolus* — Produced by parasites like Ascaris, hook worm, larvae etc.
   (c) *Fat embolus* — Generally it is produced by the fracture of the long bones. It causes obstruction to the lumen of the blood vessels by the fatty tissue, which is liberated from injured part of the long bones.
   (d) *Oily embolus* — Produced by liquid paraffin or oily injection.
   (e) *Amniotic embolus* — After delivery if droplets of amniotic fluid sucked in the uterine venous sinus, droplets covered up by fibrin shell develop emboli.
   (f) *Tissue embolus*—An embolism caused by firable placental tissue.

4. **Tumour embolus** : An embolus containing of clamps of tumour cell e.g. in Sarcoma, chronic epithellum in the blood, carcinoma in the lymphatics etc.

Q. 6.3. What are the sources of Emboli ?

They are:

(1) **Heart** : Especially *left auricle* with its appendages, *intramural part* especially in case of cardiac infract, and *vegetations of valves* in case of sub-acute bacterial endocarditis.

(2) **Arteries** : In case of anurism and atheroma of the arteries especially in case of the abdominal aorta.

(3) **Veins** : (a) *Systemic vein* — Right sided heart.
(b) *Portal vein* — Portal aorta.

Q. 6.4. What are the effects of Embolism ?

The effects of embolism depend upon the site of its occurrence; e.g. if it occurs in the coronary artery; it may produce even death, but if it occurs in a part of the body where there is collateral circulation or the part is not vital to the organism, there may not be any harmful effects. If the embolism occurs in the end arteries of the brain where there is no collateral circulation, it may produce lack of supply of the blood to the portion of the brain cause infection which may be lead to paralysis of one side of the bodv.

Q. 6.5. What are the effects of Embolus ?

1. **Septic embolus** : Septic embolus causing pyaemic abscess (pus with abscess) in the different parts of the body.
2. **Tumour cell embolus** : Causing metastatic growth.
3. **Aseptic embolus** : Nature of aseptic embolus sometimes it causes constriction and ultimately causing the necrosis of part of the body, leading to **infarct.**

Q. 6.6. What is Embolus ?

An embolus is a solid body with is carried from one part of circulatory system to distant part where it gets impacted.

7. INFARCTION

Q. 7.1. What is Infarction ? [C.U. 1972, D.M.S.78,79,80]

It is a process by means of which ischaemic necrosis of a tissue takes place due to the occlusion of end arteries of an organ.

Q. 7.2. What is Infarct ? [D.M.S. 1978,79,80]

It is ischaemic necrose part of the tissue due to obstruction of the end arteries or produced by the occlusion of the end arteries.

It is generally of 2 types : (1) **Red infarct**, and (2) **Pale infarct.**

(1) **Red infarct** : It is of red colour due to presence of blood in large quantities, and due to congestion of the part which occurs before death of the tissues. The colour is due to presence of R.B.C.s in the tissues. It generally occurs where adequated collateral circulation is present, e.g. in lungs, the pulmonary infarct is of red colour. The red infarct may also be called haemorrhage infarct.

(2) **Pale or white infarct** : It is known as anaemic infarct because the pale colour is due to lack of R.B.C.s. These infarcts are produced by arterial

occlusion, where adequate collateral circulation — is not present, e.g. infarct in the heart muscels.

Q. 7.3. What are the causes of Infarction ?

Causation :

(1) Septic embolism.
(2) Atherosclerosis with thrombosis.
(3) Atherosclerosis without thrombosis.
(4) Atherosclerosis with embolism.
(5) Aseptic embolus.

Q. 7.4. What are the various types of Infarction ?

[D.M.S. 1978,79,80]

The types are :

(1) Red or Haemorrhagic Infarction.
(2) Pale or Anaemic Infarction.

1. Red Infarction :This type of infarction generally occurs in case of soft and spongy organs e.g, Lungs infarction.

2. Pale Infarction : It occurs in case of compact muscle e.g. Infarct of the kidney.

Q. 7.5. What are the pathology of Infarction ?

Pathology of Infarction is classified under 2 heads :

1. Macroscopical.
2. Microscopical.

1. Macroscopical appearance :

Fan wedge distribution of necrotic tissue can be found on the particular part due to the occlusion of the end arteries produced by thrombosis or embolism of main artery.

Infarction gererally occurs in Lungs, Kidney, Intestine, Spleen, Brain and Retina, but rare in Liver.

2. Microscopical appearance :

Microscopically it has three demarketed areas :

(1) Zone of Infarction.

(2) Zone of Hyperaemia.
(3) Zone of Normal Tissue.

1. Zone of Infarction :

It is mainly characterised by necrosed tissues with following different changes of nucleus and cytoplasm.

(a) Different changes of nucleus :

(i) Pyknosis.
(ii) Karyrrhaxis.
(iii) Karyolysis.

(i) **Pyknosis** : It means nucleus shrunken and condensed into a small mass with nuclear details are lossed.

(ii) **Karyrrhaxis** : Nuclear chromation broken down into irregular fragments.

(iii) **Karyolysis** : In case of karyolysis chromation gradually dissolved and ultimately disappeared from that particular region.

(b) Changes of cytoplasm :

Cytoplasm becomes pale with granules, ill defined cell membrane.

2. Zone of Hyperaemia :

Hyperaemia characterised by inflammatory condition of that part with dilatation of capillaries with deposition of fibrinous exudate, lymphocytes, macrophages cells, fat cells and other tissue debris, some time glycogen are present.

3. Zone of normal tissue :

Characterised by passive congestion including full amount of R.B.C. surrounding the zone of Infarction.

Q. 7.6. What is the fate of Infarction ?

Fate or Termination :

1. Absorption by autolysis or phagocytosis in nature.
2. Calcification — Infarct part turned into clacified part, (deposition of Calcium salt).
3. Fibrosis — The part turn into fibrous tissue.
4. Softening of the part.

5. Pyaemia (pyamic abscess are seen in different parts of the organs).

Q. 7.7. What are the Sequalae of Infarct ?

The infarct may become septic due to the invasion of pyogenic organisms or it may remain bland without causing any change in its structure. The symptoms depend upon the seat of infarct, the vital or non-vital organs affected by the infarct and the complications of the infarct. Infarct in the *heart* may cause death. In the *brain*, it may cause hemiplegia, in *lungs*, it may cause symptoms of broncho-pneumonia. The pain may be present if the nerve ending are involved, and the temperature may be due to septic infarction.

8. DEGENERATION

Q. 8.1. What is Degeneration ? [D.M.S. 1977,79]

Degeneration means (Deterioration in the structure and functions of parenchymatous tissues).

Definition :

Degeneration is a pathological process in which the cell component as a whole directly affected by the toxic condition or by secondary metabolic causes. In case of degeneration the cell is primarily diseased or injured by the mechanical effect.

Accumulation of abnormal material either in the cytoplasm of the cell or intercellular ground substance occure suggesting unhealthy condition of cells.

Or

Degeneration is a retrograde process (reversible change of cell) in which cells of tissue are undergone a Biochemical changes where RNA cannot be transmitted and synthesis of mRNA is inhibited in the process of sickness, due to non-fatal injuries or adverse influences.

These injuries have essentially two effects upon the cell :

(1) *Directly toxic action.*

(2) *Secondary changes resulting from deranged intracellular metabolism, characterised morphologically by accumulation of substances normally within the affected cells.*

Q. 8.2. What is Infiltration ? [D.M.S. 1977]

Infiltration means accumulation of abnormal substances in the tissues. It is also a pathological process in which cytoplasm of normal cell filled up by abnormal quantity of the substance due to systemic disorder; resulting in cellular dysfunction.

Q. 8.3. What are the causes of degeneration ? (D.M.S. 1977, 79)

Causes :

1. Physical.
2. Chemical — (i) Exogenous.
   (ii) Endogenous.
3. Bacterial — Acute and Chronic.
4. Disorder of oxygen.

1. Physical : (a) Extreme heat.
(b) Extreme cold.
(c) X-Rays or Radium.

2. Chemical : (a) Exogenous — P_4, $CHCL_2$, As, R-OH etc.
(b) Endogenous — Metabolic products as in Jaundic or Acetone in Diabetes.

3. Bacterial : (a) Acute — Diphtheria, Pneumonia.
(b) Chronic — Tuberculosis, Syphilis etc.

4. Disorder of Oxygen : Anoxia due to Anaemia. Lack of circulation in passive venous congestion. Liver is very susceptable in this respect.

Q. 8.4. What are the differences between Degeneration and Infiltration ?

Degeneration	Infiltration
1. The cells are primarily diseased or injured by the mechanical effect.	1. The cells are not primarily diseased or injured.

2. Injury to cells preceded the abnormal accumulation.	2. An accumulation of an abnormal quantity of substance within the cytoplasm due to systemic derangements, resulting in deranged cellular function.
3. Cell component as a whole affected by bacteria or their toxins.	3. Cytoplasm only affected or filled up by abnormal quantities of the substance due to some systemic disorder.
4. Toxic action render a blockage of tRNA, and thereby ppt. of protoplasmic protein and fragmentation of chromation material is taken place.	4. Over loading of healthy cells causes injury to the cell.
5. Nucleus — atrophy and centrally placed.	5. Nucleus pushed one side or periphery of the side by the mechanical pressure of the abnormal quantities of substances (signet ring like).
6. A.T.P. is rapidly broken-down to combat the situation.	6. A.T.P. is slowly broken down.
7. Cell as a whole atrophy or degenerate.	7. No such changes take place.
8. Fate — Toxication causes Necrosis of the cells.	8. Autolysis results.

Q. 8.5. What are the various types of Degeneration ?
Or, Classify Degeneration. [D.M.S. 1979]

Various types of Degenerations are :

1. Cloudy degeneration or *Cloudy Swelling* or Albuminous degeneration.
2. Hydropic degeneration.
3. Fatty degeneration.
4. Hyaline degeneration.
5. Zenkers Hyaline degeneration.
6. Amyloid degeneration.
7. Mucoid degeneration.

8. Glycogen degeneration.

Q. 8.6. What are the types of Infiltration ?

Infiltration is of 2 types :

1. Glycogen Infiltration.

2. Fatty Infiltration.

VARIOUS TYPES OF DEGENERATION

Q. 8.7. What is meant by Cloudy Swelling ?
[D.M.S. 1975, 76, 79, 81]

1. Clody Swelling-It is the synonyms of **parenchymatous degeneration or granular degeneration or albuminous degeneration.** *It is a condition where protein of the cell becomes coagulated due to change of Electrical Polarisation, initiated by Noxious Agents.* This change is reversible to bring the cell to normal state of health. It is the mildest form of detectable illness of the cell (common cold in man). Protein are colloidal in nature but many of them can be crystallised. They are generally soluble in water. Each protein has got a particular Iso-electric point at which it is precepitated. Character of precepitation is mainly of two types — (i) **Coagulation** and (ii) **Denaturation.**

In both cases they involve intramolecular change and thereby normal synthesis of A.T.P. and other enzymes are inhibited. Cloudy Swelling is based upon this conception. So the precipitating granules are albuminous in nature and recent work has shown that the coarsely granular substances are Mitochondria, which separate from surromnding cytoplasm, when the cell is damaged. The swelling is due to increased water content of cytoplasm. In fact these changes indicate the most delicate and responsive indicator of the injury to cell.

Lesions : (i) **Macroscopic** : The affected organ (Viz. — Liver, Kidneys and sometimes Heart) is swollen, the capsule is tense and bulges out through the cut surface.

(ii) **Microscopic** : The cells are swollen, granular and Eosinophillic. Parenchyma cells of kidneys and other mentioned organs are affected. Typical changes are seen in Kidney. These changes simulate the initial changes of autolysis of the cells. The cytoplams of the cells of the tubules give a granular appearence and the Nucleous may become obscured. It is larger due to globules of Fat that may begin to appear in the cytoplasm, if it progresses to fatty degeneration.

These changes are usually encountered in early stage of Glomerulonephritis, Pyrexia, Diphtheria etc.

Q. 8.8. What is Hydropic degeneration ?

It is classed under the Cloudy Swelling, but main difference lies in imbibition of water in the cell.

As it is evident that only injuries may render a change of polarisation of cell wall so k^+ diffuses out from the cells and Na^+ enters inside the cell, thereby it attracts large amount of water inside the cell.

Lesions : It affects the protein of epithelial cells and is charcterised by vaculolisation of cell cytoplasm. In hepatic cells it may result from anaesthetics like ether (CH_5 OH-CH_4 OH), $CHCL_3$ CCI_4. The degeneration is particularly seen in the Kidneys in conditions, which seriously upset electrolyte and water balance of the body like prolonged diarrhoea, severe endocrine imbalance and other Non-specific stresses like shock leading to acute tubular Necrosis. It may be also taken place by administration of some chemicals like diethylglycol and Sulpha drugs.

Q. 8.9. What is meant by Fatty Degeneration ? Describe it in brief.
[C.U.1980,81, D.M.S. 75,76,78,81]

It is a reversible non-fatal injurious derangements in the metabolism of the cell (Transport hyperlipaemia).

Morphologically, Fatty degeneration, Fatty infiltration and Fat Phanerosis are classed under same category.

Fatty degeneration is taken place in the following organs - Liver, Heart, Kidney etc. So here it is customary to describe the Fatty changes in Liver and Heart that we very often encounter in many important ailments.

Aetiology:

(i) *Hepatoxic agents* — Poisoning of the cell enzyme.
(ii) *Chemicals* — $CHCl_2$, P_4, As, Bi, Sb, R-OH, CI-C.
(iii) *Bacterial* — Diphtheria, Spirochete like Leptospira icterohaemorrhagica, Viral like Infective Hepatitis, Yellow fever etc.

(iv) *Metabolic* —Toxomia of pregnancy, Diabetes.

(v) *Anoxia* — Lake of lipotrophic factors, too much fat going to the liver in starvation or Diabetes.

Pathogenesis and Lesions

(i) **Hepatotoxic agents:** They act by interfering with the enzyme activity of the liver cells.

As for example, we can cite an example of Alcohol

It is first oxidised in the body to form R-COH (Aldehyde), which is destroyed by aldehydes. Presence of higher aldehyde like fusil oris in Liquor is deinitely toxic to the Liver. This toxic action is aggravated by aversion to Milk (methionine) and other foods due to assciated Gastritis and poverty adds to the deprivation of Protein food in them. So it is misnomar to think that Alcohol is directly toxic to the liver.

Anoxia : The Livery has got a fix amount of Blood for nurishing its cells. So the conditions that give rise Heamapoitic disturbances can bring about anoxia, like pernicious Anaemia, Passive venous congestion — Nutmeg (painfull liver) in case of congestive cardiae failure.

Lack of Liptrophic Factors :

The main Pathogenic factors causing accumulation of Fat in the cells :

(i) Disturbances in splitting of Fat (Neutral) (N.E.F.A.) and in oxidation of higher fatty acids under the influences of various poisons like $CHCl_2$, P_4 etc.

(ii) Distrubances in the release of Fat from tissues due to disordered metabolism of phosphoilipids and to lack of choline, Methionine and others substances which exert lipotrophic action, in the food. Methionine is derived 'CH_8' group from Choline, that is to say, it is synthesised from Choline and Glycine :

CH_2 CH_2

$N{=}(CH_3)_2$ >Methl doner

HO $CH_2\,NH_2\,COOH$

Choline Glycine

Tri-glycerides present in liver, brack down the Nutral fat into Fatty acids and glycerol. This glycerol is used to be carried as phospholipides after combining with the Lipotrophic factors so lack of lipotrophic factors causes fatty changes in the liver.

Lesions in Liver :

(i) **Macroscopic view** : The liver is slighly enlarged more poler than usual soft and friable. Cut section present diffuse yellowish areas surrounded by normal livery substances.

(ii) **Microscopic lesion** : Pollygonal cells of liver lobules are distended, Fat globules appears in the cytoplasm. But in case of Fatty infiltration — Fat droplets may push the nucleous to one cornar giving a signet ring appearance. Central zone of liver is involved in chloroform poisoning, thyrotoxicosis. Midzone is infective conditions like yellow fever, peripheral zone in eclampsia or Phosphorous poisoning.

In Heart : (a) Papillar Muscles are studded with streaks of yellow Fat in Anoxic type, known as **Tobby cat appearance**.

(b) In Toxic types, like diphtheria, or in severe anaemia, Heart assumes to take a shape of flabby mass, known as **Mushrooming**.

Q. 8.10. What is Hyaline degeneration ?

It refers to a retrogressive change in cells in which cytoplasm becomes homogeneous giving appearance.

It is of two types : (a) **Cellular hyalinisation.**
(b) **Connective tissue hyalinisation.**

(a) **Cellular hyalinisation** :

It is a hetergenous group indicating simply hyaline or glassy appearance due to coagulated protein, e.g. corpora amylacea in senile Prostrate. They appear to form simply by deposition of organic material, containing acid Mucopolysaccharides. Hayaline cast in Renal tubules. These are considered to be composed of coagulated protein which posed through the glomeruli due to their abnormal character. It has, therefore got the same significance as albumin in urine.

In Liver—Russel inclusion bodies in Yellow fever, Mallory inclusion in Alcoholic Liver.

(b) Connective tissue hyalinisation :

It is caused by agglomeration and swelling of collagen as seen in Scar tissue, thickend pleura. Hyalinisation in the Blood vessels is seen in the intima and subendothelial tissue. These changes are also found in uterus or fibromyomata of uterus.

Q. 8.11. Notes on :

1. Zenkers hyaline degeneration :

This change is commonly seen in the striated muscles and two common sites of such a change are recuts abdominis and diaphragmatic muscles, particularly as a result of Toxins or excess accumulation of Lactic acid in Typhoid, Pneumonia, Diphtheria and Weils disease. Muscle cells take a coarse, clumped or homogeneously solid and dense appearance due to coagulation of the sacroplasm.

2. Amyloid degeneration : [C.U. 1980]

It represents a waxy, translucent hyaline change in the walls of the blood vessels of Spleen, Liver, Kidney.

Amyloid substances are supposed to be a Mucopolysaccharide of ptotein complex. This change is due to hyperguammaglobulinaemia. (Auto immune disorder), e.g. Sago spleen in long standing diseases.

3. Glycogen degeneration :

Abnormal glycogen deposition in side cell is known as glycogen deposition. It is found in renal tubule in Diabetes Mellitus as the process of glycogenesis is rapid in comparison with glycogenolysis. It is also found in **Vongierkes disease** due to congenital deficiency of glucose 6 phosphatase.

4. Mucoid degeneration :

Combination of protein and carbohyte form two complexes namely, Glycoprotein and Mucopolysccharide (Mucin). This type of degeneration involves the production of Mucine. It is found in Mixomatous degeneration of connective tissue tumours and in sub-cutaneous tissue in case of hypothyroidism. Epithelial muchin is found in colloid carcinoma or mucinous carcinoma.

Q. 8.12. What are the differences between Fatty Degeneration and Fatty Infiltration? [D.M.S. 1974]

	Fatty Degeneration	Fatty Infiltration
1. Definition :	It is a type of degeneration where the fat droplets are accumulated inside the cells when the cells are primarily diseased or injured by mechanical effect.	1. It is a pathological process where numerous small fat droplets accumulated inside the cell where a cell is not primarily diseased or injured.
2. Cell :	So cells are primarily diseased or injured.	2. Cells are not primarily diseased or injured.
3. Nucleus :	Atrophy and centrally placed.	3. Pushed to the periphery of the cell (No change in nucleus.)
4. Cytoplasms :	Filled up by numerous fat droplets which are originate from the component of the cells.	4. Filled up by numerous fat droplets due to systemic disorder. (Fat droplets turn into a one big fat droplets.)
5. Cause :	Bacteria or their toxins.	5. Systemic disorder or endocrine disorder.

Q. 8.13. What is Metamorphosis?

It is a condition where Fatty degeneration and Fatty infiltration occurs simultaneously in one cell.

9. TUMOUR (NEOPLASM)

Q. 9.1. What is Tumour ? [D.M.S. 1974,76,77,78,82,84]

Tumour or Neoplasm is an independent and abnormal over growth of tissue without co-ordination with that of normal tissue, and is an autonomus, uncontrolled growth of tissue, containing a mass aberrant or abnormal cells, without serving any useful purpose but is rather harmful, as it grows at the expense of the host, like a parasite; even sometimes it causes death of the subject.

Q. 9.2. Describe the nomenclature of Tumour.

Benign tumours :

Most *benign tumours* are designated histologically by attaching the suffix — *'Oma'* to the name of the cell from which the tumour arises. Thus benign tumors of fibrous tissue cell origin are termed **fibromas.** This system is useful with bone, tendons, cartilage, fat, vessels etc. *Benign epithelial tumour* are variously designated. Some are named on the basis of their microscopic pattern. Those producing gland patterns are designated as **adenomas.** Other are designated by their gross architecture. Those that from large cystic masses, as in the ovary, are referred as **cystoma** or **cyst adenomas.** Some are both papillary and cystic and are called as papillary cyst adenomas.

Malignant tumours :

Malignant tumour nomenclature, especially follows the methods use for naming benign tumours with the following additions. All malignancies are familiarly referred as **Cancer**. Maliganant neoplasms arising from mesechymal tissue are called **Sarcomas.** Malignant neoplasms of epithelial cell origin, are called **carcinomas.** If the tumours produce a glandular growth patterns, as seen on the microscopic examination, is called as **adenocarcinoma** and may be further specified according to the organ of origin.

Malignant tumours of the lymphoid origin are called *lymphomas.*

Q. 9.3. What are the main varieties of Tumour seen in the clinics? Or, How the tumours are classified ? [D.M.S. 1978, 79]

Clinically Tumours are divided into 2 broad headings :

1. Benign or Simple or Innocent.

2. Malignant.

Malignat are of 2 types:

(a) ***Sarcoma.***

(b) ***Carcinoma.***

Bengin and Malignant tumours are also divided into many subdivision according to the tissue of their origin. Generally the suffix *'Oma'* is to be added with the name of the tissue or origin in case of Benign tumour and '*Carcinoma*' and 'Sarcoma' are added with the malignant tumour or epithelial and connective tissue respectively.

Examples

Cell of Origin	Benign	Malignant
	1. Connective tissue tumour	
1. Fibrous tissue	Fibroma	Firosarcoma
2. Myxo-matous-tissue	Myxoma	Myxosarcoma
3. Fatty tissue	Lipoma	Liposarcoma
4. Cartilage	Chondroma	Chondrosarcoma
5. Bone	Osteoma	Osteosarcoma
6. Notochordal tissues.	Chordoma	Chordosarcoma
	2. Endothelial tissues	
1. Blood vessels	Haemangioma	Angiosarcoma
2. Lymph vessels	Lymphangioma	Lymphangiosarcoma
	3. Muscle tissues	
1. Smooth muscles	Leiomyoma	Leiomyosarcoma
2. Striated muscles	Rhabdomyosarcoma	
	4. Epithelial origin	
1. Squamous epi-thellium.	Papilloma	Squamous cell carcinoma
2. Adenoid tissue	Adenoma	Adenocarcinoma
	5. Nerve tissues	
1. Glial cells	Glioma	Ganglioneuroma
2. Nerve cells	Neuro blastoma	Retinoblastoma
	6. Pigmented tumours	
Naevus cell	Naevus	Melanomas
	7. Haematopoietic cells	
	No benign tumour.	Lymphomas Lymphosarcoma Hodgkins Leukemias Multiple Myeloma
	8. Special forms of epithelial tumours	
Renal cell		Hypernephrloma
Chroionic cells	—	Chorionepethalioma

9. Mixed : derived from more than one germ layer		
	Mixed tumour of salivary gland.	Malignant tumour of salivary gland.
	10. Compound	
Toti potential cells	Teratoma Dermoid	Malignant Tetratoma

Q. 9.3. What is meant by Carcinoma in Situ.

This is the condition when the malignant change in the cells is present and it has not metastasized or invade the deeper tissues. Three cytological features which indicate this condition are **nuclear change, anaplasia and loss of cell polarity**. The recognition of this condition is important for the clinician, as it is the earliers change and radicle thereby can be done. Carcinoma of he cervix is the common example. Other conditions are pagets disease of the nipple. Leukoplakia, Bowen's disease.

Q. 9.4. What are the main Characteristics of the tumours?

1. Morphological characters :
The size of the tumours varies from a pinhead to an enormous size. Mostly oval in shape and margins are clearly demarked, borders are irregular.

There are two basic components of all tumours :

(a) **Proliferating neoplastic cells, which comprise the parenchyma of the tumour.**
(b) **Supportive stroma made up of connective tissue and blood vessels.**

The parenchymal element is the most important of the two, and stromal element provides the structural support and blood supply to the parenchyma.

(i) In case of **Benign tumours** the parenchymal cells are almost resemble the normal cell of their origin, that is, they are well differentiated.

(ii) In **Malignant tumours** show various degrees of loss of differentiation, and have lost all resemblance to the normal cell.

Both these cells and their nuclei are plemorphic, varying greatly in size and shape. After the nucleus occupies the greater part of the cell, producing a nuclear cytoplasmic ratio of 1 : 1 or 1 : 2. There is increased accumulation of chromation in the nucleus, resulting in hyperchromasis or occasionally the chromatia coarsely clumped. *Multinucleated neoplastic giant cells are the most distinctive morphological features.*

2. Growth and other characters :

The tumour cells have uneasing growth and multiplication. Their growth is *autonomous*, i.e. it is not affected by external influence. It depends on the cellular activity independently. We do not know what are the exciting factors in the cells that bring about neoplastic process into activity and keeps this activity for whole life as we find that once a tumour is formed it does not stop or resolved by itself. They can grow from any kind of tissue of the body.

Generally all benign tumours grow as localised expansile masses enclosed within a fibrous membrane known as *Capsule*. But the malignant tumours almost never have the true capsules and are characterised by *infiltrative erosive growth*. The tumour extends along lines of least resistance, without necessarily maintaining contact with the central mass, erodes, and destroys normal tissue and is uninhibited by normal anatomical boundries.

Generally the tumour cells have two fold activities, namely reproduction and function. Here DNA synthesis is more. This is why it derives nourishment from adjoining tissue, so the subject is suffering from *Mal-nutritions, with cachexia.*

It arises from the existing tissues or cells of the body 'Oma**' is the suffix added to the end of that type of tissue i.e. their origin.

N.B. 1. Tumours differ from granuloma which is inflammatory in nature, and cell multiplication is also inflammatory in nature.

2. **The difference between a newgrowth from a cyst** is, while *tumour* is solid and would not yield to pressure, the cyst being filled with fluid yields to pressure.
3. **The difference between tumour and oedema** is, while tumour does not pit on pressure, oedema pits on pressure. Oedema may occur over large part of the body but the tumour is always localised.
4. **Inflammation** has redness, heat, pain and loss of function, where as all these symptoms are not found in *tumour*.
5. **The difference between tumour and hyperplasis** is, that while

Neoplasms are autonomous or independent and do not obey the law of growth, *Hyperplasia* is the result of injury and inflammation and is due to reparatory process of the tissues.

Q. 9.5. What are the factors responsible for the origin of Tumours?
(D.M.S.1977)

1. Predisposing factors—(a) Age (b) Sex
(c) Social grading (d) Diaetic errors.

(a) **Age**—The malignant tumours like carcinoma is an affections of the old age, generally after 40 years whereas sarcoma generally occurs in the earlier period of life.

(b) **Sex**—Both sexes are liable to the growth of tumours; but in females there are some organs which are more commonly affected than others, e.g., uterus, cervix and mammary glands.

(c) There are some occupations or certain habits which lead to tumour formation, e.g. chimney sweepers or habits continous smoking help to cancer formation.

2. Exciting factors—It again subdivided into following heads :
(a) *Chemical substance* : e.g. Arsenic, Pb, Hydrocarbon etc.
(b) *Physical substance* :
(i) Extreme cold and heat.
(ii) Deep ray. (iii) Radium.
(iv) Chronic irritation etc.
(c) *Inflammatory parasites* like Schistosoma haematobrium etc.

3. Genetica factors or other endogenic factors : Due to abnormal gene-developed generation after generation causes malignant neoplasm of the body e.g. Family of Napoleon Bonapart — generation after generation affected by carcinoma.

Also it has been found that there are some sex hormones which produce disordered metabolism and acts as cancer produceing substances.

Q. 9.6. What is meant by Benign and Malignant tumour ? What are their main differences ?
[C.U. 1979,82, D.M.S. 76, 77, (Dec.) 78' 81,84]

(A) Benign :

It is a new growth limited by a capsule with local expansion of the tissue without causing injury to the host or subject characterised by slow growth.

(B) Malignant :

It is also a one type of new growth characterised by absence of capsule with rapid invasion of the tissues by metastasis, causing injury to the host, even death of the subject.

*** Differences between Benign and Malignant Tumour***

(I) Macroscopic

	Bengin	**Malignant**
1. *Occurrence*	At any age	Carcinoma commonly occurs in elderly persons, sarcoma in children and in young adults.
2. *Growth*	Slow growth by expansion of the surrounding tissue.	Rapid growth with infiltration or metastasis.
3. *Capsule*	Capsulated i.e. why complete removal is possible.	Non-Capsulated i.e why complete removal is impossible.
4. *Fixity*	Absent	Present
5. *Degeneration*	Rare	Rather common
6. *Recurrence*	Not common	Common
7. *Metastasis*	Usually absent	Usually present
8. *Anaemia, Cachexia, loss of weight.*	Absent	Usually present
9. *Lymph node enlargement.*	Not enlarged	Enlarged, especially in carcinoa and malignant melanoma.

* *Metastasis*—is the process by which new abnormal cell of the primary growth implanted to the distant part of the body through the lymph chanel.

10. *Whether injurious and fatal.*	Not fatal unless it affects a vital organ e.g. Putritary adenoma.	Kills the host in a short time, unless drastic treatment is instituted. Even then 5 years survival rate may be poor.

(II) Microscopic

1. *Cell character*	No change	Changes both structural and metabolic.
2. *Representation*	Cells represent the tissue in which it grows e.g. glandular structures reproduce gland tissues, Fibrous for fibroma etc.	No true representation of same tissue.
3. *Blood vessels*	Adult type	Embryonic type
4. *Cell division* (Mitosis).	Absent	Present, Metaphase (Monaster stage), Anaphase (Diaster stage).
5. *Nucleus*	As in normal cell	Nucleus mostly larger or proportionally larger, placed in one side (eccentric).
6. *Loss of polarity*	Absent	Present
7. *Anaplasia*	Absent	Present
8. *Metaplasia cell*	Absent	Present
9. *Defferentiation*	Fully differentiated like adult cells	Undifferentiated
10. *Blood picture*	No change of WBC Normal	Leucocytosis
11. *E.S.R.*	Normal	Increased

Q. 9.7. What is Sarcoma and Carcinoma? What are the differences between them? [D.M.S. 1977,78,79,80]

Sarcoma : It is a malignant tumour originating from connective tissue implanted by blood vessels.

Carcinoma : It is also a malignant tumour derived from epithelial tissue implanted through lymph chanal.

* Differences between Sarcoma and Carcinoma *

(I) Macroscopic

	Sarcoma	Carcinoma
1. *Origin*	Connective tissue	Epitheliel tissue

2. *Age*	In early life in 2nd decade.	In latter life, after 40 years.
3. *Growth*	Rapidly growing than carcinoma.	Slowly growing

(II) Microscopic

1. *Cells*	Spherical or polygonal cells are spindle shaped or pleomorphic in character, cells are separated by the stroma i.e. surrounds individual cells.	Shows thin strands of fibrous tissue separating large mass, of spherioidal cells or polygonal cells.
2. *Cystoplasm and nuclear ratio.*	Each cell is separated by stroma, Cytoplasm and nuclear ratio is small.	Group of cells separated by stroma Large.
3. *Character of cells.*	Fair no. of cells are embryonic.	Few are embroynic.
4. *Epithalial art*	Absent	May be present
5. *Intercellular substance.*	Fibrillar stroma is present without any alveolar arrangement.	Intercellular matrix is present. Groups of cells are enclosed and separated by the stroma.
6. *Anaplasia*	More anaplastic	Cells are less Anaplastic.
7. *Differentiation*	More de-differentiated	Less de-differentiated.
8. *Inflammatory and degenerative reaction.*	More marked around the lesion.	Inflammatory and degenerative reaction are not so marked.
9. *Polarity and hyperchromic state of nucleous.*	Well marked	Not marked
10. *Mitosis*	*Anaphase* and *Telophase* are quickly taken place.	Prophase is well marked.
11. *Blood vessels*	Vessel walls are invaded by tumour	The vessels are confied to the stroma

	cells.	that separates the group of cells.
12. *Giant cells*	Presence of malignant giant cells such as osteoclastic giant cells are present.	Malignant giant cell few in number.
13. *Spreading character.*	Usually Haematogenous, Metastasis through blood vessels.	Metastasis usually by lymphatics.
	(III) X-Ray Findings	
Embolism	Cannon ball embolism is common in the chest field.	Cannon ball embolism is uncommon except Chorionic Epicthelioma.
	(IV) Clinical Findings	
(a) E.S.R.	Highly diagnostic such as Multiple Myeloma.	High
(b) W.B.C.	More lymphocytes and Polymorphos.	Plenty of poly morphos in comparison with lymphocytes.
	(V) Prognosis	
	Severe—is always formidiable.	Not worst in early stage.
	Less Radio sensitive.	Radio sensitive

Q. 9.7. Some important Carcinoma and Sarcoma.

(I) Carcinoma

1. Squamous cell carcinoma :

This usually occurs in the Skin and Stratified Mucous surfaces containing Squamous epithelium, namely, Mouth, Lip, Tongue, Pharynx, Osephagus, Cardiac end of the stomach and rectum, Upper air passage, Larynx and Cervix Uteri. They might also arise as a process of Metaplasia from bronchogenic Carcinoma, and Calumnar cells, of the Gall bladder.

Microscopically—It consists of Strands or Columns of Poly gonal cells infiltrating into the deeper tissue with breach of the basement membrane. As the cells grow in sheets and columns, the central older cells become differentiated, Keratinised resembling the cells of Stratum Corneum forming cell nests or epithelial perl; around the lesion, degenerative and inflammatory reaction are present.

2. Basal Cell Carcinoma (or Rodent ulcer). [C.U. 1982, 84]

Rodent ulcer arises from the Basal Layer of skin, hair follicles or sweat gland etc. *Microscopically*, the Basal Cells proliferate to form masses of small closely packed columnar cells with rounded masses projecting downwards into the corium associated with Lymphocytes from the ulcerated area. The growth commonly occurs on the face some where above the line drawn from the tragus of the ear to angle of the mouth.

(II) Sarcoma

1. Angioma

These are usually of three types :

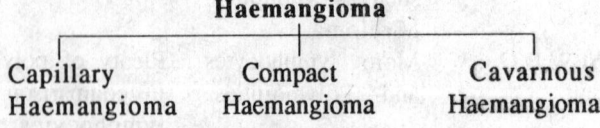

Haemangioma

- Capillary Haemangioma
- Compact Haemangioma
- Cavarnous Haemangioma

*** Cavarnous Haemangioma**

They have the structure of erectile tissues, being composed of large blood spaces, which are separated from one another by scanty connective tissue stroma.

****Capillary Haemangioma:**Tumour consists of a mesh work of endothelium, forming irregular channels of variable size and contain red blood corpuscles in the lumen.

2. Classification of Sarcoma:

Sarcomas may be classified from:

(i) ***Histological or Cytological point of view***

(a) Round cells sarcoma
(b) Spindle cell sarcoma
(c) Mixed cell sarcoma
(d) Giant cell sarcoma

(ii) According to the Origin of tissue e.g. Fibrosarcoma from fibrous tissue.

(iii) ***Modern classification***

(a) Differentiated.

(b) Undifferentiated.

Though malignant changes of Embryonal cell is classed under carcinoma, yet classification is made as they show rapid Metastasis.

Embryonal Carcinoma

Teratoma | Teratocarcinoma | Testicular Adenocarcinoma of infancy

Chorionepithelioma

Q. 9.8. Write short notes on: (1) Anaplasia, (2) Metaplasia, (3) Dedifferentiation, (4) Metastasis. [C.U. 1979, D.M.S. 74,75,79]

1. Anaplasia :

It denotes reversion of the cell into more primitive embryonic or undifferentiated type.

Such cells have the potentiality of greater growth and multiplication but less capacity for specialised function.

2. Metaplasia : Metaplasia is a form of abnormal regeneration, in which a type of cell, different from one normally found in a given location is produced e.g. Squamus epithelium may replace columnar epithelium or bone may replace fibrous connective tissue. It is subdivided into two:

(a) *Epithelial Metaplasia* : Chronic inflammation. Vit. A deficiency, Neoplasia.

(b) *Connective Tissue Metaplasia* : Found in Osteogenic sarcoma.

Apart from that there are other types too. Such as endothelial Metaplasia, False Metaplaia Cysts etc.

3. De-Differentiation : It indicates that cell which has reached maturity undergoes reversion of evolution to embryonic type of cell that differentiates into normal adult cell.

4. Metastasis : It is the dissemination of a tumour to the distal parts of the body from the site of primary growth. This is a characteristic feature of Malignant tumour which widely in their ability to Metastasis. Some grow to a great size before any matastaisis is seen, whereas others, when still small, invade the Lymphatic and Blood vessels to produce Metastasis e.g. Melanoma of the skin. Metastasis is usually of three types:

(a) *Lymphatic*—This is seen in all types of Carcinoma specially. But sarcoma may invade Lympatics as its power of invasion is greater in comparison to carcinoma.

(b) *Haematogenic*—It is specially for Sarcoma that produce cannon ball emboli in chest field.

(c) *Direct Implanation*.—Metastasis from tumours can take place by penetrating the serous cavities or meningeal spaces e.g. Krukenbergs tumour from stomach to ovary.

Q. 9.9. How are the Tumours (Neoplasm) spread ? [C.U.1979,82]

The power and method of spread constitute the main feature of the tumour. A tumour may be spread by any one of the following methods or combination thereof :

1. *By infiltration*
2. *By lypathatics*
3. *By blood vessels*
4. *Along the natural passages*
5. *Through serous cavities*
6. *By innoculation.*

1. By Infiltration of the tissue spaces :

This is one of the chief characteristics of a *malignant tumours*, where tumour cells invade through intercellular substance by a lymph flow or by blood vessels. The cancer cells are amoeboid and motile. The cells of the benign tumours and normal tissues are incapable of movement because they are firmly anchored to one another by cells adhesiveness. Cancer cells are free because of greatly reduced adhesiveness. This turn seems to be due to deficiency of calcium in the cell membrane. It has also been suggested that the invasiveness of cancer cell is due to hyaluronidase which breaks down the resistance of the viscid ground substance.

2. By Lymphatics: [C.U. 1979]

Tumour cells can readily enter lymphatic channels. They may extend also these channels by permeation or they may be carried both to regional and distant nodes by lymphatic embolism. The lymphatic system provides the most common pathways for *metastatic dissemination of carcinomas*. *Sarcomas* also use this route.

The pattern of lymphatic involvement in any malignancy is dependent upon the natural routes of drainage of the primary site of origin of the cancer. Thus the *bronchogenic carcinoma* metastasiza first to the tracheo-bronchial nodes and then to the mediastinum, while carcinoma of the *breast* usually involves first the axillary and internal mammary nodes.

The lymphatic spread of carcinoma is primarily embolic. All the lymph from the abdominal organs reach the thoracic duct, which finally open into the left jugulary vein and so metastasis into the organs through blood occurs.

3. By blood vessels :

Cancer cells may reach the blood either by way of the thoracic duct or by direct invasions of the blood vessels. The veins are invaded with great readiness, but the arteries very rarely. The chief reason for this striking difference appears to be the fact that lymphatic frequently from plexus reaching to the sub-endothelial region, this is not true in cases of arteries. A thrombus forms over the eroded endothelium and this is invaded by tumour cells. This becomes detached and forms tumour emboli, that are likely to result in the metastasis. Kidneys, the endocrine glands, particularly the adrenals, and the bone marrow are favoured lodgements of the arterial emboli. The lings, liver and axial bones are the sites for the venous metastasis. This distribution reflects the large volume of venous drainage channeled through each of these organs. *Sarcomas* commonly spread by the this method.

4. By natural passages :

Tumour cells may be carried along such passages as the bronchus, bowel and ureter. They become implanted on the epithelial surface and form a new growth. This might explain the simultaneous occurrence of the same type of tumour in the renal pelvis and the bladder.

5. Through serous cavities :

This method is known as transcelomic spread, and in the explanation given for the metastasis from the stomach to the ovaries. Small implantations on the peritoneum can often be traced between stomach and ovary.

6. By inoculation :

Transfer of tumour cell by inoculation into the surrounding tissue may occur in the course of an operation for cancer.

Instruments, glavaves which may be contaminated by cutting into the tumour to obtain biopsy, may be transplanted in the surrounding areas of skin.

N.B. : Metastasis—The ability to spread, both locally and to a distance place is one of the most important characteristics of malignant tumour.

Generally the following factors modify the metastasis:

(a) Size of the tumour.
(b) Blood and lymphatic supply of the organ.
(c) Size of the emboli.
(d) Capacity of the cancer to Metastasis.

Q. 9.10. What is meant by Metastasis?

[C.U. 1979, D.M.S. 74,75,79,82,84]

It is a process by which an abnormal growth develop on the distal part of the body from primary new growth through lymph channla or blood vessels.

Or, It is an implantation of a tumour cell to the distal part of the body from the site of the primary new growth through blood vessels or lymph channal. [It is an important characteristic point of malignancy].

N.B. Also see page —283.

Q. 9.11. Discuss the Laboratory diagnosis of Tumours.

The various methods of diagnosis are as follows :

(1) *Histological diagnosis*
(2) *Cytological diagnosis*
(3) *Peripheral blood studies*
(4) *Hormone and enzyme studies.*

1. Histological diagnosis :

Histological examination is the most important valid method of diagnosis. In small tumours *biopsy* is done excision type and in the large tumours *subtotal* or *incisional* biopsy is done. There are many methods available for further study of this section. The classis and time honoured method is to *embed in the paraffin and stain with Haematoxylin and Eosim.* This requires 24 hours. Techniques are available, which permit more rapid paraffin embedding and sectioning giving adequate expendient preparation within four hours. The most rapid method is to *prepare frozen sections* which makes the slides available for study within few minutes and diagnostic accurancy of 90% to 95% is obtained. The frozen section technique is the invaluable particularly in the case of breast tumours, when the surgeon is operating on the case and he wants to ascertain the nature of the tumour and immediately institute appropriate measures.

Needle biopsy or *Aspiration biopsy* is useful in certain cases and the technique has many advantages, as it requires little preparation and no anaesthesia, biopsy can be performed on an outpatient or on office basis. The limitations are that it is a blind procedure and the nodule or part may easily be missed and only gives a small part of the larger scene and sometimes interpretition is difficult.

2. Cytological diagnosis :

Cancer cells lose sickness or adhesiveness, characteristic of normal cells, so that they tend to be cast off or exfoliated from a surface very eaisly early in the disease. These cells are found in exudates, secretions, washings and scrapings. Its greatest value is at present in cancer of the cervix and bronchus. It is also used for suspected Cancer of stomach, ureter, bladder and prostate, It has got immense importance in early cancers, where the lesion is easily overlooked with ordinary methods of investigation.

3. Peripheral blood studies :

A number of haematologic techniques have been reported as having some value in the diagnosis of cancer. The cancer cells are desquamated into the blood at the site of the neoplasm and are identifiable in properly stained sediments or concentrates of the circulating blood. Usually, too few cells are present to permit their discovery in a routine blood smear. By special techniques, tumour cells have found circulating in the blood in approximately 10—80% of cases of established neoplasia.

4. Hormone and enzyme studies :

Hormone and enzyme studies may be useful, in the diagnosis of cancer. The elaboration of acid phosphatase by prostatic tumour metastatic to bone provides an important clue to the diagnosis of these neoplasms. Similarly, finding of chorionic gonadotrophin in the urine or serum of a male is indicative of choriocarcinoma usually in the testis. Abnormally high levels in the female, as above those attributable to pregnancy again provide important clues the presence of hydationiform mole or choriocarcinoma.

10. JAUNDICE

Q. 10.1. What is Jaundice ? {C.U. 1980, D.M.S. 74, 77 (Dec.)}

It is a syndrome characterised by yellowish discolouration of the skin, sclera, and other mucous membrane of the body due to hyper bilirubinaemia.

Normal blood bilirubin content is 1/400,000 to 1/1000,000, i.e. 0.2-0.5 units, a unit being 1/200,000 or 0.5 mg percent. The renal threshold is 1/50,000 or 4 units or 2 mg percent. Clinically manifestation of Jaundice occurs when 1/80,000 is exceeded, but when hyper bilirubinaemia is below the level there is no yellow staining of the tissues (**Latent Jaundice**) as is cancer and cirrhosis of the liver and pernicious anaemia.

Q.10.2. What are the various types of Jaundice seen in clinics ? (C.U. 1980)

(A) According to McNee's

Clinically Jaundice are of 3 types :

1. **Haemolytic.**
2. **Obstructive.**
3. **Toxic.**

(B) According to Richs Jaundice are of 3 types :

1. **Retention Jaundice.**
2. **Regurgitation Jaundice.**
3. **Mixed Jaundice.**

1. Haemolytic Jaundice-(Pre-hepatic Jaundice)

This is due to increased bilirubin in the plasma with excessive breakdown of R.B.C. due to some toxic effect; resulting in :

(i) excess bilirubin in plasma.
(ii) presence of stercobilinogen in faeces.
(iii) persence of urobilinogen in urine.

Causes :

This generally occur in malaria, black water fever, alcoholic family jaundice, incompletible blood transfusion, snake bite, icterus neonatorum, paxorysmal haemoglobinuria and acute streptococcal infections.

Clinical manifestions :

The conjunctivae being rarely affected, the staining colour is lemon yellow, splenomegaly is frequent, the liver is enlarged or normal, anaemia profound, the sedimentation rate of the RBC increased, **Vanden Bergh's test** is indirect.

2. Obstructive Jaundice (Post-hepatic Jaundice).

It is due to obstruction of passage of conjucated bilirubin from liver cell to the intestine. It is mainly due to the obstruction of extrahepatic origin, and some times due to intrahepatic obstruction. It is also known as cholestasis.

Causes :

(a) Extra-hepatic :

1. Blockage of common bile duct by gallstone, congenital stenosis, growth stricture etc.
2. Obstruction of ampula of vater due to carcinoma.
3. Obstruction at the pancreas due to origin of cancer at the head of the pancreas by mechanical pressure.
4. Formation of lymph node at portahepatis.
5. Parasitic obstruction at the common bile duct (Ascaris lumbricoides).

(b) Intra-hepatic :

1. Tumour inside the liver cell.
2. Carcinoma at the lobule of the liver.

Clinical manifestations :

In obstructive Jaundice, the onset is stormy, the **conjunctivae are more pigmented than the skin, the colour being dirty yellow,** pruritus is severe, the liver is enlarged, the stools bulky whitish and **Vanden Bergh's test** is direct immediate positive.

In this case-(i) Increased amount of bilirubin in plasma:

(ii) Absence of stercobilinogen in stool (so whitish stool).

(iii) Urolibinogen absence in urine.

3. Toxic Jaundice (Hepatic Jaundice) :

It is due to some toxin produced by certain virus or some by injections (chloropromazine).

Causes : It is found in catarrhal jaundice, weil's disease, infective hepatitis, chemical poisonings, bacterial infections (pneumonia, typhoid) and drug toxicity.

Clinical manifestations : The onset is quiet, *the skin is affected before the conjunctiva, the colour being orange-yellow*; pruritus is slight, the liver is enlarged or dormal, Vanden *Bergh's test show delayed direct* response *or biphasic.*

(B) Arnold Rich classifies Jaundice as :

1. *Retention Jaundice* i.e., a form of jaundice due to the inability of the liver to dispose of the bilirubin provided by the circulating blood.
2. *Regurgitative Jaundice*, i.e., a jaundice in which the whole bile accumulates and is returned to the circulating blood.
3. *Mixed Jaundice*, being a combination of both.

Q. 10.3. What is Latent Jaundice ?

It is a condition where increase bilirution in blood without any clinical manifestations of Jaundice. In this case inner cells completely turn into yellowish greenish except cells of brain matter. Generally it is seen in case of bilirubin content of blood is above 2 to 3 mg/100 ml.

Q. 10.4. What is meant by Reaction of Jaundice (Vanden Bergh Reaction)?

Pathologically reaction of Jaundice classified under following heads:

(a) *Direct Vanden Bergh Reaction.*
(b) *Indirect Vanden Bergh Reaction.*
(c) *Biphasis Vanden Bergh Reaction.*

In obstructive Jaundice—Vanden Bergh test is direct and prompt.
In Haemolytic Jaundice—Vanden Bergh test is indirect.
In Toxic or infective Jaundice—Where there is parenchymatous liver damage—Vanden Bergh test is delayed direct or biphasic.

Q. 10.5. What is the test done to determine the type of Jaundice? Or, What is Vanden Bergh test? How it is done?

[C.U. 1980 (Sup.) D.M.S. 77 (Dec)]

Vanden Bergh Test :

This test helps in detection of bile pigment in blood serum. There are three types of reactions :

(a) Direct, (b) Biphasic, (c) Indirect.

Two solutions are used in this test :

Solution I :	Sulphanilic acid	0.1 gm.
	Concentrated HCI	1.5 ml.
	Dist. water	100 ml.
Solution II :	Sodium nitrate	0.5 gm.
	Water	100 ml.

Procedure :

25 ml. of No. I solution is mixed with 0.75 ml. of No. II solution : *Diazo-reagent*. Then 1 ml. of serum is taken in a small test tube and to it equal amount of Diazo-reagnet is added, any one of the following reactions may be occurred.

1. Direct reactions :

(a) *Immediate or Prompt—A bluish violet* colour immediately appears (with in 10—30 seconds).

(b) *Delayed—Reddish* colour appears which gradually becomes violet and this takes from 5—15 minutes or even half an hour.

2. Biphasic reaction: A reddish colour appears promptly and after much longer time becomes violet.

3. Indirect reaction : At first 1 ml. of serum is treated with 2 ml. of 9% alcohol. It is shaken and centrifuged. 1 ml. of supernatant fluid is taken and to it 0.25 ml. of Diazoreagent is added. *A reddish-violet* colour appears immediately.

Conclusions:

Vanden Bergh test is direct and prompt—*Obstractive Jaundice*.

Vanden Bergh test indirect—*Haenmolytic Jaundice*.

Vanden Bergh test is delayed direct or biphasic—*Toxic or infective Jaundice* where there is parenchymatous liver damage.

[N.B.: Q. How will you investigate a case of Jaundice in the laboratory ?] [C.U. 1980 (Sup)]

Q. 10.6. What are the differences between Obstructive, Toxic and Haemolytic Jaundice?

	Obstructive	Toxic or defective	Haemolytic
Onset	Stormy	Quiet	Chronic
Colour of skin	Yellow, orange or greenish.	Yellow, orange or greenish.	Light yellow, 'lemon yellow'
Distribution of pigment	Seen in conjunctiva before skin.	Seen in skin before Conjunctiva.	Conjunctivae rarely affected.
Irritation of skin	Usually severe	May be present	Not present.
Colour of stool	Pale	Normal of pale	Normal
Urine	Bile pigments present.	Often no bile pigments Urobilin present	No bile pigments Urobilin present
Liver	Large or very large	Large, normal or small	A little large or round
Gall bladder	May be palpable	Not palpable	Not palpable
Spleen	Rarely palpable	Rarely palpable	Often palpable
Anaemia	May or may not present	Usually not severe	Severe
Sedimental rate	Usually normal	Normal or increased	Much increased
Serum alkaline phosphatase	Increased	Little increased	Little increased
Turbidity test	Negative	Positive	Variable
Albumin and globulin ratio.	Normal	Low albumin, raised gamma-globulin	Normal
Prothombin level	Normal until later disease.	Decreased	Normal, fragility of red cells may be increased.
Vanden Bergh reaction (serum bilirbubin)	Steadly raising serum bilirubin and direct reaction.	Moderate serum billi-rubin and indirect reaction.	High serum bilirubin and no direct reaction.

Q. 10.7. What are the Physio-pathogenesis of Jaundice ?

The bile pigments involved are bilirubin, biliverdin, the urobilinogens, and the urobilinoid pigments. These natural bile pigments derived from the catabolism of heme; sources include the Hb and non-Hb heme of degenerating RBCs, RBC precursors in the marrow, and heme proteins of liver and other tissues. There is no evidence for the direct synthesis of bilirubin from heme precursors.

Bilirubin is a pigmented organic anion closely related to porphyrins and other tetrapyrroles. As an insoluble waste product of heme catabolism, it must be converted to water soluble products for excretion. This transformation is over all purpose of bilirubin metabolism, which takes place in the five major steps. Abnormalities at any of the following steps can result in Jaundice :

1. Formation : About 250 to 350 mg of bilirubin are formed daily, and 80 to 85 percent is derived from the breakdown of senescent RBCs. The remaining 15 to 20 percent of the pigment arises from other heme proteins primarily located in the bone marrow and the liver. The hene moiety of Hb is degraded to iron and the intermediate product, biliverdin by the microsomal enzyme heme oxygenase.

The biliverdin produced in converted to bilirubin available supernatant enzyme, biliverdin reductage.

Little information is available concerning the specific reactions leading from non-Hlb heme to bilirubin. One of the major areas of interest, however, involves the **early labeled bilirubin** that bilirubin which is synthesized from heme other than that of the circulating RBCs. Early labeled bilirubin comprises 10 to 20 percent of bilirubin secreted under normal circumstances, but upto 80 percent of that secreted by patients with pernicious anaemia, thalacemia, and erythropoitic porphyria. Early labeled bilirubin is heterogeneous; the first major component arises from noneryth ropoietic heme, has its origin primarily in the liver, and is related in part of the turnover of heme — containing enzymes in the liver. The second major component is crythropoietic in origin and includes both Hb and non-Hb heme.

2. Plasma transport :

Bilirubin, which is insoluble in water, is transported in the plasma bound to albumin. Although the binding is light, it is weakend under certain conditions, such as acidosis, and there is competition for the binding sites, for examples, by certain antibiotiotics, thyroxine, and free fatty acids. This circulating unconjugated (in direct-reacting) bilirubin cannot difuse across cell membranes other than those in the liver and, therefore, does not appear in the urine.

3. Hapatic uptake :

The details of bilirubin uptake by liver have not been worked out, the process is rapid, does not involve the uptake of serum albumin, and probably involves active transport. The role of ligandin (Y protein) and other intracellular binding proteins remains to be defined.

4. Conjugation :

Free bilirubin is concentrated in the liver and then conjugated with glucuronic acid to from bilirubin diglucuronide , or conjugated ("direct-reacting") bilirubin. This reaction, catalyzed by the microsomal enzyme glocoronyl transferase, renders to pigment water soluble. Bilirubin conjugates other than the diglucuronide are also formed but their significance is uncertain.

5. Biliary excretion :

Conjugated bilirubin is secreted into the bile canaliculus alongwith the other constituents of bile. This process is complex and can be affected by the presence of other organic anions or drugs. In the gut, the pigment is deconjugated and reduced by the bacterial flora to various compounds collectively called stercobilinogens. Most of these are excreted in the faeces, but substantial amounts are absorbed and re-excreted in bile; small amounts reach the urine as urobilinogen. The Kidney can also excrete bilirubin diglucuronide, but not unconjugated bilirubin. Renal excretion of the bile pigments is not important normally but may become so with deep Jaundice.

So from the above discussion it is seen that—*increased formation, impaired hepatic uptake*, or *decreased conjugation* cause unconjugated hyperbilirubinemia. Impaired biliary excretion also produces conjugated byperbilirubinemia. In practice, however, hepatic diseases and biliary obstruction usually create multiple defects, resulting in a mixed hyperbilirubinemia. In most patients with obvious hepatobiliary disease, bilirubin fractionation is, therefore, of little diagnostic value.

Haemolysis and several uncommon disorders of bilirubin metarbolism produce jaundice in the absence of demonstratble liver disease.

11. ANAEMIA

Q. 11.1. What is Anaemia ?

Anaemia is a condition in which the blood is deficient either in quantity or in quality—the latter due either to diminution of the amount of haemoglobin (*oligochromaemia*) or to diminution in the number of the red cells (*oligocythaemia*).

Q. 11.2. Classify Anaemias. [C.U. 1979,80 (Sup.)

Or, Discuss the classification of Anaemias.

Classification of Anaemias

Morphological	Haematological	Aetiological
1. Mcrocytoc anaemia.	1. Microcytic hyprochromic.	1. Haemorrhagic anaemia.
2. Normocytic anaemia.	2. Macrocytic hyperchromic.	2. Haemolytic
3. Microcytic anaemia.		3. Dyshaemopoietic.
4. Hyrochromic microcytic anaemia.		

*** Clinical**

1. *Deficiency anaemia.*
   e.g. Iron deficiency anaemia,
   Anti-anaemia, principle deficiency anaemia, etc.
2. *APlastic Anaemia* (Destruction of bone marrow).
3. *Post-haemorrhagic anaemia.*
4. *Haemolytic anaemia.*

Q. 11.3. What are the common causes of Anaemia ?

[C.U. 1979 80 (Sup.)]

- ANAEMIA
  - Haemorrhagic
    - Trauma.
    - Haemorrhoids.
    - Metrorrhagia.
    - Haemophillia.
    - Uterine Fibroid.
    - Ancylostomiasis etc.
  - Haemolytic
    - Malaria.
    - Drugs.
    - Snake Venoms etc.
  - Dyshaemopoietic
    - Aplastic.
    - Pernicious.
    - Sprue.
    - Nutritional deficiencies like Vit B_{12}. Folic acid, Iron etc.

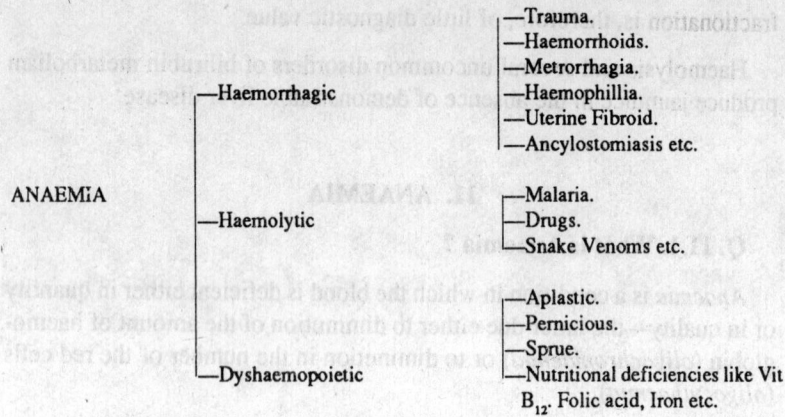

Q. 11.4. How will you investigate a case of Iron deficiency anaemias?
[C.U. 1980 (Sup.) 82]

Iron Deficiency Anaemia

Iron deficiency anaemia is the commonest human ailment and is easily treatable. Though commonly hypochronic in nature, it is not synonymous with hypochronic anaemia.

Investigations

(I) *To establish the severity of Iron deficiency.*

(II) *To determine the cause of iron deficiency.*

(I) To establish the severity of Iron deficiency (Laboratory tests) :

1. Haemoglobin, haematocrit, MCHC are reduced.
2. Peripheral smear will reveal hypochromia and microcytosis. Occasional target cells, anisocytosis and poikilocytosis may be present. Reticulocyte count is normal, leucocytes and platelets are normal.
3. Serum iron is reduced, iron binding capacity is increased and transferrin is saturation less than 15-20 percent.
4. Bone marrow shows micronormoblast with ragged margins. Marrow iron is diminished.
5. Gastic hypochlorhydia, mild malabsorption findings are not uncommon in severe iron dificiency anaemias.

(II) To determine the cause of Iron deficiency :

Nutritional deficiency forms the commonest etiology of the Iron deficiency anaemia. But number of investigations will be needed to rule out the coexisting factors.

Stool examination for ancylostomiasis, whiph worms, amoebiasis and occults blood, *proctoscopy* for piles, *sigmoidoscopy* for malignancy, *Barium swallow, Barium meal and upper gut scopy* for cases of esophageal varices, peptic ulcer and gastic carcinoma, *radiological studies* of lungs and Urinary tract for haemoptysis and haematuria, proper *Gynecological check up* in female patients and finally *coagulation studies and urinary haemosiderin estimation* may be needed.

12. IMMUNITY

Q. 12.1. What is Immunity? [D.M.S. 1974,76,77,78,81]

The word "**immunis**" means 'exempt'. The term immunity signifies all those properties of the host which confer resistance to a specific infectious agent. So the immunity is the ability of the body to resist or overcome infection. The state of resistance is indicated either by the failure of the individual to develop the diseaseupon exposure or insome cases by the demonstration of specific immuned bodies (antibodies) in the blood which are considered effective against the invading organism.

So the term **immunity implies resistance or non-susceptibility to a disease or any organisms naturally or artificially acquired.**

It may be against the organisms (antibacterial) or antiviral or the toxin liberated by them (antitoxic).

Immunity may be:

(1) **Natural or congenital** i.e. **from birth.**

(2) **Acquired—(a) Active**—by suffering from disease or by vaccination.

(b) Passive—by serum.

** **Natural** are of following types—(a) **Species**—Rats of diphtheria, Fowl to tetanus, and goat, Horse to tuberculosis.

(b) **Racial**—Negroes to yellow fever, Jews to tuberculosis.

(c) **Individual**—In smallpox, influenza etc.

* Haematological Pictures in Different Types of Anaemia *

	M.C.D.	M.C.V.	Vanden Bergh	Colour Index	Gastric analysis by fractional test meal	Total R.B.C. count	Total W.B.C. count	Immature blood cells	Hb	Platelet count
Pernicious anaemia (Vit B_{12})	Raised above 8 μ.	Raised 100 μ or more	Positive indirect	1 or above 1 i.e., high	Free HCI absent even after injection of histamin .01 mg. per kg. of body wt.	Diminished much	Diminished, relative or absolute lympho-cytosis	Megaloblast Normoblast Myelocyte	Redu-ced much	Redu-ced much
Anaemia of pregnancy (Macrocytic due to Vit B_{12} or Folic acid)	High normal	Ditto	Ditto	Ditto	Usually no achlorhydria which if present is reversible	Reduced	Leucocy-sis ±	Ditto	Reduced	Reduced slightly
Aplastic anaemia (Inhibition of bone marrow).	Normal	Normal	Normal	1 (normal)	Normal	Reduced markedly	Reduced markedly	Absent		Reduced
Idiopathic microcytic hypochromic anaemia (Iron).	Reduced	Reduced	Normal	Very low upto 0.3	Achlorhydria		Normal	Normo-blasts	Reduced very much.	Normal
After acute haemorrhage.	Normal then after a few days reduced.	Normal after few days reduced	Normal	Low	Normal	Reduced	Normal after initial leucocyto-cytosis	Normo-blasts	Reduce-ced	Normal
Chronic haemorrha-gic anaemia	Reduced	Reduced		Very low		Slightly reduced latter much reduced	Leucopenia later normal	No megalo-eythro-blast	Much reduced	Redu-ced

Q. 12.1(A). What are the different types of immunity? [D.M.S. 1974,76,78,81]

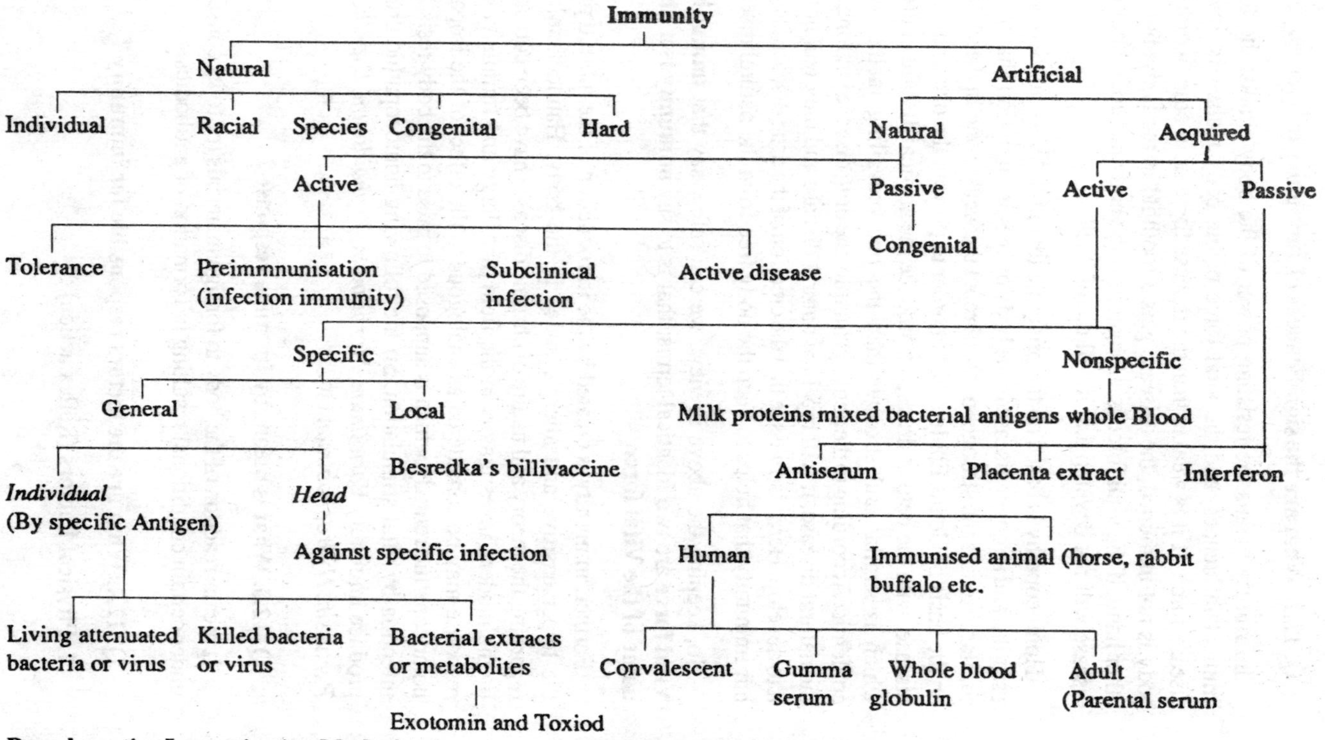

Done by active Immunization Methods. **Done by Passive Immunization Methods.**

Q. 12.2. What are the significances of Immunity in homoeopathy?

Immunity means the resisting power of the body against the foreign inimical influences, and the vital force of the body resists the invading disease force. If it is weaker than the disease force or in other words if the body is not immuned, the disease gets a foothold in the body; but on the other hand, if the vital force is stronger or if the body has got immunity the disease will not develop and it will die of itself.

Homoeopathy is based on the principle that in order to cure we produce a similar and stronger disease in the body on the presumption that out of the similar diseases the stronger one will repel the weaker one.In the same way, on the basis of Genus Epidemicus in order to prevent the occurrence of the disease, with the help of drugs, we produce the artifical disease in the body which is similar and stronger than the one prevailing in the form of epidemic. According to the above principle, the drug disease is stronger than the natural disease, it will repel the natural disease and they will not allow it to develop. Here also we see that the creation of the drug disease is nothing but immunity that helps to keep the body free from the natural disease.

So, keeping the above in view, we can safely say that **immunity** and **Vital force** are two identical terms; that is to say **immunity is a physical name of the Vital force.**

Further, immunity is created by the introduction of the morbid produce the hypersensitive and allergic states in the body. Hahnemann's ideas regarding the theory and nature of chronic diseases have been corroborated by the modern investigators in the field of Allergy and Immunity type of response may be considered as analogous to the effect of the isopathic or homoeopathic remedy which is supposed to raise to the body resistance to infection by vital stimulation. So the following homoeopathic drugs can produce immunity *Variolinum, Morbilinum, Typhoidinum, Diphtherinum, Pertussin, Hydrophobinum* etc.

Q. 12.3. What is meant by Immune response ?

It means reaction of the body to foreign materials (or to its constituents, under certain conditions) resulting in formation of antibodies.

Q. 12.4. What are the factors responsible for immunity ?

1. **Phvsical Factors** (Reflex action) :

(a) Integrity of skin and living epithelium of skin and stratified squamous epithelium.

(b) The living epithelium of respiratory and alimentary tract secrete thick tenecious mucus which provides a protective coating, so that bacteria can penetrate with difficulty. The ciliated epithelium of respiratory tract by their ciliary movement helps of expel out foreign bodies, bacteria get entangles due to its stickiness and they are expelled out. This is why, lowering of muco-ciliary resistance of respiratory tract due to any factor will predispose to bacterial infection.

(c) The acid sweat liberated by skin helps to keep the skin free from infection. In other words the sweat acts as anto-sterilising agents.

2. Chemical Factors :

(a) *Gastric Juice*—HCI content of stomach has a high bacterial action and it protects against infection of alimentary canal.

(b) *Lysozyme*— It has a bacteriocidal action and present in all secretion and excretion of the body except urine, sweat and C.S.F. It is present in maximum concentration in lachrimal secretion and cartilages. The conjunctiva is normally kept free from bacterial infection as it is bathed in lysozyme.

3. Celulo-Humoral Mechanisms :

Cellular Mechanism—The various—phagocytic cells of the system help in the process of phagocytosis of bacteria and latter on undergoes intracellular lysis. The following are the phagocytic cells:

(i) Cells of circulating blood—Polymorphos and Monocytes.

(ii) Cells in the tissue—These tissue cells concerned in phagocytosis and are of 2 types:

(I) Fixed called of particular organs:

(a) *Kuffer's cells of the Liver.*
(b) *Endothelial cells of bone marrow.*
(c) *Cells living in the sinus of the lymph gland.*

(II) Wandering cells—are also histocytes tissue and they are mononuclear cells.

**Actions of cellular components which help in immunity are :

(a) The cells liberate proteolytic enzyme which produce healing and immunity against infection.
(b) The cells also concerned with the formation of complement *Opsonin*—which add to defensive force.

(b) Humoral Mechanism:

(i) *Bacterial element in blood*—There are some bacteriocidal substances present normally in serum e.g. L-lysin, Lukin, Plakin etc.

(ii) *Antibodies like*—Agglutinin, Bacteriotropin etc, are produced in the serum which defensive against infection.

(iii) *Artificial immunity.*

This Immuinity results by artificial means. It is of 2 types, viz.,

(a) Active and (b) Passive.

*** How Immunisation are done for an Individual and Community ?**

1. ACTIVE ARTIFICIAL MEANS

This immunity results from a course of Specific vaccination or by infection e.g. T.A.B.C. Vaccine, Plague, Autovaccine etc.

Vaccines (including toxoids)

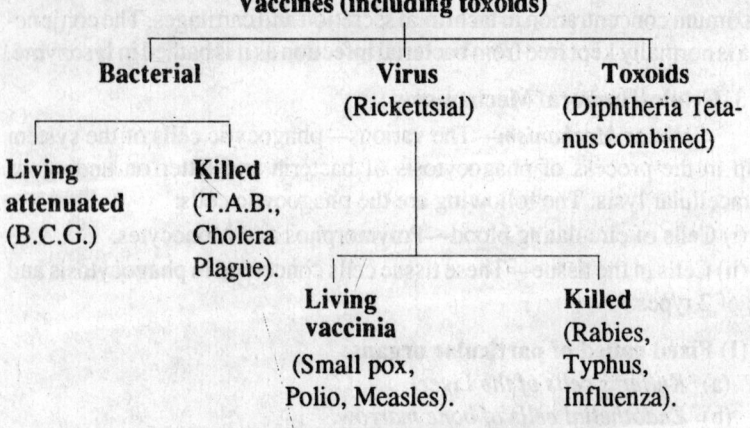

- **Bacterial**
  - **Living attenuated** (B.C.G.)
  - **Killed** (T.A.B., Cholera Plague).
- **Virus** (Rickettsial)
  - **Living vaccinia** (Small pox, Polio, Measles).
  - **Killed** (Rabies, Typhus, Influenza).
- **Toxoids** (Diphtheria Tetanus combined)

2. PASSIVE ARTIFICIAL MEANS

(a) **Serum Theraphy**—Readymade antibodies are supplied to the person through the serum. The serum used for passive immunity may be either of the following types:

(i) *Antitoxic serum*—Against Diphtheria, Tetanus, Gasgangrenes acts by neutrialisation of exotoxin liberated by bacteria with body.

(ii) *Antibacterial serum*—Against Pneumonia and eningococcus infections. Acts by destruction of bacteria and thereby preventing increase of endotoxin.

(iii) *Convalcent or antiviral serum* is also used against infection of Smallpox or Ant. polimyelitis etc.

(iv) *Bacteriophage therapy*—Recently passive immunity also be induced by bacteriophase therapy.

[N.B. Q. What do you meant by artificial immunity ? Describe the various methods by which it can be produced in a man.]

Q. 12.5. What is meant by Active Immunity and Passive Immunity? What are the differences between them? [D.M.S. 1974,77,78]

Active Immunity :

This type of acquired immunity produced by an individual due to introduction of micro-organism or their toxins in the body. The body cells take part in formation of antibodies to protect the individual e.g. smallpox vaccination, prophylactic inoculation of typhoid fevers.

Passive Immunity :

The person is immunised by prepared antibodies and the body cells do not take active part in production of immunity, e.g. Anti-diphtheric serum, Antitetanic serum.

Differences

Active Immunity	Passive Immunity
1. It is produced by cellular activity of individual. It is not borrowed or preformed.	1. It is always preformed or borrowed and not related cellular activity of a person.
2. Produced by: (i) Suffering from the disease. (ii) Useing vaccine. (iii) Repeated subclinical infection.	2. Produced by : (i) Inheritance. (ii) Serum therapy.
3. Takes 8 to 10 days to develop.	3. No time is lost. Immunity develops as soon as serum therapy is instituted.
4. During first 8 to 10 days the person is more susceptible and has no antibody.	4. No such negative phase, as the effect is immediate.

5. It is long lasting.	5. Duration is very short.
6. Reaction is severe and it may be local or general.	6. Reaction negligible except that due to protein shock.
7. Main use in prophylactic.	7. Main use in threapeutic.
8. Cannot be inherited.	8. Can be inherited from mother.

Q. 12.6. What is meant by Antigen?

The term **antigen** is used to describe any material usually of a complex nature, that stimulates a specific bodily immunity because the body recognises it as foreign. More than one component of the structural pattern of an antigen can be recognized by the immunological system as foreign; each component so recognises is known as an *antigenic determinate*. An antigen can be modified by the addition of a simple chemical group, which acts as an antigenic determinant and is called Hapten (Greek Haptain, to grasp).

So, *an antigen is a substance which, when introduced into the tissue of an animal, stimulates the formation of specific neutralizing substance or antibody, with which it reacts specifically in some detectable (observable) way.*

Or, *An antigen is a substance which, when introduced into the body of a susceptible antimal, leads to an immnue response producting a specific change—so that when the substance (antigen) is introduced on a subsequent occasion, the response obtained is altogether differ from that in the first time.*

Various antigens are:

1. According to antigenic constituents :

(a) *True antigens or Immunogens*—Higher molecular weight proteins having antigenic property de-novo.

(b) *Haptens* or *incomplete antigens*—Low molecular weight, non-protein substances, having little or no antigenic properties; but they acquire antigenic property when they combine with proteins to form new-antigens.

2. According to antigenic specificity :

(a) Species specific antigens.
(b) Organs specific antigens.
(c) Heterophile antigens.

(d) Allo antigens.
(e) Auto antigens.

Q. 12.7. What is meant by Antibodies ?

An antibody is a specialized protein (called an immunoglobulin) *that is liable to combine especially with an antigen.* After antibodies are released from the cell in which they are synthesized they enter body fluids and are responsible for specific protective properties, sometimes called humoral immunity, that are present, especially in blood. Antibodies also cause certain forms of hyperactivity or hypersensitivity to antigens. Other hypersensitivity reactions are caused by the mechanisms of cell-mediated immunity i.e. a manifestation of specific immunity that is not attributable to antibodies circulating in the blood stream but is the result of the action of certain cells (lymphocytes) reacting directly with an antigen and requiring the co-operation of scavenging cells called macrophages to extert some of their effects.

So an antibody is a specific substance produced in response to introduction of a specific antigen into the tissues of an animal, and which can react specifically with that antigen in some detectable (observable) ways.

An antibody is specific in its action. Specificity of an antibody depends on chemical structure of the individual immunoglobulins.

Various Antibodies:

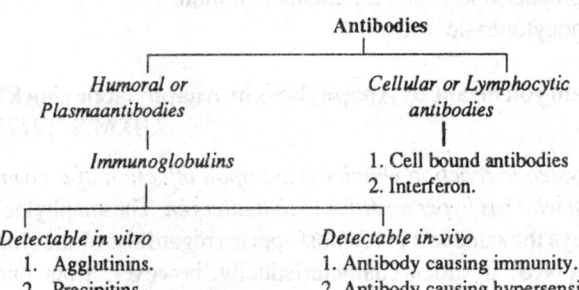

Antibodies

- *Humoral or Plasmaantibodies*
  - *Immunoglobulins*
    - *Detectable in vitro*
      1. Agglutinins.
      2. Precipitins.
      3. Amboceptors or lysins.
      4. Opsonins.
      5. Blocking antibodies.
      6. Neutralising antibodies:
         (i) anti-toxins.
         (ii) anti-enzymes.
    - *Detectable in-vivo*
      1. Antibody causing immunity.
      2. Antibody causing hypersensitivity.
- *Cellular or Lymphocytic antibodies*
  1. Cell bound antibodies
  2. Interferon.

Q. 12.8. What do you meant by Antigen-antibody reactions or Serological reactions?

Serology is study of reactions between antigen and antibodies. It attempts to qualitate these reactions by keeping one reagent constant and diluting the other.

Antigen-antibody reactions or Serological reaction are used to identify antigen or antibodies if either of these reagent is known. They are also employed to estimate the relative quantity of these antigens and antibodies. Thus the level or titre of antibodies in the serum or man or animal can be determined by mean of known antigens and conclusions can be drown regarding past contact of the host with the antigen. This is particularly valuable in the diagnosis of infection of certain forms of hypersensitivity. Conversely by means of known antibodies, the various antigens of a micro-organisms or other biological material which characterise it may be identified. The various methods used for demonstrating antibodies are as follows :

1. Precipitation reactions.
2. Agglutination reactions.
3. Toxin-Antitoxin reaction.
4. Bactericidal and lytic reaction.
5. Complement Fixation reaction.
6. Nutralisation reactions.
7. Immobilization test for Treponema pallidum.
8. Opisonocytophasic tests.

Q. 12.9. What do you meant by Anaphylaxis or Anaphylactic shock? [D.M.S. 1977]

It is an acute systemic reaction which occurs upon infection of a given allergen into a host which is hypersensitive to that allergen. The anaphylactic reaction is always the same in a given host species regardless of the type of of antigen involved. It varies characteristically, however, from one species to another. The reaction is specific and second dose of allergen of a different nature from a different animal will not produce any symptoms. *Anaphylaxis is an antigen antibody reactian in which antigen is called anaphylactogen and antibody as anaphylactin. This is a form of immediate allergic or hyper sensitivity reaction.*

The following conditions are necessary to produce anaphy laxis—

(i) *Sensitizing injection*—An adequate sensitizing dose of antigen is required.

(ii) *A Waiting period*— 2 to 3 weeks.

(iii) *Eliciting injection*—The rapid intravenous or intracardic injection of massive dose (0.1—10 mg of protein) the same antigen as was used for sensitizing injection].

13. AIDS
(Acquired Immuno Deficiency Syndrome)

Few disases in recent times have aroused as much fear and attention as AIDS. Though scientists have succeeded in isolating and 'figer-printing' the dreaded virus HTLV III as probable killer—direct evidence of causality has yet to be produced. Over 17,000 cases have already been reported in the US, half of which have been fatal. France has reported 300 cases, Great Britain 184, and West Germany 160. In Central Africa it is widely prevalent in Zaire, Ruanda, Burundi, Kenya, Uganda and Tanzania. In Aisa AIDS has yet to made its appearance. The news of AIDS being detected in our country (India) has created an unnecessary and unwarranted fear in minds of the people. The six cases detected in Madras are not full blown cases of AIDS. In fact, none of the six patients seen to have developed any sings and symptoms of AIDS even though tests have confirmed that all of them of are positive for AIDS virus antibodies.

Q. 13.1. What is AIDS ?

AIDS (Acquired Immuno Deficiency Syndrome) is an illness in which the body's immune system (i.e. natural defence against infection and disease) is destroyed to a great extent. Body has an army to cope with germs from outside as well as from those who have turned against the body like Cancer cells. Because of 'AIDS' the body is not able to fight against diseases and he comes defenceless. Such a person becomes susceptible to 'opportunistic infection' with those organisms which do not cause disease in normal healthy persons and may develop diseases such as pneumonia, white patchs inside the mouth and nodules in the skin.

Q. 13.2. What causes AIDS ?

AIDS is caused by a virus (probable Virus HTLV III (Human T-cell Lymphoma Laukaemia Virus.) which infects cells in the blood.

Not every one with the virus develops AIDS or even falls sick.

Very few get full-blown disease only about 10 out of 100 persons on the average who have the virus develop the syndrome, about 25 persons have mild symptoms and the remaining are free from symptoms.

Q. 13.4. How do diagnosis AIDS ?

AIDS is difficult to diagnose. The diagnosis is based upon a spectrum of signs, symptoms and various laboratory parameters. Blood tests is a complex one.

Q. 13.5. What are the early signs and symptoms of AIDS ?

(i) Significant and unexplained weight loss.
(ii) Swollen glands.
(iii) Fever and night sweats and malaise.
(iv) Persistent watery diarrhoea.
(v) Oral or/and oesophageal candidasis.

Having any of these signs and symptoms necessarily confirm the diagnosis of AIDS. They may occur in other diseases as well.

Q. 13. 6. What is the Incubation period ?

The incubation period is the time before the entry of germs and appearance of symptoms and signs of the diseases. The mean incubation period is about 29 months in adults and about 12 months in children, however, some cases with shorter incubation periods or longer incubation periods upto five years have been reported.

Q. 13.7. Who are the Groups "at risk" ?

1. Homosexual men having a large number of different sexual partners.
2. Drug users who use common syringes of injecting drugs.
3. People who receive transfusions of blood or blood products i.e. haemophiliaes and person with coagulation disorders.
4. Babies born to mothers with AIDS.

Treatment :

Various medicines have been tried in the treatment of AIDS but relatively little success. Antiboitics used to treat specific infection, are the only treatment that ameliorates the symptoms of AIDS. Scientist are now investigating the definite causes of this disease and its proper treatment.

Conclusions:

There is no magic bullet for the treatment of AIDS, however, we must inform citizens that our great enemies are **"The Virus, Ignorance and Blatant Prejudice".**

14. PEPTIC ULCER

Q. 14.1. What are the different sites of peptic ulcer ?

1. Gastric ulcer— occuring in relation to lesser curvature and its adjacent anterior and posterior surfaces which normally corresponds with the food canal.
2. Duodenal ulcer—occuring in the 1st part of duodenum commonly on its anterior surface.
3. Gastrojejunal ulcers following gastrojejunostomy.
4. Peptic ulcers in Mekel's diverticulum.
5. In the terminal (introgastric part) of the oesophagus.

14.2. Describe the morbid anatomy of Gastric ulcer.

1. Site : Commonest site is in the region of lesser curvature and its adjacent surfaces at least 2" above the pyloric end ulcer may be situated in the pylorus.

2. Number : Usually single. In 5 to 10% of cases it may be multiple.

3. Size : Usually less than 1" in diameter (gastric ulcers having diameter larger than 1" should be taken to be ulcerative type of carcinoma).

4. Shape : Usually it is funnel shaped. Superficial ulcers may be oval or round in shape.

5. Floor : It is always deep, usually formed by the serous coat. The muscle coat at the floor is always destroyed and there is a circular gap in muscle coat. The floor feels indurated.

6. Corresponding serous coat : It looks pearly white in colour, hard and cartilagenous to feel (hence it is said that G.U. are better palpated than seen from outside). The thickened serous coat is puckared and tags of omentum. Adjacent coats of intestine etc. are usually seen adherent to it.

7. Margin : They are always steep or may be sloping. The cardiac end of the ulcer is steeper than its pyloric end.

14.3. Microscopical appearance of Gastric Ulcer :

A progressive chronic gastric ulcer has the following features :

1. Most superficially a zone of acute inflammatory cells consisting of polymorphs, mononuclear cells and there is breach in the continuity of mucosal line.
2. The muscle coat at the site.
3. A zone of fibrous tissue proliferation at the base of the ulcer.
4. The vessels show endarteritis obliterans.
5. The muscle fibres spread out in fanwise manner from the periphery of the ulcer and ultimately fuse with the muscularis mucosa.

14.4. Healing of Peptic Ulcer :

Once the ulcer becomes chronic it shows better tendency for healing. Healing is retarded because of the following factors :

1. The part is constantly exposed to irritant acid gastric juice which sets up irritation.

2. Necrotic slough present at the base of the ulcer covers, the granulation tissue and provides no footing for the growing epithelium. The dense layer of scar tissue interfers with healing preventing approximation of the edges of the ulcer.

3. Endarteritis oblierans of the vessels interfere with blood supply so that the part becomes more and more devitalised.

Because of all these factors gastric ulcer once formed becomes gradually progressive. It may show some amount of healing just to recur within a short period.

14.5. Difference between Ulcerative type of carcinoma and Gastric ulcer undergoing malignant change.

Ulcerative Type of Carcinoma i.e. Cancer Ulcer	G.U. Showing Malignant Change i.e. Ulcer Cancer
1. Site usually at the pyloric	1. Usual site is lesser curvature

region.	and its anterior and posterior surfaces about 2-4" above the pyloric region.
2. **Size** — Diameter of the ulcer is always larger than 1".	2. **Size** — It is usually less than 1".
3. The condition of the muscle coat at the floor — muscle fibres are present but are infiltrated with yellowish white streaks of tumour tissue producing gramentation of the muscle coat.	3. Muscle coat at the region is completely destroyed and there is a circular gap or deficiency in it.
4. Regional lymph glands — are involved. They are enlarged, hard to feel.	4. Less involved except in a late case where the glands have the features of metastatic lymph node.

Microscopical :

A chronic gastric ulcer undergoing secondary carcinomatous change will show the following positive features :

1. It is the edge of the ulcer which is carcinomatous, not the base. So loops of malignant cells are present only at the edge and are seen infiltrating into the healthy area.
2. Complete destruction of underlying muscle coat.
3. Dense scar tissue at the floor.
4. Endarteritis of blood vessels.

All these features are not seen in ulcerative type of carcinoma. Tissue taken from any part of the ulcer will show presence of carcinoma.

14.6. Complications of Peptic ulcer :

1. Haemorrhage : Both haematemasis and malaena may be the result. It is due to erosin of the blood vessels caused by desperation of the necrotic slough during formation of ulcer. Haematemasis is a feature of gastric ulcer usually whereas malaena is a feature of duodenal ulcer.

2. Perforation : This is very common as the ulcers are very deep seated, floor being formed by the serous coat. The peritonitis resulting from perforation is at first non-infective and sterile but later on there is invariable bacterial infection due to reflex inbinition of gastric and secretion. The perforation may be either complete or may be leaking in type when there is slow leakage of contents into the periforeum. Such leaking perforation is often closed by mental adhesion.

3. **Perigastric adhesion** : Adhesions are quite common with the pancreas, the greater omentum, liver, transverse colon etc. Due to retraction of these fibrous bands the stomach may get distorted in its shape.

4. **Pyloric obstruction** : This is usually seen in duodenal ulcer when the duodenal bulb gets deformed, distorted. Gastric ulcer deep situated no doubt may give rise rarely to pyloric obstruction.

5. **Honour glass deformity** : This is invariably seen during healing up of gastric ulcer. The dense ring of scar tissue formed divides the stomach into two segments. The pyloric segment is usually smaller than the cardiac one. The communication between these two sacs through the narrow opening is never situated at the lowest point, because it is the greater curvature which is approximated on to the corresponding part of the lesser curvature at the site.

N.B. : Malignancy :

This is never seen in duodenal ulcer. The frequency of malignant change in gastric ulcer usually seen in 5—25% of cases. About the diagnosis of malignant change there is lot of controversy. Some consider the presence of distored proliferated glands present in deeper coats in the stomach will be diagnostic of malignant change, others hold that such appearance of glands may be the usual feature of gastric ulcer undergoing healing and according to latter view limited number of cases of gastric ulcer (5% only) show real malignant change.

15. CARCINOMA OF STOMACH

This is the most malignant tumour often in male. It is dangerous because of its rapidity of growth, deep seated position, insidious onset.

Incidence of the disease is most common in Spain, Holland etc. which is explained by Hust on the basis of dietary defect in people of these countries. The important predisposing factors :

Chronic gastritis, gastric ulcer are worth considered. Excessive smoking, use of alcohol, intake of hot heavily spiced foodstuff, orel sepsis etc.

predispose the disease by precinitation gastritis.

15.1. Site of origin :

About 60% of gastric carcinoma arise from the pyloric region, 20% from the lesser curvature and cardiac end and rest from greater curvature.

15.2. Types of gastric carcinoma. (Naked Eye Classification)

1. *Ulcerative type.*
2. *Proliferative or papillary type.*
3. *Mucoid or colloid type.*
4. *Infiltration type :*
   (a) Localised or anular type.
   (b) Diffused or leather bottle type or linitus plastica.

1. Ulcerative type :

Very common in pyloric region although no part of the stomach is exempted the ulcer possesses the features of malignant ulcers — edge of which are raised, rolled out, erected; base of the ulcer feels hard and indurated. The diameter of ulcer is usually longer than 1". The depth of the ulcer extends to the submucuous coat but in advanced cases the depth may extend on the serous coat. Both local and distal spreads are very marked in this type.

Cut section shows marked thickening of the wall of ulcers c scattered yellow areas of necrotic tissue.

2. Proliferative type :

Commonly occurs in the body of the stomach where it projects as a massive, bulky, soft, cauliflowers like growth and when present in pyloric region it precipitates pyloric obstruction due to its bulky size.

As the growth is very soft, superficial ulceration and necrosis is very common. It is very commonly secondarily infected leading to marked cochexia. The local spread in the wall of the stomach is not so marked as in previous type.

3. Colloid or Mucoid type :

This should not be considered as a special type, becuase it represents the change of mucoid degeneration on the other types of gastric caroinoma. The growth as a rule starts from the pyloric region and c̄ in a short period it involves the surface paritoneum and cause adhesion to surrounding structures like liver, spleen, omentum etc. is very common. The growth is translucent and c̄ the above structure the tumour is included in a gelatinous casing.

4. Infiltrative type :

(i) Annular variety :

This occurs in the pyloric region where hard, whitish growth is seen to encircle the pyloric region is in the form of dense annular ring.

The part of stomach above the growth is markedly dilated and hypertrophied and pyloric obstruction is very common in this type over the localised area of growth, the stomach feels markedly hard due to fibrous thickness and cuts c̄ resistance.

(ii) Diffuse type :

Growth starts in the pylorus and proceeds upwards and in established cases the whole stomach right from pylorus to cardiac end is affected, spread is absolutely localised to the stomach wall. Distal metastasis is late and rare (Beast malignant form of gastric carinoma).

Growth never extends to duodenum. The stomach itself is thickened, rigid and grossly shrunken and atrophied so much so, that the length of organ may be reduced to 4" only. (Normally 12") and the capacity of the organ may be reduced to 4 oz only (Normal being 40-50 oz).

The mucous membrane of the stomach is hypertrophied and shown prominent rugosity. It is congested, oadematous c superficial ulceration. Cut section through the stomach wall shows whitish streaks of malignant growth passing into deeper part of stomach causing segmentation of the muscle coat which is characteristic.

In the pyloric region from where the growth originates, an ulcer may be present which is probably the starting point. The serous coat of stomach is thickened and nearly white in colour.

15.3. Microscopic variety :

1. Adeno-caroninoma :

Tumours show numerous irregular imperfectly formed acini or gland — like structures lined by many layers of deep stained columner cells showing malignant character. The basement membrane of many cells is broken due to invasion of these malignant cells. The glands are separated by thin scanty stroma.

2. Carcinoma simplex :

Here the pattern of glandular structure is not at all reproduced. The tumour consists of solid irregular group of speroidel cells showing evidence of malignancy and individual groups separated by fibrous stroma. Depending on stroma and cells, of two types :

(i) Scirrhous type :

When clump of malignant cells are small and these are separated by excessive fibrous stroma.

(ii) Encephaloid type :

Which is the most malignant form and tumour shows large solid groups of cells separated by thin strands of stroma.

3. Colloid caroinoma :

The tumour cells become round due to mucoid degeneration showing c nodules pushed towards the periphery. These so-called signar ring cells showing malignant characteristics of nuclei are characteristic. Evidence of mucoid degeneration is also seen is stroma or supporting tissue of the tumour.

4. Epidermoid carcinoma-Rare variety :

It originates either from the lower end of oesophagus or it may be seen when the growth is superimposed on mucosa stomach undergoing squamous metaplasia.

15.4. How spreads ?

Gastric Carcinoma

1. Local spread :

In the wall of the stomach. This is marked in the infiltrating variety, leather bottle type, though to some extent it is also seen in other types.

Local spread occurs both by the process of infiltration and by way of Lymphatics. Lymphatic spread occurs mostly in submucous coat and evidence is seen far beyond the actual ulcer called growth and even more distinctly there is evidence of microscoprical spread. This local spread.

down or upwards from the pylorous will be causing either pyloric obstruction or oesophageal obstruction in many cases.

2. Distant spread : This takes place by :

(a) A simple process of infiltration as a result of which adjacent structures like greater omentum, liver, head or pancreas are commonly involved. Rarely the spleen or transvers colon may be affected.

(b) Spread via Blood stream:
This is rather rare and late in appearance. Spread by way of blood vessels will cause metastasis in lungs, bones, brain and kidney.

(c) Spread by transcoelomic implantation :
When the growth involves the serous coat of the organ many of the malignant cells fall off and drop down into the peritoneal cavity. These are later on deposited on the structures of pelvic floor involving both ovaries (This metastatic carcinoma of varies is called kruchenbergis tumour), the broad ligaments and other structures of pelvic floor.

(d) Spread to lymph glands :
This is the commonest mode of spread and occurs quite early. The glands involved will very accordingly to the site of primary growth. When the growth is situated in the pylorus or lesser curvature due to lymphatic spread there is affection of:

(i) Lower coronary group of glands situated inbetween the layers of the lesser omentum in relation of destal part of the lesser curvature. From these glands there is further spread to upper coronary glands and to glands of coeliac exis and paraortic glands. By retrograde spread from glands in coeliac exis there may be affection of glands at portahepatis from where the liver may be involved.

(ii) In some cases there is spread to pyloric and subpyloric glands occuring inbetween it and the head of the pancreas. From these glands there is affection of the supra paucreatic glands and the root of the mesentry these later group of glands when enlarged due to metastasis may be mechanically pressing duodenal obstruction.

In rare cases where the growth is situated near the greater curvature there is affection of gastro-epiploric group of gland situated in between the layers of gastrocolic ligament in the greater omentum. These glands subsequently drain into the pyloric and subpyloric group of glands so that further spread will be like that mentioned above.

16. CARCINOMA OF LIVER

(I) Primary :

Primary carcinoma of liver includes :

1. *That originating from liver cells which is called Hepatoma.*
2. *That originating from lining epithelium of biliary passage is called cholangioma.*

(A) Hepatoma or primary liver cell carcinoma :

The incidence of this type of tumour is becoming far more common than gas previously thought.

In the past all carcinoma of liver were practically though to be secondary but detail and careful study have revealed that hepatoma are common.

Hepatoma constitutes about 92% of primary liver carcinoma and extremely common in male above 40 years. (Males are affected in 96% of cases).

Etiology

It has been suggested that the tumour originates from hyperplastic and regenerated liver lobules in cases of portal cirrhosis where the process of hyperplasia goes far beyond the healthy limit. This is why in more than 90% of cases hepatoma are associated with cirrhosis of liver. The disease is extremely common in South Africa, Gava, Malay etc. where the diet is specially deficient in case in riboflavia. Experimental evidence also shows that such tumour of liver may be experimentally produced in the liver of mice by treatment c azodyes, if the diet is made deficient in cassin and ribo flavin.

(a) Naked eye examination:

1. Liver is small and atrophic because of cirrhotic change (Here describe the appearance of cirrhosis of liver). Cut section will show a solitary massive growth with irregular infiltration into the surrounding liver tissue. There is absence of fibrous capsule. The growth very commonly shows necrosis and haemorrhage. Besides the main growth, the outline of the liver tissue may show a few scattered nodules of growth.

2. Rarely throughout the liver tissue there are multiple scattered nodules of growth. This is supposed to be due to multicentric origin of the tumour.

(b) Microscopical examination :

1. There are irregular solid groups of large deepstain malignant cells which appear to the polyhedyal in shape.

The cells are arranged in the form of interlacing strands but rarely they show alveolar arrangement.

2. Presence of tumour giant cells.

3. Tissues near the growth commonly show evidence of necrosis and haemorrhage.

4. Besides the tumour proper the rest of the liver tissue will show the picture of cortal cirrhosis microscopically.

(B) Cholangioma : This is another form of primary liver carcinoma which is rather rare (8%). The tumour in this case originates from the lining epithelium of biliary passage.

Naked eye examination :

Liver shows multiple scattered small nodules of growth which are usually bite staired. Liver is not at all shruken or atrophic as the disease is not related to portal cirrhosis. On the other hand the size is either normal or enlarged.

Microscope :

The picture is one of adenocarcinoma. The tumour giant cell is usually absent.

(II) Secondary Carcionoma of Liver :

This is the most commonest type of liver carcinoma because liver is the size of metastasis from primary growth elsewhere in the system very commonly.

Metastatic carcinoma may originate by :

1. **The process of infiltration :** From the carcinoma of the head of pancreas, pylorus of stomach, gall bladder and transverse colon. Liver shows firm adhesion c those structure as the growth infiltrates by sending claw like process.

2. Way of lymphatics: From the growth occuring in its organs mentioned above.

3. Way of portal vein : This is the commonest route by which the liver is involved and about 50% of liver carcinoma originate in this way. Primary growth in these cases is either in the stomach or lower and of oesophagus, rectum and other parts of the large gut.

4. Way of hepatic artery:

This mode of origin is rather rare, and primary growth in these cases in the lung, uterus, prostrate, kidney, breast, bones etc.

Naked eye examination :

Liver is usually enlarged and cut section shows multiple localised nodules of varying sizes c clear out outline. The nodule is either bile stained or they are deeply stained and haemorrhagic.

They are very firm when palpated through the rest of healthy liver tissue. There is no zone of fibrosis surrounding the nodules and the nodules occur both on the surface and in the liver tissue substance (of Gumma of Livers).

Central part of the nodules often undergo necrosis as it is deprived of the blood supply, as a result of which the central part is depressed which is called *umbelicution.*

The multiple character of growth is due to invasion of large tributaries of portal vein due to which there is spread througout the organ. The haemorrhagic areas c in the nodules look dark red or black.

Microscope :

There is typical picture of secondary liver carcinoma.

The appearance of tumour will very according to the nature of the primary growth, from which there has been a spread to the liver. We either get adeno-carcinoma or spheroidal cell carconoma like scirrhous or encephaloid variety.

17. LOBAR PNEUMONIA

It is a process of consolidation or solidification of lung, alveoli, lobar in distribution. The air present within the alveoli is absorbed and replaced by collection of inflammatory exudate.

17.1. Etiology

A. Predisposing Cause :

(1) Young adults suddenly exposed to chill and cold.
(2) Trauma of the chest with or without fracture of rib.
(3) As a complication of chronic debilitarory disease like subacute nephritis, chronic Kala-azar. Diabetes Mellitus.
(4) In chronic alcoholism.
(5) Any cause of prolonged fatigue.

In all these conditions the normal mucocilliary resistance of the respiratory tract is broken so that organisms inhaled can easily enter the depth of the alveoli.

B. Exciting Cause:

Causative Bacteria :

(1) Pneumococcus in about 95 p.c. of cases. Infection of type I and type II pneumococcal infection is commnest and that by type II though rare cause fatal type of infection. Infection by type IV is very rare.

(2) Friedlander's Pneumobacillus in about 5% cases.

17.2. Pathogensis

Under the condition of lowered mucocilliary resistance, the causative organism can pass down through the respiratory tract, ultimately reaching the alveoli the route of infection is debatable. It was so long believed that pneumococci inhaled lower down the air passage, thus pass from the wall of the brochi by means of lymphatics of interstitial tissues of lung—ultimately reaching the wall of the alveoli (Backdoor Theory). But recent idea is that the organisms are directly inhaled into the depth of the alveoli and initially there is massive collection of oedema fluid in which the pneumococci actively multiply lying embodded within a thick plug of mucous. Phagocytic cells of the body cannot reach the area because of the aggression toxin liberated by pneumococci. During the process of coughing a wave is set within the oedema fluid which passes from one alveoli to the adjacent one through minute pores present in the septum called "Intra-alveolar pores of cohn". In this way there is progressive spread in infection from one alveoli to the other and the spread is also guided by the posture of the patient and the action of gravity, the process of collection of the inflammatory exudate is only intercepted by that of interlobar septum. This explains the lobar distribution of the disease. In case of massive infection organisms may overflow into circulation causing septicaemia, and by subsequent localisation in different organs it may cause purulent lesion like meningitis, endocarditis, pericarditis, arthritis etc.

The process of healing consists of removal of the inflammatory exudate and this process is so complete that it usually leaves behind no complication. It is so because there is no necrosis of lung parenchyma proper in case of lobar pneumonia (cf. Broncho-pneumonia). At first the exudate is liquified by proteclytic enzyma liberated by disintegrated polymorph and bacteria. This liquified substances is subsequently removed by:

(1) *Major part is coughed out as expectoration.*

(2) *Partly carried by the phagocytic cells to the regional lymph node later on to blood stream.*

(3) *Part of it undergoes simple process of diffusion in the blood vessels present in the wall of the alveoli.*

17.3. Pathology :

The disease passes through the successive stage of congestion, Red hepatisation, Grey hepatisation and resolution. Lesion starts from the hilum and progress towards the periphery. This is so because tissue at different depth of the same loby may be passing through different stages.

1. **Stage of Congestion**: 1-2 days. Only change is marked dilatation of vessels in wall of the alveoli and the alveoli themselves contain oedema fluid.

2. **Stage of red Hepatisation**: 3-5 days. N.E. Appearance. The affected lobe is voluminous, yellowish brown in colour, firm and solid to feel. The pleura on the surface is thickened due to fibrinous deposition.

(a) **Cut surface** : Dry and granular cut section sinks in the water.
(b) **Microscopical App.**: All alveoli are filled up with acute inflammatory exudate, consisting of mainly R.B.C., few polymorphs and plenty of fibrin flakes i.e., no gap between the exudate and the wall of the alveoli. The most important characteristic of the exudate is that it looks very fresh with clear and alveolar septa are thickened due to oedema, congestionby the same type of cells.

3. Stage of Grey Hepatisation: 5th - 7th day.

a) N.E. App.: Changes are like the previous stage c̄ the following exceptions:

(i) The colour of the lobe is greyish yellow.

(ii) Cut surface is moist because degeneration starts in constituent of the exudate at this stage.

b) Microscopic App.: The exudate filling up the alveoli is composed of plenty of polymorph, a few mononuclear phagocytic cells, a few R.B.C. and amorphous fibrin. The fresh character of it is altogether lost so that cellular outline appears hazy and the nuclei are indistinct. There is usually a gap between the exudate and the wall of the alveoli.

4. Stage of Resolution: 7th day onwards.

(a) *N.E. Appearance* : The affected lobe presents a translucent, jelly like appearance and the cut section is very moist. The regional lymph nodes are markedly enlarged.

(b) *Microscopic Appearance*: The cellular constituent of the exudate show evidence of necrosis and liquifaction. There is edvent of large phagecytic cells derived from R.E. system. They are so-called septal cells.

18. BRONCHOPNEUMONIA

Here the process of consolidation is patchy in nature and essential lesion is inflammation of bronchocle.

Causative Bacteria: (1) Streptococcus haemolyticus.
(2) Staphylo aurous or albus.
(3) Pneumo aurous albus.
(4) Haemophilus influenzae.
(5) Friodlanders pneumobacillus.
(6) Virus.

18.1. Etiology and Types :

1. **Primary bronchopneumonia**: Mostly seen in children. Children are commonly affected because of: (a) short and wide bronchial tree which facilitates easy entry of organism, (b) poor cough reflex sc that the various irritants cannot be expectorated cut, (c) delicate mucous lining so that ciliary action or resistance is easily broken.

2. **Secondary Bronchopneumonia**: This usually follows either of the

following primary conditions:

(a) *Inhalation group* — When septic material after operation in the throat is inhaled into the depth of the lung.
(b) *Aspiration* — Septic material from either bronchiectatic cavity or lung abscess may be aspirated down the bronchopneumonia indistant lung tissue.
(c) *In disease* — Commonly follows acute infective fevers like diphtheria, measles, whooping cough etc.
(d) It may also follow chronic debilitating disease like ports cirrhosis, diabetes, S.A. nephritis and chronic nephritis, kala azar etc.

18.2. Pathogensis : When the mucociliary resistance is lowered the causative organisms are inhaled in the depth of the lung tissue and primary change is bronchiolitis. This will lead to obstruction in the bronchiole and surrounding alveoli will undergo absorption collapse whereas those situated paripherally will show compensatory emphysema. To start with the disease is bilateral and the patchy process of consolidation alternated with collapse and emphysema will be scattered all through the lung tissue.

As there is necrosis of the lung tissue proper like bronchiole alveoli etc., the disease heals up by replacement fibrosis and the fibrosed bronchicle easily dilates out resulting in bronchiectasis. As the process of healing is delayed, there is ample time for the exudate to be organised so that pulmonary fibrosis is also a possibility.

18.3. Pathology : Both lungs show patchy areas of consolidation which will be firm to — feel and the cut section of the affected lung will sink in water. There are also scattered areas of collapse which are deep purple in colour and slightly depressed from surface of the lung. The trachcheobronchial lymph nodes are enlarged.

Microscopic Appearance :

(1) *Area of Bronchiolitis* : The lining mucous membrane of the affected bronchiole is narrowed and desquamated into the lumen. The lumen also contains acute bronchiole is markedly thickened due to congestion, inflammatory oedema and infiltration by acute inflammatory cells.
(2) Surrounding alveoli are consolidated as is evident by collection as is evident by collection of inflammatory exudate within the
(3) Alveoli situated more distally are markedly dilated c thinned out

septum ruptured at places.

(4) The most periperally situated alveoli are normal.

19. PULMONARY TUBERCULOSIS

Types of lesion 2 :

1. Primary type or childhood type.

2. Reinfection or Adult type.

1. Primary lesion : This is seen in children and rarely in adult living in hilly regions or rural areas may have same type of lesion because since their childhood they do not come in contact c̄ tuberculous patient with the result that they behave as cases of primary infection.

Lesions of primary type essentially consists in formation of primary complex which have the following components:

(i) A caseous parinchymatons (lung focus). This is very small ½ - 1 cm. in diameter seen in any lobe of lung though common in rt. middle lobe it is usually solitary but 2-3 foci may be present. It is always supleural in position and deparated from the rest of the lung tissue by a fibrous capsuls.

(ii) Caseous Glandular Focus — The draining lymph glands are result enlarged and caseous and at times glandular and as focus may be larger than original lung focus.

(iii) The intervening Lymphatics — connecting caseous lung tracheobronchial glands. These also show tuberculous in the wall of these lymphatics.

In primary lesion the lung focus is called Ghon's focus may show focus may show scattered tiny tube rqles.

19.1. Fate of primary lesion : This will depend on the dose of infection and resistance on the part of the host.

(a) If resistance is good both lung and glandular foci may heal up by :

(i) Encapsulation and fibrosis.

(ii) Calcification and even oesification.

Massive radiography of children show such clacified foci is more than 92% of cases. The bacilli may remain viatis even when buroied c in the calcified mass. Even when lesion heals up it leaves behind the phenomena of allergy and immunity as future of events in the child's life will be decided by the balance between these two resultant processes.

(b) If resistance is poor as compared to infection the child will develop progressive primary lesion. This is invariable fatal and the usual compilation of which will be as follows:

(i) Either caseous lung or a glandular foucus burst into a blood vessels and pouring out numerous bacilli is circulation. The child will thus develop miliary tuberculosis.

(ii) The process of caseation may be scattered rapidly although the lung tissue as a result of either bronchogenic spread or via lymphatic. The caseous foci becomes confluent so that ultimately whole lobe may appear to be caseous or the process may be patchy also.

(Acute caseous pneumonia or sronchopneumonia). At some places solid caseous area may show softening and breakdown with the formation of acute type of cavities.

Thus child of primary tuberculosis will either recover completely from the process and share the resultant of allergy and immunity or it will invariable die of progressive primary lesion. Usually complication being generalised tuberculous or acute caseous pneumonia. Unlike tuberculosis of adult it does not show a chronic source and also there is never formation of chronic fibrolic cavities as in adults.

20. ADULT TYPE OF TUBERCULOSIS

Mode of Infection :

(1) **Exogenous:** There is fresh inhalation of massive dose of bacilli sufficient enough to break through the body resistance of the host.

(2) **Endogenous:** Some believe that infection may be due to flaring up and spread from the arrested primary lesion in case of devitalised condition.

20.1. Site of lesion : In contract to childhood type upper lobe of right lung is the commonest site. Rt. lung is more affected possibly because the rt. bronchus is almost direct continuation of tracher, so organisms once inhaled are easily carried down to Rt. bronchus and this is mainly due to *peculiarity of Rt. pulmonary artery* which is long and narrow wind round the nerte-divides-into many branches before entering through hilum.

Apical distribution of the lesion is difficult to explain. It has been suggested that the apical region has always restricted movements so that the part cannot be effectively bathed c blood and tissue fluid. More a tinfactory explanation is that normally pulmonary arterial pressure is minimum at the apex, specially in erect posture. Hence the apex has less supply of blood which meansless formation of tissue fluid so that antibody produced in the system cannot reach the area in adequate concentration. Thus condition becomes ideal for bacterial growth. Proof in favour of this hypothesis may be seen in cases of pulmonary tuberculosis, hypertension apical distribution of the lesion is difficult to explain.

20.2. Type of Lesion :

Besides dose of infection and resistance of the host types of adult tuberculosis is dependent on the balance between allergy and immunity confered during primary infection in childhood. Adult tuberculosis accordingly may be of following types :

(i) Fibroid type of lesion — where immunity predominates.
(ii) Fibrocaseous type — Commonest type seen in cases where there is a nice balance between allergy and immunity.
(iii) Acute caseous pneumonia.so-called galloping crisis.
(iv) Acute miliary tuberculosis.

The best two types are associated — marked allergic response and at the same time body resistance is much lowered.

1. Fibroid type of Tuberculosis : The lung feels firms and indurated due to pleural adhesion with the parieties. The scar is black due to arrest of carbon particles in the lymphatics which are strangulated by fibroid bands. There may be evidence of calcification when chalky white deposits are seen in the region. Cut section shows irregular bonds of fibrous tissue traversing through lung tissue.

2. Microscopically : The area shows marked proliferation of fibrous tissue c infiltration of Epithelod cells and lymphocytes. There is little or no caseation and giant cells are usually absent. Bluish granules of calcification may also be seen in Haematoxylin of Eosin stain.

3. Fbrocaseous type :

1. This type of lesion is seen when there is balance between allergy and immunity. Lesions are as follows:

(a) Caseous area undergoes softening and liquifaction and this liquified product is subsequently removed through draining bronchus leaving behind a cavity.

(b) Due to invasion of bronchioles by tubercular granulation tissue there is obstruction and consequent collapse of many alveoli. This exerts a pulling force which helps in increasing the size of the cavity.

(c) Due to obstruction there is some amount of bronchiectatic changes and due to this tuberculous bronchiectasis the cavity has a clear — cut sharp outline.

(d) Partly also there is retraction and shortening of the peribroncheclic fibrolic bands which contribute to the increase in size of the cavity.

In fibrocaseous tuberculosis the lining wall of the cavity is also caseous. There is absence of congestion in wall is usually smooth and fibrolic. The cavity is either empty or may be partly filled up with liquified caseous material. The vessels passing through the cavity usually show some neurysmal dilatation and due to lack of support they usually give way to severe haemoptysis.

2. Besides the cavity the adjacent lung tissue shows caseous areas of varying size. Some of these areas may show breakdown and later on inflammation of cavities.

3. The lung tissue also shows scattered tubercles greyish white in colour.

4. The evidence of fibrosis is not only seen in the wall cut section show numerous fibrolic bands passing through the frame work of lung.

5. The blood vessels and bronchi are also thickened and extensive adhesion c the parioties and diaphragm Lymph glands are usually spread.

***Microscopically :**

This type shows the usual histological picuture of tuberculosis c structureless hemogenous pink stained caseous area, infiltration of epitheloid cells giant cells (Langhans type), Lymphocytes and peripheral fibrolic proliferation. Adjacent alveloi shows presence of exudate within their lumen and distant alveoli show emphysema.

4. Acute caseous Pneumonia :

In this type not only the body resistance is poor but also allergy predominates for more as comapared to immunity which is practically none existing. The essential lesion is massive caseasion. There are numerous caseousfoci scattered although the lobe of the lung which developes due to spread via lymphatics and partly through broncholar tree. The caseous foci later on becomes confluent so that ultimately the whole lobe is converted into structureless caseous mass. The area may show breakdown at places formation of small acute cavities with raggesd necrotic wall.

The lumph glands are also enlarged and casecus. There is no evidence of fibrosis in cut section and then pleura is not much thickened. The disease runs a dramatic course and death is invariably due to massive tuberculous toxin.

Microscopically :

Caseation is extensive infiltration of epitheloid cells and lymphocytes. Giant cells are usually absent and there is no fibrobleastic proliforation. Caseous necrosis is 80 perfect that even elastic tissue stain does not reveal presence of such tissue in contrast to fibrocaseous type.

5. Acute Miliary Tuberculosis :

This results from rupture of caseous lung or glandular focus into blood vessels showing numerous bacilli in circulation when the foci ruptures into a branch of pulmonary artery we get miliary tuberculosis of lung only whereas when the rupture occurs into a trubutary of pulmonary vein — generalised miliary tuberculosis occurs.

Both lungs shows numerous tubercles scattered throughout the lung and they are of uniform size. To start with they are translucent and greyish white in colour but when caseation supervenes this becomes opaque and yellow. There is no congestion around these tuberculosis s and there is no evidence of fibrosis of lung tissue. The disease is invariable fatal and is associated with numerous tubercle in other visceras like spleen, intestine, liver, brain etc. Usual complication of which is that the patient dies of tuberculous meningitis.

Microscopically : There is area of multiple scattered tubercle in the inter alveolar septum. Alveoli themselves are altogether free. The tubercle in the septum do not show any giant cell and fibroblastic proliferation is absent.

*** N.B. Malignant Tumours of Lung**

A. Primary : (1) Bronchogenic carcinoma.
(2) Sarcoma — very rare.

B. Secondary : (1) Secondary carcinoma of lung.
(2) Sarcoma.
(3) Malignant melanoma.
(4) Chorion epithelioma.
(5) Hyper nephroma.

21. BRONCHOGENIC CARCINOMA

The incidence of Bronchogenic carcinoma of lung is probably far more than that was considered so long. In the past many of these tumours were diagnosed as sarcoma. But the improved technique of examination has shown conclusively that their nature is carcinoma.

Of the various predisposing factors excessive smoking is the most important. It is also believed that diseases like influenza, tuberculosis etc. may also predispose.

Hilar type : Commonest type appears as large greyish white growth arising from bronchial wall near the hilum of the lung. The lumph glands are also involved due to metastasis and enlarged glands along with growth casts shadow in X-Ray. It is origin from the concluded from the fact that there is either fibrous thickening in the bronchial wall (Annular type of growth) or rarely there may be white roughening of bronchial mucosa. The growth often projects into the lumen of bronchus as papillary mass precipitating obstruction or bronchocele.

Peripheral type of growth : This is evident as a small circumscribed mass in the extreme periphery of the lung almost subpleural in position. The growth occurs from the lining mucosa of finer ramification of bronchial tree. This type is ideal for surgical removal. The lung tissue surrounding the growth shown small nedules which are to be considered at secondary metastasis within the lung tissue as a result of lymphatic spread.

Miliary type: Small multiple scattered nodules of growth which resemble very much miliary tuberculosis of lung. The exact differentiation can be made by microscopical examination only.

Diffuse pneumonic type of growth: Such picture is seen when the growth within the lung spread very rapidly either by way of lymphatics or following the wall of bronchial tree throughout the entire lobe of the lung. The individual masses of growth becomes confluent later on so that it resembles the picture of pneumonic consolidation.

Associated Lung Changes :

The picture of Bronchogenic carcinoma is completely over shadowed by the secondary lung changes which the growth itself has produced. Such changes bronchiectatis collapse of lung, lung abscess, Pleural effusion. Bronchiectasis is due to bronchial obstruction and partly due to the lumen (ii) partly by pressure by the metastatic lymph node.

Collapse Atelectasis :

(1) Partly due so bronchial obstruction.

(2) Partly due to pressure by the fluid collected in the pleural cavity when the growth undergoes necrosis and breakdown and later on bacterial infection superimposed on it. The growth may be converted into a lung abscess.

B. Microscopical Varieties :

This may be of following types:

(a) **Adenocarinoma** :When the picture is one of numerous gland like spaces lined by many layers of malignant cells along c̄ invasion of basement membrane.

(b) **Medullary Carcinoma:** Here the large solid masses of malignant cells are arranged in groups and the individual groups are separated by thin fibrous stands of fibrous tissue. The picture of the gland is not reproduced.

(c) **Alvestar Carcinoma :** The names has been given on belief that malig tumour cells crep along the wall of bronchi and reaching the alveoli they provide the cellular outline of the alveoli but truly speaking this tumour has nothing to do with alveolar cells. They may be considered as secondary adenocarcinoma.

2. Epidermoid Carcinoma: This occurs when bronchial mucous membrane undergoes squamous metaphysis.

3. Anaplastic type of care: These group of tumours are even microscopically confused c sarcoma but careful examination shows presence of stroma inbetween the group of cells and not between the individual cells. Depending on the cell type aplastic carcinoma may be of following types:

(i) Spindle celled type.

(ii) Round celled type.

(iii) Oat celled type.
(iv) The most malig. form of bronchogenic carcinoma.

22. GLOMERULUNEPHRITIS

According to Valhard and Fahr the process passes through 3 successive stages. It starts as acute and passing through the subacute stage ultimately terminate as chronic. Though there are three stages they are not sharply demarcated and considerable overlapping may occur between the 3 stages.

22.1. Aetiology : The accepted view is that the condition results from allergy or lymph hypersen activeness kidney tissue to infection by B-haemolytic streptococci. The primary focus is usually situated in the throat and tonsil. The allergic basis of the disease is supported by the following facts:

(1) Proliferative character at the lesion.
(2) Absence of organisms of the site of lesion.
(3) Interval of 1-2 weeks lapsing between the throat infection and development of nephritis.
(4) In experimental animals identical lesions could be produced by infection of Masugis.

Nephrotoxic serum (serum prepared in one animal by injection of kidney tissues of another species of animal. If the latter animal receives injection of serum prepared in this way same type of lesion as seen in glomerulonephritis can be produced. This also proves that the basis of the disease is antigen antibody reaction in the kidney tissue itself which makes it hypersensitive.

(I) Acute Nephritis

Naked eye appearance—Both kidneys are enlarged, surface smooth, capsule strips off easily. In cut section the cortex is swollen up and looks pale as compared to the medulla.

M.C. Changes are mostly seen in glomeruli and to some extent in the tubules. Blood vessels or interstitial tissue usually escape.

1. Glomerular change—Majority of glomerali look enlarged and marked cellular changes are seen in all components of the glomeruli.

(a) *Change in the glumerular capilliary tuft:* Each glomerular capillery is narrowly lined by endethelial cells on the inner side and epithelial cells on the outer side which in the periphery becomes continuous c the lining cells there are two basement membrane, which are separated by few connecting cells. In acute phase there is marked proliferation of the endothelial cells and to some extent of the epithelial cells because of swelling and proliferation of the endothelium there is almost complete blockage of the capillary. Hence marked oliguria. The glomeruli infiltrate c good number of plymorphs which are also seen in between the two basement membrane.

(b) *Change in the capsular space:* There is compous exudation into the space of plasma, fibrins, polymorphs, R.B.C. and epithelial cells which are ultimately voided through urine.

(c) *Change in Bowman's capsuls*: The epithelial lining cells of Bowman's capsuls also show proliferation and fuse c the proliferated epithelial cells of the glomerular capillaries. The ultimate result is the glomerulus consists of cells all condensed together.

2. Tubular change : This is negligible so far as the dysfunction of the kidney is concerned in the disease. As tubulas have to depend for their blood supply on the glomeruli, occlusion of glomerular vessels will naturally lead to secondary degeneration like cloudy swelling, fatty degeneration of the lining cells of the tubulus.

*** Fate of acute nephritis :**

(1) In about 85% of cases there is complete resolutions, so much so that in future no structural abnormality could be detected.

(2) About 5% of cases will die of (a) hypertension and left ventricular failure, (b) hypertension excaphalopathy, (c) anaemia.

(3) In about 10% of cases the albuminuria persists and the disease passes to the subacute phase ultimately terminating into chronic. Usually after 6-8 weeks. It goes to subacute phase.

(II) SUBACUTE NEPHRITIS :

Naked eye appearance:

Both kidneys are enlarged and pale or white (large white kidney) capsuls strips as usual. Surface smooth, consistency is soft. In cut section the cortex is thinned and looks markedly pale as compared to medulla. The cortex may be traversed by yellow streaks or lines which represent lipoid deposit.

(a) M.E.

(1) Glomerular change : This will show a junctional phase—some glomeruli will show proliferative changes of the previous stage and some will show hyalinisation and scar of the chronic stage. The remaining glomeruli show compensatory hypertrophy. The space between the basement membrane is markedly increased due to deposition of protein layer by layer (hence the other name of the disease is membranous nephritis). Cellular infiltration in the glomeruli is much less marked as compared to acute. The capsular space now contains few R.B.C., pus cells, fair number of epithelial cells and copious protein materials. The lining cells of the Bowman's capsule still show proliferative changes but it is limited to a particular corner in the form of a cresent. These epithetial crescents are diagnostic of this phase though rarely they may be seen in S.A. bacterial endocarditis and kidney of malignant hypertension.

(2) Tubular change : They are very prominent and is seen most in cells of convoluted tubules. There is massive collection of neutral fat cholestord and its osters in the lining cells of convoluted tubules which can as demonstrated by special method of staining like sudan III scarlet red and blood vessels and interstitinal tissue do not show any change.

Fate of S.A. Nephritis :

(1) About 95% die of intercurrent infection. Infection is so common because massive albuminia causes hypo protinemia with the result that re-globulin content is much lower. This causes poor antibody response and hence the infection is often fatal.

(2) The rest passes on the the salerotic stage of chronic nephritis is resultant hypertension renal failure.

(III) Chronic Nephritis :

(a) Naked eye appearance:

Both kidneys are smaller atrophic capsule is thickened adherent to underlying cortex so that where stripped off there is decortication. The surface is granular may show retention cysts. Consistency is firm. Peritophic and paranephric fat is increased. In cut section there is marked atrophy of cortex which may be only 1 mm. wide. The normal cortical rays or lines show a distorted appearance.

(b) M.E. : Changes are seen in all forms components of the kidney.

1. Glomerular change :

(a) Majority show complete hylinisation. They are converted into structureless eosinstained homogenous mass. These may ultimately fuse c the interstitial tissues all being involved in fibrotic mass.

(b) Others show hypertrophy and they appear even more cellular.

2. Tubular change :

(a) Some tubules show extreme atrophy. They are small lined by flattened epithelium.

(b) Others are hypertrophic and lined by cubical epithelinum. These hypertrophied tubules may fuse forming large masses which project on the surface and they are the cause of granularity on the surface.

3. Change in blood vessels :

There is marked thickening of the blood vessels of kidney due to associated hypertension. Smaller vessels show hyaline degeneration, larger ones show elastosis. The effect of all these is to produce endarteritis.

4. Change in interstitial tissue :

This is increased in amounts and show proliferation of fibro us tissue scattered collection of inflammatory cells. Contractors of these fibrous tissue in the underlying kidney parenchyma causes the depressions in between the granules on the surface.

Character of Urine in Different Types of Nephritis

Physical Exam.	Acute	Sub-acute	Chronic
(a) Quantity	5-10 oz	15-20 oz	60-80 oz
(b) Sp. gr.	1025-1030	1025	more often fixed at 1010
(c) Appearance	Smokey or there may be frank haematuria.	Straw colour	pale straw
2. Chemical Exam.			
Albumin	Marked albuminuria 0.5-1%	Copious 2-3% or more	Trace

3. M.E.

(a) Pus cells	Fair numbers	A few or occasional	Nil.
(b) R.B.C.	Plenty	A few or occasional	Usually absent unless there is haematuria due to hypertension.
(c) Cast	Blood cast - Both R.B.C. or leukocytic cast are diagnostic .	Fatty cast are diagnostic through granular cast are also seen.	

N.B.: Epithelial cast, epithelial cells or hyaline cast may be present in any stage or Nephritis Hyaline casts. are found in normal urine.

4. Blood Bio-chemistry.

1. Protein	Normal except in the later part when it may be slightly low.	Marked hypoprotinaemia c̄ reversion of Albumin and globulin ratio. Oedema develops when protein level goes below 4 gm%.	Normal.
2. Cholesteral	Normal.	Increased, may be 300 mg% or more	Normal
3. Urea or N.P.N.	Slightly raised 50-60 mg%	Normal	Markedly raised may be 100 mg%

Fate of chronic nephritis :

Invariably fatal. The usual causes of death are :

(1) Uraemia.
(2) Hypertension and left ventricular failure.
(3) Cerebro-vascular accidents and coronary thrombosis.
(4) Intercurrent infection, specially respiratory tract.

22.2. Ellis concept of nephritis :

Ellis and his associates followed 600 cases of nephritis for about 20 years of which 200 could be post-mortemed. From the study be concluded that there are two different types of nephritis differing from each other in aetiology, mode of onset, clinical picture;and prognosis, this differing from the idea held by volhard and Far who considered nephritis to be a single disease having 3 successive stages of acute, subacute and chronic. According to Ellis there are distinct types 2 (1) *Type—nephritis* follows one to two weeks after sore throat. The onset sudden with haematuria and there is great constitutional disturbance like fever, vomiting etc. This corresponds c usual acute nephritis or the lesions are essentially proliferative. The fate is like that of acute nephritis c the exception that about 10% of cases passes directly into the chronic stage without passing through the nephrotic stage.

Type II Nephritis :

Aetiology is not known. Onset is insidious. There is never great constitutional disorder. The patient only shows copious albuminuria or hypoproteinaemia. This corresponds to so-called subacute nephritis the fate is identical. The main lesion is in the basement membre of glumrular capillaries which is markedly thickened due to deposition of protein and the picture is nothing but chronic membraneous nephritis. Through such hyperpermeable glomeruli there is massive leakage of protein. 95% cases die as usual of infection and 5% develop hypertension.

Change in kidney in hypertension :

In benign hypertension: In about 75% of cases the kidney looks smooth, only in long standing cases characteristic picture of granular contracted kidney is seen.

Microscopically the kidney looks exactly like that of chronic nephritis. The differentiation between the two is often impossible. The points which may be of help for differenting are the following:

Chronic Nephritis	Arterias chronotic Kidney
1. Size of kidney — less so.	1. More shrunken and atrophic
2. Size of the granules on the surface smaller.	2. Granules are larger
3. Appearance of kidney not so red looking as cortical atrophy is less marked.	3. As there is marked cortical atrophy the blood present within the underlying vessels will impart a redflush to the whole kidney.
4. Cut section — No such thickened and gaping vessels seen.	4. Section of gaping blood vessels is often seen specially and the base of pyramids.

Even microscopically it is very difficult to differentiate between the two conditions. Same types of changes in the glomerulus in the tubercular in the blood vessels and in interstetial tissue are seen. The only point which may be taken as suggestive or Chronic nephritis. presence of inflammatory cells in the conu.t. grame work of kidney may also point to chronic nephritis.

Change in malignant hypertension. As the temp of the process is very quick granular contracted kidney as seen in benign hypertension is very rare. The kidney is often enlarged surface is smoothend shows large blotchy haemorrhage both on the surface and also in the kidney substance.

Microscopically the change is essential vascular. Both cellular hyperplasia and necrotising arteriolitis are seen in the blood veseels (See chapter on vascular changes in hypertension). Involvement of kidney parenchyma is not a prominent feature. When present it is evident as :

(a) Areas of focal glomerulitis.

(b) Dilatation of the tubules.

It is the vascular lesion which is most important in causing uraemia which is the commonest cause of death.

23. NEPHROSIS

Previously the main lesion in nephritis was thought to be tubular degeneration but idea of the present moment is that though tubular changes are very prominent yet it is the glomelular lesion which has the main role in the genesis of the process. Now-a-days nephrosis is classified into two big groups depending on the structure mainly involved:

(1) Glomerulonephrosis :

This is the main cause of nephrotic syndrome which is characterised by massive oedema or anasarca, copious albuminuria marked hypoproteinaemia hypercholesterolaemia, normal cardio vascular findings in absence of renal insufficiency or azotaemia.

(2) Tuberbonephrosis :

Unlike the previous variety here the essential lesion is in the tubercles and it is characterised by oliguria or anuria. And terminal azotaemia. The lesion starts in the lower part of the nephron voz., loop of Henb, its ascending limb or in second convoluted tubules and hence it is often referred to as lower nephron nephrosis. This term is not so popular because in progress of the process it also involves the upper nephrosis.

23.1. Glomerulenephrosis :

The process in often characterised by nephrotic syndrome and changes are most important in the glomeruli. They are all made hyperpermeable so that protein of blood leak into the capsular spaces. The process includes the following diseases:

1. Lipoid nephrosis.
2. Amyloid nephrosis.
3. Intercapillary glomerulosclerosis. Seen in diabetes mallitus.
4. Nephroduct sclerosis seen in disseminated lupus erythematosue.
5. Nephrosis of pregnancy and texaemias of preganancy (Eclampsia).

(A) Lipoid Nephrosis :

1. *Glomerular change* :

The main lesion is thickening of basement membrane of glemerular capiliary tuft due to deposition of protein layer by layer (chr. membranous nephosis). This glomerular change is diffused and uniform so that practically noglomeruli are spared. The lesion is same as in S.A. nephritis or type 11 nephritis of Ellis because of which the disease is now synonymous c S.A. nephritis. It is because of this glomerular change that they are made hyperpermeable allowing basement membrane is thickened there is no occlusion of glomerular capillary tuft, in fact they are dilated.

2. *Tubular change* :

Microscopically this is always evident and lining epithelial cells of the tubules contain droplets of lipoid deposit in the tubules there may be seen yellow streaks or lines traversing the cortex.

(B) Amyloid Nephrosis :

The kidney is large and pale and presents similar appearance as seen in large white kidney of S.A. nephritis. The only point of difference being is the peculiar translucent waxy appearance in cut section and firm feel. Areas of amyloid look dark brown c application of iodine.

Microscopically structureless homogenous lesion stained amyloid at 3 sites :

(a) If the glomerular capillary tuft. There is increasing deposition of amyloid in between the basement membrane and capillary endothelium. The result is there is gradual occlusion of glomerul c subsequent atropy of kidney parenchyma or hypertension. It may terminate in granular contracted kidney.

(b) In the wall of blood vessels causing gradual thickening and occlusion of the vessels.

2. In the interstitial tissue :

Tubular changes will occur due to ischaemia caused by occlusion of glomeruli. The lining epithelial cells show hyaline and fatty droplets due to degeneration and at times their lumen may contain large homogeneous casts called colloid casts which are voided c urine.

(C) Nephrosis in diabetes mellitus or inter capillary glomerulo sclerosis. (Kiemmelstcist wilson lesion): True diabetic lesion is evident as:

1. Nodular type seen in about 33% of cases and is diagnostic and it is seen as a localised well defined homogeneous hyaline mass in the centre of the glomerulus and is produced by increase in intercapillary conn. T. Some consider these to be due to splitting up of capillary basement membrane. Others think them to be resulting fromexidation of plasma and fibrin in between the glomerular capillaries due to fat emboli plugging such vessels. Fat embolism results probably from liver.

2. *Diffuse*: Here the whole glomerulus from the hilum to the periphery becomes fibrillary and hyaline. This is not diagnostic and probably results from deposition of fibrinogen lipoid from the blood.

In addition to these two other changes may be seen in diabetes :

(a) Fibrin cap :

Hyaline material is deposition inbetween basement membrane capsular endothelium and the material gives staining reaction for fibrin.

(b) Capsular drop :

It is lipocarbohydrateprotein camphor deposited under the parieptal layer of doithelinum.

Wireloop sclerosis

The glomerular capillary membrane show patchy areas of thickening and it results from lupus erythematosus.

(D) Nephrosis in Pregnancy :

The main change is odema occuring in a space between two basement membranes of glomeruli because of which becomes thickened. Also there is swelling of capillary endothelium. This causes occlususion of glomeruli c̄ subsequent development of hypertension uraemia.

23.2. Tubulonphrosis :

The tubules are most affected in this group in contrast to this the glomeruli are practically spread. Two distinct varieties aetiologically different from each other are included under this group.

1. Toxic group caused by exogenous poisons like mercury, arsenic, carbon tetrachlor etc. When they are excreted via the kidney. The posion gets concentrated after reabsorption of water electrolytes by the tubule; thus exerting its harmful effect on the proximal part of the tubule which at first comes in contact c it. In 2-3 days the living epithelial cells are perfectly necrosed, desquamated into the lumen precipitating blockage. In about a week this collection within the lumen may clear up leaving behind the bare named tubules through when the glomerular filtrate readily passes into interstitial tissue hence fail to reach the urinary bladder causing persistence of oliguria or anuria.

2. Anoxic or Ischaemic group :

Practically speaking two different varieties of conditions belong to this:

(a) Conditions where anoxia or ischaemia is the only factor. This includes shock, burn, haemorrhage, trauma, intestinal obstrn. dehydration from any other cause etc. They are collectively known as 'shock kidney'.

(b) Conditions where both ischaemia action of toxins of unknown nature have a role. This includes incomparible blood transfusion, earnst syndrome and black water fever etc. The lesion in the anoxic group is most marked, at the boundary zone between cortex medulla involving the loop of Henle its ascending limb and its ocrtical extension called second convoluted tubule. Because this area receives blood supply last of all hence is very susceptible to ischaemia of even slight degree. In this belief the term lower nephron nephrosis was given but though initially it is so in no time it involves the proximal part also.

Naked appearance of Kidney :

Both kidneys are enlarged look markedly pale. Cut section presents a characteristic appearance in the form of marked pallor, swelling of cortex in contracts to the medulla which is intensely congested.

M.E :

1. Tubules show necrosis of lining cells which when desquated occupy the central whole of the lumen.
2. Collection of inflammatory cells like lymphocytes, plasma cells and few polymorphs inbetween the tubules.
3. There is granulomatious lesions in the intertitial tissue resulting from rupture of tubular contents.
4. The veins in the neighbourhood may show thrombosis due to rupture of tubular content into such vein.
5. Caste both pigmented nonpigmented may occupy the lumen of the tubules.
6. The vessels in the medulla are intensely congested.

Pathogenesis of anoxic nephrosis :

The exact mechanism is not known. Trueta suggested that in all these conditions renal, specially cortical ischaemia results from shunt or by passing of blood directly into the medulla without passing through the cortex by way of juxtamedullary glomerulus (Truetas shunt.). Others believe that cortical ischaemia is due to vasoconstriction of renal vessels in response to nervous hormonal factors. Whatever be the actual cause of cortical ischaemia once it is there it will certainly lead to tubular degeneration blockage causing rise of pressure once this blockage is there a viscious cycle is established because rise of pressure within the tubules means more exudation into interstitial tissue which will cause further obstruction rise of pressure. In this way there will be more and more exudation c leakage of glomerular filtrate into interstitial tissue so that no or little urine can reach the bladder. Thus there will be oliguria or anuria c terminal renal failure.

Bright's disease - This includes inflammatory (non-suppurative) degenerative and vascular disorders of the Kidney.

Inflammatory group - This includes glomerulonephritis and chronic pyelonephritis. The lesion involves kidney parenchyma proper.

Degenerative group - The lesion is mainly seen in the tubules (nephrosis). According to severity Bright classified nephrosis into 4 groups:-

(a) Mild or lateral - usually seen in acute infections.
(b) Lipoid
(c) Amyloid
(d) Necrotising - This is the severest form of nephrosis usually caused by heavy metal poisoning.

Vascular group: The following are included:

(a) Benign nephrosclerosis or primary contracted kidney.
(b) Malignant nephrosclerosis seen in malignant hypertension.
(c) Senile of antheromatous kidney caused by atheroma of renal vessels.

Classification of nephritis:-

It may be primarily of two types:

(1) **Parenchymatous** - Where kidneys tissue proper is involved.

(2) **Interstitial** - Inflammatory changes and collection of inflammatory cells are seen in the interstitial frame work of the kidney tissue, without any involvement of kidney tissue proper. Usually seen in acute infective fevers.

Parenchymatons group may either be diffuse or focal. Diffuse nephritis may again be either acute, subacute or. chronic. The focal glomerulonephritis may be either embolic (as seen in S.s. bacterial endocarditis) or non-embolic caused by infective fevers like diphtheria, scarlet fever, pneumonia etc.

PART - IV

SPOT LIGHT

WHAT TO BE DONE ?

(I) For Practical Examination

1. Urine

1. Test for Sugar

Experiments	*Observation*	*Inference*
(i) **Fehling's Test :** Equal volumes (1 ml) of Fehling's solution No. 1 and Fehling's solution 2 are taken in a test tube, mixed and shaken. The solution was warmed to make a clear solution. Then 2 c.c. urine was mixed with it and shaken then boiled.	(i) Red precipitrate at the test tube.	(i) Sugar present
(ii) **Benedicts test :** 5 ml. Benedict's solution was taken in a test tube then 10 drops urine is added to it, boiled vigorously for two minutes and then cooled.	(ii) Red, yellow or green ppt.	(ii) Sugar present.

2. Test for Aceton

Experiments	*Observation*	*Inference*
(i) **Rothera's Sodium Nitroprusside test :** A few ml.(4 ml. of urine was taken in a test tube	(i) A deep violet per-	(ii) Aceton is present.

and it was saturated with Ammonium sulphate crystal then a few drops of freshly prepared Sodium Nitropruside solution was mixed with it and it was shaken, then a few drops strong. Ammonia solution (liquor ammonia fort) was poured carefully along the side of the test tube.	manganate ring appears at the junction of the two solution.	

3. Bile Test

Experiments	*Observation*	*Inference*
A few ml. of urine (5 ml.) was taken in a test tube. A small amount of finely powdered flowers of Sulphur is sprinkled into it.	Sulphur powder sinks.	Bile is present.

4. Test for Albumin

Experiments	*Observation*	*Inference*
(a) Heat test :		
Urine is taken 2/3 rd of the test tube. It was heated in the upper portion holding the test tube in a slanting way.	Haziness appears at the site of heating.	Albumin may be present.
A few drops of dilute Acetic Acid was added.	Haziness disappears.	Albumin present
(b) Hellar's Nitric Acid test:		
A few ml. of urine was taken in a test tube then cold concentrated Nitirc Acid was trickle down with a pipette by the side of the test tube	A white ring appears at the junction of the urine and Nitric. acid.	Albumin present

holding the tube in a slanting way. It was now erected.

CROSS QUESTIONS

****Q. 1. Name some conditions where sugar is present in Urine ?**

1. Diabetes Mellitus.
2. Hyperthroidism.
3. Hyperpitutarism.
4. Suprarenal ootex tumours..
5. Renal glycosuria due to lowering of renal threshold.
6. Alimentary glycosuria.
7. Temporary glycosuria resulting from :
   (a) Cerebral injuries, haemorrhage and tumours.
   (b) Alcoholic subject.
   (c) Pancreatic disease.
   (d) After general anasthesia.
   (e) During pregnancy.

****Q. 2. Name some conditions where Acetone is present in Urine ?**

1. In case of Diabetes mellitus and Coma.
2. In case of prolonged starvation of Carbohydrates due to :
   (a) Gastric ulcer, cancer.
   (b) Oesophageal stenosis.
   (c) Intestinal obstruction.
   (d) Cachexia resulting from tuberculosis, malignant diseases, Malaria and Syphilis.
   (e) Persistant vomiting of pregnancy.
   (f) Cyclical vomiting of children.
   (g) Infantile diarrhoea and vomiting.
3. Uraemia.
4. Eclampsia.
5. Delayed chloroform poisoning etc.

**** Q. 3. Name some diseases where Bile is present in Urine.**

1. Obstructive and Toxaemic Jaundice.
2. Yellow fever.

****Q. 4. Name some conditions where Albumen is present in Urine.**

1. *Temporary or functional.*
2. *Permanent or organic.*

1. *Temporary Albuminuria in cases of:*

(a) Dyspepsia : due to functional hepatic disorder, over eating, over exertion, nervous, overstrain (Anxiety, fear etc.), Anaemia.

(b) Drugs : Alcohol, Turpentine etc.

(c) Temporary renal congestion.

2. *Permanent Albuminuria in cases of :*

(a) Active and Passive renal congestion.

(b) Acute and Chronic rephritis of all forms, and waxy kidney.

(c) Syphilis, tuberculosis and gout.

(d) Chronic poisoning e.g. Lead, Arsenic, Phosphorus etc.

(e) Jaundice.

(f) Toximia of pregnancy.

(g) Congestive cardiac failure.

2. STAINING

1. LEISHMAN'S STAIN

Q. Draw a proper blood film. Stain it with Leishman's method of staining.

Requirements :

(i) A pair of clean and grease free glass slide.

(ii) Tray with bridges.

(iii) Leishman's stain solution.

(iv) Distilled water.

(v) Spirit lamp.

(vi) Pricking needle.

(vii) Cotton, etc.

Procedure

(i) Preparation of proper blood film :

A proper blood film was prepared on the clean and grease free glass slide and it was dried in air.

(ii) Staining :

A few drops of Leishman's stain solution was poured over the film, it was waited for (1/2 to 1 minute) 50 seconds. Equal volume of distilled water was poured over the film, it was waited for (12 to 15 minutes) 12 minutes then washed by running water and dried in air.

It is now ready to be examined under the oil emersion lens of microscope.

CROSS QUESTION

Q. 1. Why we stain blood film?
Or, What we may get on the blood film after staining with Leishman's method ?

1. To observe any alteration of size and shape of RBC.
2. For differential count (D.C.) of WBC.
3. For average counting of platelets.
4. Any other organisms which are present in blood, like parasites and bacteria.

Q. 2. What are the parasites and bactaria seen in Blood ?

(a) Parasites :
1. Malaria parasites (within RBC) [pl. vivax, pl. falciparun, pl. ovale, pl. malariae].
2. Microfilaria (between the cell).
3. L.D. bodies (Leishmania donovani) inside the monocyte.

(b) Bacteria :
1. Pasteurella pestis (plague bacillus).
2. Spirilum minus (rat bite fever).

2. ACID FAST STAIN

Q. Draw a proper film and stain it with Ziehe Neelson method of stain.

Requirements:
(i) A clean and grease free glass slide.
(ii) Tray with bridges.
(iii) Brooms stick.
(iv) Spirit lamp or Bunsen's burner.

(v) Carbol fuchsin solution.
(vi) 20% Sulphuric acid ($H_2 SO_4$).
(vii) Methylene blue solution.
(viii) Cotton etc.

Procedure:

(i) *Preparation of a proper film* : A film was prepared on the clean and grease free glass slide with the material (name of the specimen) supplied with the help of a broom stick. It was dried in air.
(ii) *Fixation of the film* : It was fixed by passing over the flame of the spirit lamp or bunsen's burner (as supplied).
(iii) *Stain and mordanting* : Steaming carbol fuchsin solution was poured over the film (5 ml approx.), wait for 10 minutes.
(iv) Decolourisation : It was decolourised with 20% $H_2 SO_4$ (unit a faint pink colour comes).
(v) Counter Stain : It was counter stain with Methylene Blue solution. A few drops of Methylene blue solution was poured over the film, wait for 1 minute.
(vi) It was washed by running tap water and then it was dried in air. It was now ready to be examined under the oil emersion lens of microscope.

CROSS QUESTIONS

Q. 1. What do you mean by Acid fast organisms ? Why they so-called?

Acid fast organisms mean that can stand their stained in mineral acid and alcohol. *M. tuberculosis* and *M. leprae* and *Segma bacillus* are Acid fast as they retain staining by carbol fuchisn when treated by $H_2 SO_4$.

Q. 2. What do you mean by non-acid fast organisms ?

Those organisms which discharge the staining colour (Red) while washing with 20% H_2SO_4 but takes the counter stain colour (Methylene colour-Blue) are known as Non-acid fast organism.

Q. 3. What sort of stain it is ?

Differential method of stain.

Q. 4. Why it is so called ?

Because we can differentiate Acid fast organism from Non-acid fast organism in slide.

Q. 5. What makes the organism acid fast ?

Those organisms which contain Mycolic Acid (Mycol) in their outer coat retained the staining colour.

Q. 6. Why you have chosen carbol fuchsin for staining ?

For better penetration of bacterial envelop i.e. Mycolic acid layer.

Q. 7. In Carbol fuchi which stains the film and which is the mordant ?

Basic Fuschin Stain the film and Carbolic acid act as Mordanting agent.

Q. 8. Why 20% H_2SO_4 is used ?

Excess carbol fuchsion is washed out by using 20% H_2SO_4. If strong or conc, acid is used entire smear will be washed out, so 20% H_2SO_4 is used.

Q. 9. Give the Morphological differences between M. tuberculosis and M. leprae.

M. Tuberculosis : The slender, beaded rod shaped bacilli with slighty curved appearance, single or pair in amount. **M. Lepare** is arranged in bundles just like match sticks in a match box. They are within a shell — called Lepra shell.

3. GRAM'S STAINING

Q. Draw a proper film and stain it with gram method of staining ?

Requirements:

(i) A clean and grease free glass slide.
(ii) Tray with bridges.
(iii) Brooms stick.
(iv) Gention Violet sol.
(v) Gram's Iodin sol.
(vi) Absolute alcohol.

(vii) Saffranin sol.
(viii) Spirit lamp or Bunsen's burner (as supplied), cotton etc.

Procedure:

(i) *Preparation of a proper film* : A film was prepared with the material (name of the specimen) supplied with the help of a Broom stick at the centre of the clean and grease free glass slide. It is dried in air.
(ii) *Fixation* : It was fixed by passing over the flame of a spirit lamp or Bunsen's burner (as supplied).
(iii) *Staining* : It was stain with gention voilet sol. was poured over the film and wait for 1/2-1 minutes.
(iv) *Mordanting* : Gram's Iodin sol. was flooded over the film, wait for 1-2 minutes.
(v) *Decolourisation* : It was decolourised with absolute alcohol.
(vi) *Counter staining* : It was counter stained with Saffranin solution. A few drops of Safflramin sol. was poured over the film wait for 1 minute.
(vii) It was washed by running tap water and then it was dried in air. Now it was ready to be examined under the oil emersion lens of microscope.

CROSS QUESTIONS

Q. 1. What we do gram staining ?

To place the whole group of bacteria in 2 groups or to classify bacteria into gram + ve and gram — ve groups.

Q. 2. What do you mean by gram positive organism ?

Those organism which retain the staining colour (Gention violet colour—Violet) inspite of subsequent washing with absolute alcohol are known as Gram positive organism.

Q. 3. What are the gram negative organism ? Why they so called?

Those organism which discharge the staining colour while washing with abosolute but take the counter stain colour (Saffranin colour—Red) are known as negative organism.

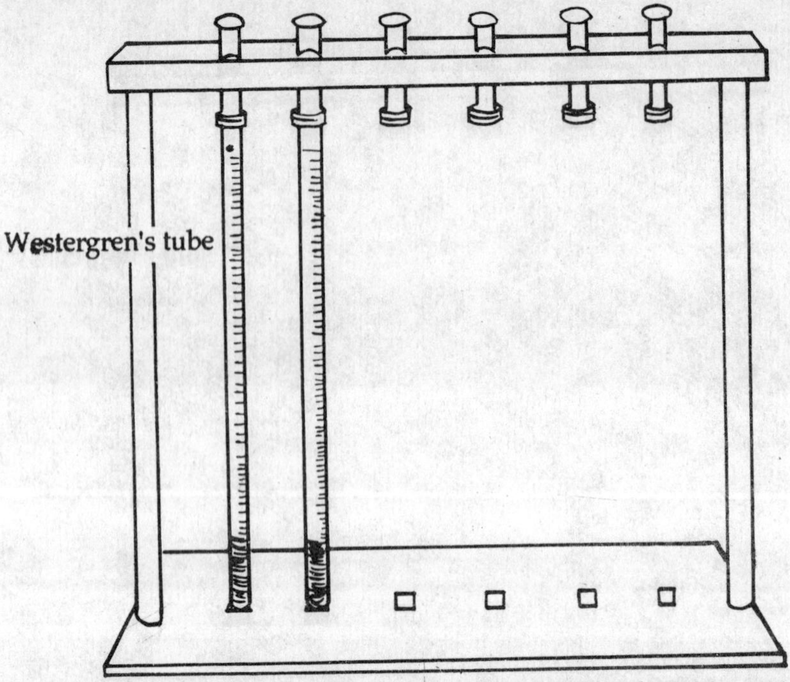

Erythrocyte Sedimentation Rate Tube (E.S.R. Tube with rack)

Q. 4. Name some gram positive and negative cocci.

All cocci are gram positive except Neissaria groups e.g. Streptococci, Staphyllococci and Pneumococci are gram positive and Gonococci and meningococci are gram negative.

Q. 5. Name some gram positive and gram negative bacili ?

All bacillus are gram negative except Mycobacterium tuberculosis and Mycoleprae.

Q. 6. What makes the organism gram positiveness ?

Due to presence of Magnesium salt of R.N.A. (Ribo Nucleic Acid).

Q. 7. What is the role of iodine ?

Iodine has a mordanting action. It fixes the stain by reducing porocity of cell wall and making bacterial protoplasm acidic.

I. FOR ORAL

Instrumentation

(i) Erythrocyte Sedimentation. Rate Tube (Westergreen).
(ii) Haemocytometer. (iii) Haemoglobinometer.
(iv) Urinometer. (v) Doremus Ureometer.
(vi) Esbach's Albuminometer. (vii) Lumbar Puncture Needle.
(viii) Sterral Puncture Needle. (ix) Dreyer's Copper Rack.

1. ERYTHROCYTE SEDIMENTATION RATE TUBE
Syn. E.S.R. Tube with rack :

Description : It is a hollow glass tube open at both ends, Approx. length 300 mm and internal diameter 2.5 mm. There is some graduation and marking as from above downwards 0, 20, 40, 60....180, but graduated upto 200. It is graduated in (mm.) The capacity of the tube from 0 to 200 is 1 ml.

Calculation : Let R_1 mm may be the 1st hour reading and R_2 be the 2nd hour reading. Therefore, mean E.S.R. will be.

$$\frac{R_1 + \dfrac{R_2 - R_1}{2}}{2} \text{ per hour.}$$

CROSS QUESTIONS

Q. 1. What are the uses of this instrument ?

(i) To know the prognosis of the disease.
(ii) To corroborate our clinical findings.

Q. 2. What are the normal E.S.R. ?

(i) New born baby — 0.5 mm. per hour.
(ii) Children — 3 to 10 mm. per hour.
(iii) Male — 2 to 10 mm. per hour.
(iv) Female — 5 to 15 mm. per hour.

Q. 3. Name some conditions in which E.S.R. is high ?

Physiological : Duirng menstrual period, late month of pregnancy and after child brith.

Diseases : Tuberculosis, Severe anaemia, Rheumatic fever, Rheumatiod arthritis, Malignant disease, other collagen disorders etc.

Q. 4. Name some conditions in which E.S.R. in low ?

Congestive cardiac failure, Polycythaemia, whooping cough etc.

Q. 5. What factors control the E.S.R. ?

(i) Specific gravity of plasma.
(ii) Viscosity of plasma.
(iii) R.B.C. volume and amount of haemoglobin.
(iv) Clamping of R.B.C. into bigger massess.

Q. 6. What is function of Sodium citrate ?

It will act as anti-coagulant.

2. HAEMOCYTOMETER

This instrument is used for counting the total number of R.B.C. and the total and differential count of W.B.C. per cu. mm. of blood.

It consist of : (i) A speical glass slide (counting chamber), (ii) One graduated pipette for R.B.C. count, (iii) Another pipette for W.B.C. count, (iv) One cover glass.

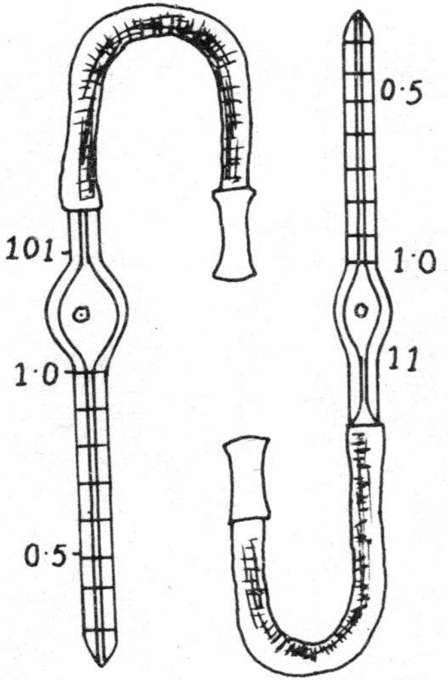

R.B.C. Pipette W.B.C. Pipette

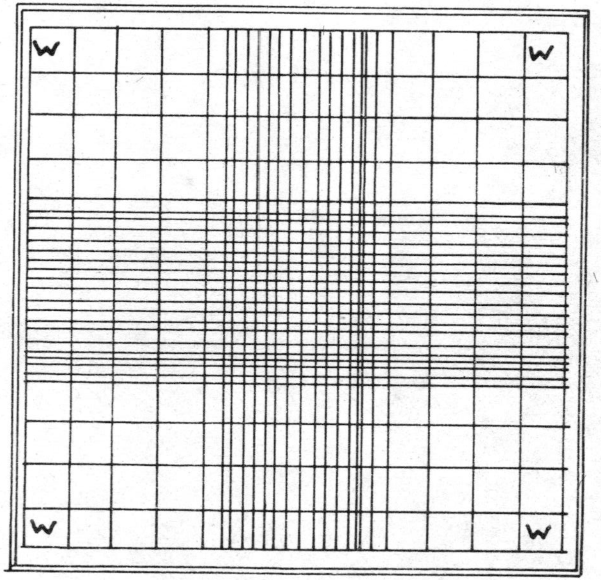

Counting chamber

HAEMOCYTOMETER

1. R.B.C. Pipette

Indentification : The bulb is large and bead inside is red in colour. The markings are 0.5, 1.0 and 11. Two markings 0.5 and 1 are present on the stem of the pipette and 3rd mark 11, is placed just above the bulb.

Uses : To find out T.C. of R.B.C. per cu mm., and also W.B.C. in leukaemia.

2. W.B.C. Pipette

Indentification : The blub is smaller and the bead inside is white in colour. Markings are 0.5, 1.0 and 11.

Uses : To find out T.C. of W.B.C., and also to find out the cell count of serous fluid and semen for the total count of Spermatozoea.

CROSS QUESTIONS

Q. 1. What is normal T.C. of R.B.C. ?

5.0 million/cu. mm. of blood, in male and 4.5. million/cu.mm. of blood in female.

Q. 2. What is R.B.C. fluid ?

The different types of R.B.C. fluids are as follows:

(a) **Hoyem's fluid** : It is made up of (i) Mercuric chloride 0.5. gm., (ii) Sodium chloride : 1 gm, (iii) Sodium sulphate 5 gm. (iv) Distilled water -200 ml.

(b) **Toisson's fluid**-It is made up of (i) Mathyl Violet 0.25 gm. (ii) Sodium chloride 1 gm., (iii) Sodium sulphate 8 gm, (iv) Neutral Glycerin 30 ml., (v) Distilled water 160 ml.

(c) Normal saline.

Q. 3. What is the normal T.C. of W.B.C. ?

It is 6000—8000 per cu. mm. of blood.

Q. 4. What is W.B.C. fluid ?

It contains (i) Glacial acetic acid 2 ml., (ii) Gention violet sol. (1% aqueous)-1ml, (iii) Distilled water 100 ml.

****Q. 5. What is Leucocytosis?**

It is a condition when total count of W.B.C. goes above 10,000 per cu. mm. in the blood and the W.B.C. cell are fully matured.

Q. 6. What are the common causes of Lecocytosis ?

Causes of it are (1) *Infective*, e.g. *Pyogenic Infection* like Tonsilitis, or Osteomyelitis, Appendicitis etc.

2. Non Infective :

(i) Any case of tissue injury or necrosis.
(ii) Leukaemia and Leukaemoib reaction.
(iii) Spirochaetal infection.
(iv) Burn.
(v) Severe haemorrhage.
(vi) Acute gout.
(vii) Intestinal haemorrhage.
(viii) Tropical eosinophilia.
(ix) Malignant tumours like sarcoma.

Q. 7. What is Leucopenia ?

It is a condition when the total count of W.B.C. is less than 5000 cu. mm. in blood.

Q. 8 What are common causes of Leucopenia ?

Causes:

1. ***Infective condition*** : Tuberculosis, Typhoid, and Virus infection.
2. ***Blood disorders*** : Aplastic anaemia, Aleukaemic leucoemia.
3. ***Poisons*** : Arsenic, X-Ray.
4. ***Bone marrow disease*** : Neoplastic deposit.

Q. 9. What is the normal D.C. of W.B.C. ?

The different percentage of W.B.C. are:

(i) Neutrophil (60—70%), (ii) Eosinophil (1—60%), (iii) Basophil (0.1%), (iv) Lymphocytes both large and small (20—30%), (v) Monocytes (4—8%).

Q. 10. What is the average ratio of T.C. of W.B.C. and T.C. of R.B.C.

It is about 1 : 700.

****Q. 11. What is Pancytopaenia ?**

The condition where all the forms elements of blood (the T.C. of W.B.C., T.C. of R.B.C. and T.C. of platelets) are diminished known as pancytopaenia. Seen in cases of :

1. Aplastic anaemia, 2. Alukaeamic leukoemia, 3. Splenomegaly, 4. Kala azar, 5. Pernicious anaemia, 6. Miliary tuberculosis.

****Q. 12. What is leucoemia ? What are its causes ?**

When the W.B.C. count increased above normal count sometimes ranging 50,000 to 1 lakh per cu. ml. of blood but the W.B.C. cells are immature are called Leucoemia.

Causes : Neoplasm, Malignant neoplasm-carcinoma, sarcoma.

****Q. 13. What is meant by polymorpho nuclear leucocytosis ? Whom it is seen ?**

Polymopho Nuclear Leucocytosis : Increased percentage of Neutrophil. Seen in cases of - Acute infection, Tonsilitis and all types of inflammation.

****Q. 14. What is meant by eosinophilia ? Where it is seen ?**

Eosinophilia : Increased percentage of Eosinophil.

Seen in cases of :

1. **Allergic condition** : Food, drugs and synthetic products.
2. **Skin disease** : Eczema, Urticaria etc.
3. **Parasites** : Filariasis, Helminthesiasis, Ascariasis.
4. **Blood disorders** : Leukoemia.
5. **Lungs disorders** : Chronic Bronchitis, Asthma, Eosinophilic lungs.
6. **Other conditions**-Malignant disease e.g. sarcoma, carcinoma. Chronic osteomyelitis, Hodgkin disease, In administration of drugs — like Camphor, Chronic. sulphate etc.

****Q.15. What do you mean by basophilia ? Where it is found ?**

Basophilia : Increased percentage of Basophil.

Seen in cases of - (i) Basophilic leucoemia.
(ii) Early stage of Hodgkin disease.
(iii) Chronic myeloid leucoemia.

****Q. 16. What do you meant by lymphocytosis ? Where it is seen ?**

Lymphocytosis : Increased percentage of Lymphocytes.

Seen in cases of :

1. Physiologically in infants:
2. Pathologically in cases of:
   (a) Infection like Influenza. Hooping cough, Measles.
   (b) Blood disorders like Leukoemia and other cases are Diabetes and Hypothyrodism.

****Q. 17. What is monocytosis ?**

Monocytosis : Increased percentage of Monocyte.

Seen in cases of : (i) Tuberculosis.
(ii) Typhoid fever.
(iii) Ulcerative colitis.
(iv) Lymphosarcoma.
(v) Sympathetic opthalmia.

3. HAEMOGLOBINOMETER

This instrument consists of : (i) Comparator box, (ii) One graduated tube, (iii) One capillary pipette and (iv) One glass rod.

Use : Determination of percentage of haemoglobin in the blood.

CROSS QUESTIONS

Q. 1. What is the normal Hb% ?

It is 14.5 gm./100 ml. of blood.

Q. 2. What is haemolysis ?

It is the process when haemoglobin is coming out from matured R.B.C. when it is put into hypotonic solution.

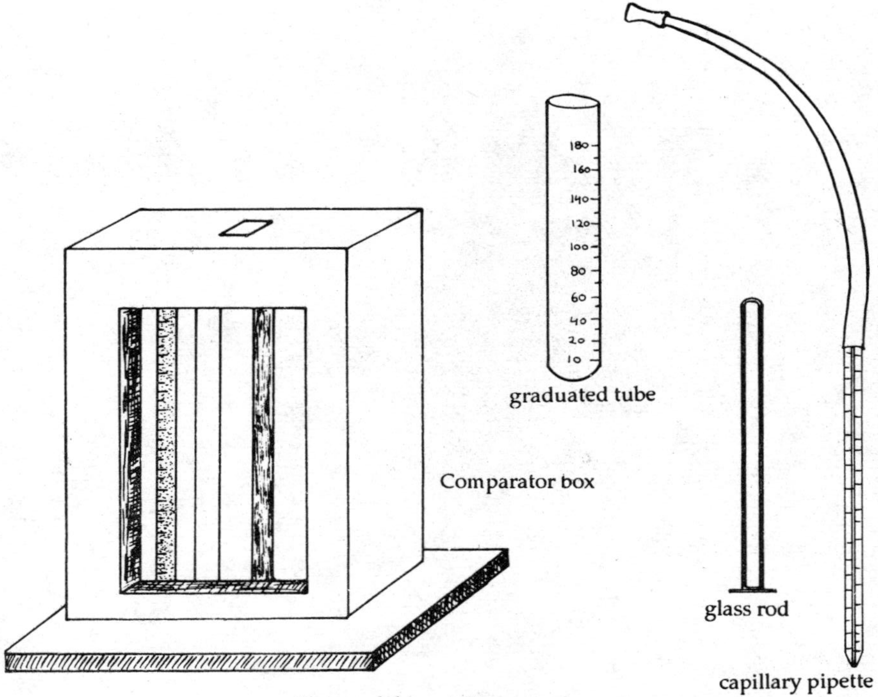

Haemoglobinometer

Q. 3. What is haemoglobin ?

Haemoglobin is a conjugated protein containing basic protein globuin (histone) united with four prosthetic haem groups.

Q. 4. What are the functions of haemoglobin ?

(i) Essentials are O_2 Carriage and CO_2 transport.
(ii) It is one the buffers of blood and thus helps to maintain acid base balance.
(iii) Bile pigment, Stool pigment and Urine pigments are formed from it.
(iv) Estimation of E.S.R.

Q. 5. What is Anaemia ?

Qualitative or quantitative reduction of circulating R.B.C. or of the percentage of haemoglobin concentration.

Q. 6. What is N_{10}. Hcl ?

It means that 10 ml. of concentrated hydrochloric acid is dissolved in a litre of distilled water.

Q. 7. What is Thalassaemia ?

This is transmitted by Mandelian inheritance, where Foetal Haemoglobin may be 40 to 100% or it may be absent.

Q. 8. What is sikle cell Anaemia ?

Where Haemoglobin is carried on a single gene so that two genes from a parent may be either in a Haemozygous or hetero zygous manner. Here type and Haemoglobin is prominantly present.

Q. 9. What is Anaemia ?

Anaemia is a qualitative and quantitative dimunution of Hb R.B.C. in blood.

Q. 10. What are the various types of Anaemia ?

Anaemia may be due to :

(i) Blood loss in the form of acute or chronic haemorrhage.
(ii) Lack of essential factors for the formation either of Haemoglobin

itself or the red cells stroma (Dyshaemo poeitic anaemias). Such factors include iron, Vit B_{12}, Folic acid, Vitamin c protein and thyroxine. Defficiency anaemies such as. Iron defficiency, Folic and acid difficiency anaemias.

(iii) Bone marrow failure : Aplastic, hypoplastic anaemias due to lack of Erythroprotein, the action of drugs or irradiation and unknown causes (Idiopathic).

(iv) In filtration of the bone marrow : Secondary carcinoma, Leukemia, Myclomatosis or with fibrous or bone as in Myelosclerosis.

(v) Increased cell destruction : Haemolytic anaemia.

(vi) Miscellaneous anaemias occuring in the course of other diseases : (Secondary anaemias).

Q. 11. What is packed cell volume ?

The volume of the packed R.B.C. is known as packed cell volume (P.C.V.)

Normal value in Male : 40 to 50%.

Normal value in Female : 37 to 47%,

****Q. 12. What is colour index ?**

Colour index is $\frac{\text{Hb\%}}{\text{R.B.C.\%}}$. Normal value is '1'.

Q. 13. What is M.C.V. (Mean Corpuscular Volume) ?

$$\text{M.C.V.} = \frac{\text{P.C.V. in ml./1000 ml. of blood}}{\text{R.B.C. in million/ cu. mm.}}$$

Normal value = 76 to 96 cu.μ ± 7.

Q. 14. What is M.C.H. (Mean Corpuscular Haemoglobin) ?

$$\text{M.C.H.} = \frac{\text{Hb in gm./1000 ml. of blood}}{\text{R.B.C. in Million/cu. mm.}}$$

Normal Value = (27 to 32 mmg).

Q. 15. What is mean corpuscular haemoglobin concentration (M.C.H.C.)

$$\text{M.C.H.C.} = \frac{\text{Hb in gram\%}}{\text{P.C.V.\%}} \times 100$$

Normal — 32 to 36% ± 3

Q. 16. What is normal bleeding time ?

The Normal value is 2 to 4 min.

Q. 17. What is clotting time ?

Normal value is 6 to 10 min.

4. URINOMETER

Identification : The instrument has got a mercury filled bulb at the bottom. The idea is to keep the instrument erect in the fluid. There is a constriction above the blub. The graduation in the stem is 1000 to 1060 above downwards.

Use : To measure the specific gravity of urine.

CROSS QUESTIONS

Q. 1. What is the normal sp. gragvity of urine ?

It is 1010 to 1020.

Q. 2. When the sp. gr. of urine is high ?

In (i) Acute Nephritis, (ii) Diabetes mellitus, (iii) Dehydration.

Q. 3. When the sq. gr. of urine is low ?

In (i) Diabetes incipidus, (ii) Chronic Nephritis, (iii) Functional nervous disorder.

Q. 4. What are the differences between diabetes mellitus and incipidus ?

Diabetes Mellitus	Diabetes Incipidus
Sp. gr. increase	Sp. gr. decrease
Sugar present in urine	Sugar absent in urine

Q. 5. What is diabetes mellitus ?

It is a condition of glyosuria accompanied with hyper glyceamia.

Q. 6. What is glycosuria ?

It is a condition when glucose is found in urine.

Q. 7. What is hyper glyceamia ?

It is a condition when the blood sugar level is above 120 mg. per 100 ml. of blood.

Q. 8. What is daily excretion of urine ?

It is 1.5 litre (approx.)

Q. 9. What is the characteristic of sp. gr. in chronic nephritis?

Sp. gr. of urine in chronic nephritis is fixed below 1010 irrespective of fluid intake or output.

5. DOREMUS UREOMETER

Indentification : It is a 'V' shaped tube. It consists of a graduated bulb. Closed at the top and open at the bulbous extremity. There is a side tube, open at the top provided with the glass topper at the bottom. The side tube is graduated in ml. and is meant for the urine to be examined. The larger divisions at the upper protion of the bulb are marked as 0.01, 0.02 and 0.03. Each larger division is again graduated in tenths and represents so many grams of urea per ml. of the urine utilised in the test. Each smaller division represents 0.001 gm. of urea.

CROSS QUESTIONS

Q. 1. What is the normal percentage of urea?

It is 2-5-30%.

Q. 2. What is the daily execution of urea ?

25-40 gms.

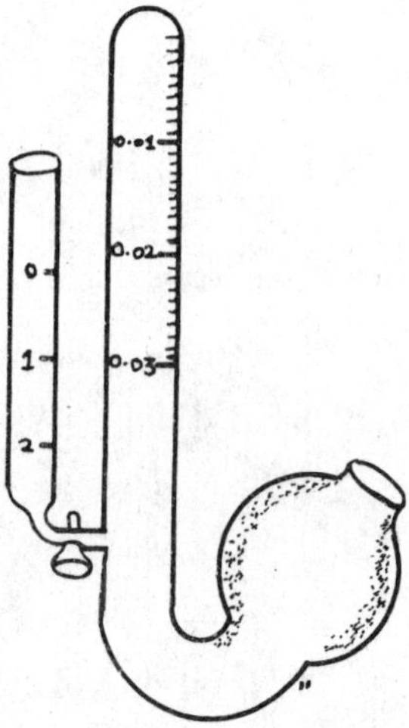

Doremus Ureometer

Q. 3. What is the importance of the urea test ?

Percentage of urea in urine indicates kidney function. If it is below 25% there is impairment of kidney function and in a suspected case of ureamia, it is 1.5% the prognosis of the patient is very bad.

Q. 4. What is sodium hypobromide solution ?

The Sodium hypobromide solution consists of 23 ml. of 30% caustic soda and 2 ml. of bromine. The solution is prepared immediately before use.

****Q. 5 What are the conditions, where urea increased or decreased in Urine ?**

Increased : (1) Intake of much protein food, (2) Fevers, (3) Diabetic coma, (4) Poisoning of Phosphorous and arsenic, (5) During resolution of pneumonia, (6) During absorption of lung exudates. (7) Severe burn, (8) Servere surgical shock.

Decreased : (1) Acidosis, (2) Uraemia, (3) Kidney disease, (4) Severe diseases of liver, (5) Intake of less protein food or water.

Q. 6. What is urea clearance vlaue ?

$$\text{Standard clearance} = \frac{U \times Vu}{B}$$

U = Urea in mgm. per c.c.
V = Volume of urine in c.c./min
B = Blood urea in mgm%

Q. 7. What is ketone bodies ?

These are formed by the oxidation of Fatty acids. These are as follows — Aceto acetic acid, B Hydroxy Butric acid, Acetone.

These are found in : (i) Diabetes Mellitus.
(ii) Starvation etc.

Q. 8. What is the normal value of the uric acid in blood ?

Blood contains 1-3 m.g.m. uric acid 100 c.c. Average is 2 m.gm.

Q. 9. What is Normal value of Creatinine ?

7-2 mg. 100 c.c. of blood.

Q. 10. What is Normal value of Creatine ?

10 mg.m./100 c.c. of the Blood.

Q. 11. What is Ammonia Coefficient ?

Normal 5%

$$\frac{\text{Ammonia } N_2 \text{ in urine}}{\text{Total } N_2 \text{ in urine}} \times 100$$

In acidisis — It is raised.
In alcalosis — It is decreased.

6. ESBACH'S ALBUMINOMETER

Identification: It is an elongated thick glass tube filled with a rubber cork. There are some graduation and markings. Markings are 1,2,3...12 indicating gm. per litre and 'U' for urine and 'R' for reagent. It is kept in a wooden stand and in vertical position.

Use : It is required for quantative estimation of Albumin in urine.

CROSS QUESTIONS

Q. 1. What is the normal percentage of Albumin in urine ?

It is nil.

Q. 2.In which body fluid we may got Albumin ?

In blood and Cerebro Spinal Fluid.

Q. 3. What are the composition of Esbach's reagent ?

Picric acid — 10 gm. Citric acid — 20 gm. and distilled water upto 1000 ml.

Q. 4. What is the function of Picric acid ?

It causes precipitation by reacting with protein.

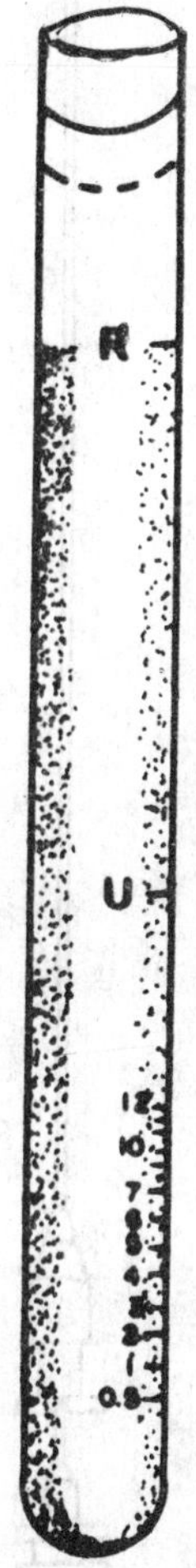

Esbach's Albuminometer

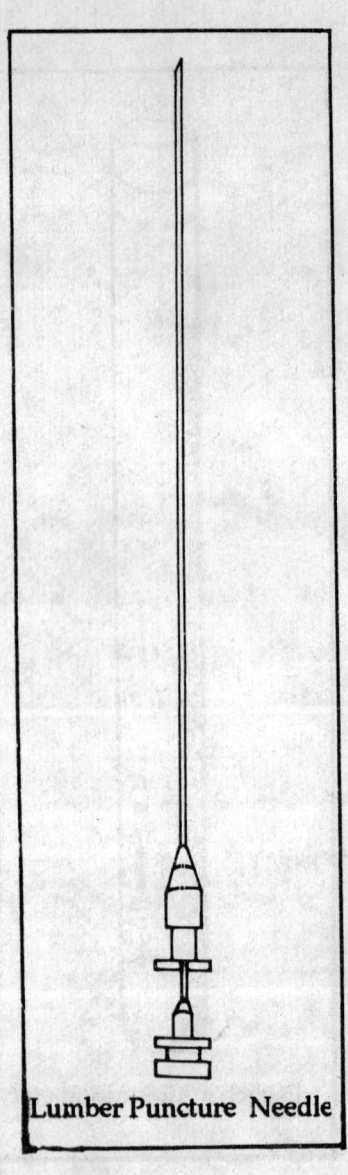

Lumber Puncture Needle

Q. 5. What is the function of Citric acid ?

It maintains the acid reaction.

****Q. 6. What are the causes of Albuminuria ?**

See Page 342.

Q. 7. Can you use Esbach's Albuminometer for other purposes ?

Yes, for quantitative estimation of protein in any fluid it can be used.

Q. 8. Why Albumin is not present in urine normally ?

Filtering pores of kidney allow only those substances which molecular weight is less than 70,000. The molecular weight of Albumin is 70,000. So it cannot pass through these pores.

7. LUMBAR PUNCTURE NEEDLE

Parts : (i) Needle, (ii) Stillet (No mobile guard).
Site : Between 3rd and 4th Lumbar Vertebrae.
***Uses** : (i) **Diagnostic** — Meningitis, internal haemorrhage.
(ii) **To relive the intra** — cranial tension.
(iii) **Anaesthestic** — Prior to operations elsewhere in vertebrae.
(iv) **Prognostic** — Prognosis of disease.

CROSS QUESTIONS

Q. 1. What is the normal colour of C.S.F. ? What are the condition when colour will be changed ?

Normally it is as colourless as distilled water. Canary yellow colour suggests intercranial haemorrhage. Greenish or grayish yellow colour suggest meningitis.

Q. 2. What is the normal pressure of C.S.F. ?

The normal pressure of C.S.F. becomes 60 to 150 mm. of water. Or one drop per second.

8. STERNAL PUNCTURE NEEDLE

Parts: (i) Mobile guard.
(ii) Needle with pore.
(iii) Stillets.

****Uses :**

Diagnostic : Kala azar, Leukaemia, Anaemia and Polychythaemia.

Prognosis : To know the efficacy of the disease.

9. DREYER'S RACK FOR WIDAL TEST

It is an agglutination reaction in which the unknown antibodies (H,O) developed in patient's serum during inflection is indentified with the help of known standard antigenic suspension in presence of electrolytic Sodium Chloride Positive result is evidenced by clumping or flacculation.

Uses :

The widal test is used for disgnosis of enteric group of fever.

Procedure :

3 ml. of blood is collected from the patient by puncturing his cubital vein. It is then allowed to clot in a dry test tube. Serum is separated and diluted 1/10 in normal saline.

Arranged of Dreyer's tubes in Dreyer's rack

There are six rows of tubes. Each row consisting of six tubes. Two rows (H, O) are each for S. Typhi, S. paratyphi A and S. paratyphi B. Serum is taken in these tubes in following manner :

10 drops are taken in first tube.

5 drops in second, 3 drops in the 3rd.

Two drops in the fourth and one drop in the fifth tube. The sixth tube of each row serve as control and serum is not taken in them. Normal Saline is added low to each tube in such a manner that Saline and Serum together become 10 drops in each tube. Now 15 drops of known Standard antigenic suspension of Th, To, Ah, Ao, Bh. Bo. in normal Saline is added in each tube. The rack along with these tubes is now kept in water-bath in 56° C. for 4 hours. Each tube is then examined for presence of visible clumping. Positive tubes show a deposite at bottom and clear supernated fluid at top. Sixth tube (acting as control) of each row must not show clumping. But if

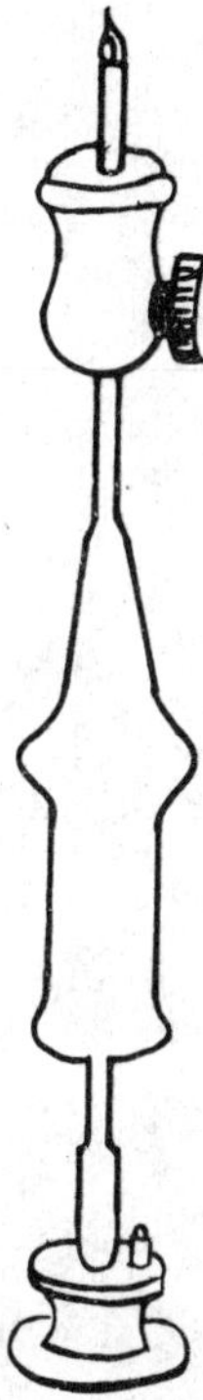

Sternal Puncture Needle

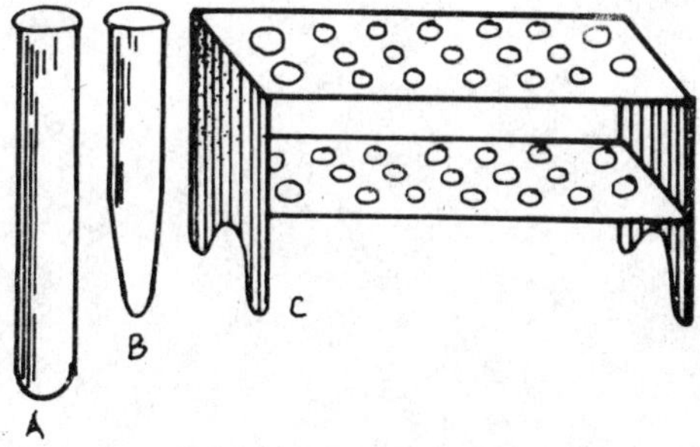

Dreyer's Rack For Widal Test

A. Dilution tube.
B. Agglutination tube.
C. Dreyer's rack.

clumping is seen in the control tubes due to agglutination, the test is to be discarded. The tube with maximum dilution showing positive clumpting is called agglutination titre.

II. FOR ORAL

(I) BACTERIOLOGY

Q. 1. What do you mean by bacteria ?

These are unicellular, Microscopic organisms without any cholorophyl.

Q. 2. What are the types of bacteria ?

Two types:

(i) **Higher bacteria :** Those which are divided by branching.

(ii) **Lower bacteria :** Those which are divided by binary fission. They include coccus, bacillus and spirallae.

Q. 3. What is coccus ?

Spherical shaped bacteria is called coccus.

Q. 4. What is bacillus ?

Rod shaped bacteria is called bacillus.

Q. 5. What is spiralae ?

Curved shaped bacteria is called spiralae.

Q. 6. What are types of spiralae ?

These are of two types:

(i) **Spirallum** : When there is a more than one curvature e.g. Spirallum minus.

(ii) **Spirochaeta** : When there are multiple curvature e.g. Treponema pallidum.

Q. 7. What are gram negative and gram positive bacterias ?

Those bacteria lose violet iodine combination in the presence of alcohol is called gram-negative.

And those which hold the violet dye called gram-positive.

Q. 8. Name some gram-positive, gram-negative cocci.

Gram-positive : Streptococcus, Staphylococcus, Pneumococcus.
Gram-negative : Gonococcus, Meningococcus.

Q. 9. Name some gram-positive, gram negative bacili.

Gram-positive : B. Diphteriae, Cl. Tetani, Cl. Welchi.
Gram-negative : B.Coli, B. Cholerae, B. Dysenteriae.

Q. 10. What is the other name of diphtheria bacillus ? How will you make the diagnosis of diphtheria ?

The other name of Diphtheria is Klebs Loffler Bacillus.
Diagnosis : (a) Clinical (b) Laboratory identification of bacteria, from lesion by:

(i) Director examination of smear by Neisser's Stain.
(ii) Cultural methods.
(iii) Fermentations test, etc.

Differentiation from Diphteroids by Schick's test.

Q. 11. What is Toxin, Exotoxin and Endotoxin ?

Toxin : It is a substance produced by the organism.
Exotoxin : It is a toxic substance produced by the living organism.
Endotoxin : It is a toxic substance produced only after the death or destruction of an organism.

Q. 12. What are the bacterias which have exotoxin ?

Cl. Tetani Cl. Welchi, C. Diphtheria, Stereptococcus and Stophylococcus.

Q. 13. What are the bacterias which have endotoxin ?

Pneumococcus, B. Typhosus, Gonococcus and Meningococcus.

Q. 14. What is toxiemia ?

It is the presence of only exotoxinin circulation.

Q. 15. What is Bacteraemia ?

It is the presence of bacteria in circulation.

Q. 16. What is septicaemia ?

When the organism multiply in circulation the condition is known as septicaemia.

Q. 17. What is pyaemia ?

When the septicaemia is complicated with embolic abscess to different parts of the body is known as Pyaemia.

Q.18. What are the acid fast organism ? Why they are so called ?

M. leprae, M. Tuberculosis and Smegma bacillus.

They retain the stain of Carbol fuchsion when subsequently treated with H_2SO_4. So they are called acid fast ogranism.

Q. 19. Who discovered the tubercular bacillus ?

Robert Koch (in 1882) discovered the tubercular bacillus.

The toxin of M. Tuberculosis forms minute nodules which are called tubercles consisting of central caseation eqetheloid cell, bacteria, giant cell etc.

Q. 20. What is toxoid ?

It is toxin molecule which has lost irreversably its toxicity but retains the antigenicity and ability to unite with specific antitoxins.

Q. 21. What is an antibiotic ?

An antibiotic is a substance manufactured by one type of micro organism which will kill or inhibit the growth of the others, when administered in small dose.

Q. 22. What are the uses of toxoid in prevention of diseases ?

It is used as active artificial immunity e.g. Tetanus toxoid to prevent tetanus.

Q. 23. What are Dysentery bacillus ? Name them.

Shiggella shigae, Sh. flexneri, Sh. boydi etc.

Q. 24. Name some motile bacteria ? Why are they motile ?

B. coli, V. cholera, Salmonella typhi. They are motile due to presence of flagella.

Q. 25. What is coma bacillus ?

Coma bacillus is cholera bacillus i.e. vibrio cholerae as they have on permanent curvature looking like coma.

Q. 26. Who discovered coma bacillus ?

Robert Koch (in 1883).

Q. 27. How would you diagnosis a case of typhoid according to weeks.

	Blood Culture (B)	Agglutination (A)	Stool (S)	Urine (U)
1st week	+	–	–	–
2nd week	±	+	±	–
3rd week	–	+	+	+
4th week				

Q 28. What is agglutination ?

A reaction in which particles (as R . B. C. or bacteria) suspended in a liquid collects into clumps and which occurs, especially as a serologic response to a specific antibody.

Q. 29. What is Widal test ? When is it done ?

It is serological agglutination test with known antigenic preparation done for identification of diseases like typhoid, paratyphoid A, paratyphoid B.

It is done in 2nd week of fever or afterwards in a case of continuous type of fever.

Q. 30. What is gonorrhoea ?

It is an infection of the mucous membrane of genito-urinary tract by Neisseria Gonorrhoea.

Q. 31. What is syphilis ?

This is chronic infection caused by Treponema pallidum.

Q. 32. What is the capsule of the bacteria ?

It is mucilagenous envelop surrounding the bacteria body.

Q. 33. Name some capsular bacteria ?

Cl. Welchii, Pneumococcus, H. influenza etc.

Q. 34. What is the utility of capsule ?

It is related to the virulence of the bacteria as it hampers the process of phagocytosis and acts as a safeguard for bacteria. Capsulated bacteria are more virulent than non-capsulated one.

Q. 35. What is flagellum ?

It is a thick hair-like contractile protoplasmic process arising either from the bacterial membrane or from just underneath it.

Q. 36. What is antiseptic ?

These are the chemical substances as sufficiently non-toxic for superficial application to living tissue which either kill micro-organism or present their growth.

Q. 37. What is antiserum ?

Serum containing antibody is called antiserum ?

Q. 38. What are types of antiserum ?

These are three types :

(i) **Antitoxic Serum** : This contains antibodies which are produced against diseases e.g. Tetanus.

(ii) **Antibacterial serum** : This contains antibodies against endotoxin of bacteria e.g. Menigococcal serum.

(iii) **Antiviral serum** : This contains antibodies against virus.

Q. 39. What is Symbiosis ?

It is a state when two organisms grow together to their mutual benefit.

Q. 40. What is Vector ?

Vector is the carrier of diseases when they are transmitted to man.

Q. 41. What is Virus ?

Viruses are minute ultramicroscopic organisms causing various diseases like Smallpox, Measles etc.

Q. 42. What is Viraemia ?

The presence of virus in Circulation.

Q. 43. What do you mean by Pathogen ?

Pathogen is an organism which produces disease.

Q. 44. What is Aerobe ?

A micro-organism which requires air as free oxygen for the maintenance of life e.g. Staphylococci.

Q. 45. What is Anaerobe ?

A micro-organism which can only grow without free oxygen is anaerobe.

Q. 46. What is Facultative anaerobe ?

When the bacteria are aerobic but can also grow in anaerobic condition, they are facultative anerobe.

Q. 47. What is an obligatory anaerobe ?

When the bacteria do not grow even in presence of O_2.

Q. 48. What is Spirocheates ? Name diseases cause by them.

Spirocheates is a spiral shaped bacteria. Diseases caused by them :

(i) T. Pallidum — Produce Syphilis.

(ii) Leptospira ectero haemorrhagica — Epiemic jaundice (weil's disease).

(iii) Spirillum minus — Rat bite fever.

(iv) S. Vincent — Vincent's angina.

(II) PARASITOLOGY

Q. 1. What is Parasitology ?

It is a branch of science which deals with the study of the organism that live temporarily or permanently on or within the organisms.

Q. 2. What is Parasite ?

Parasite is an organism which obtains food or shelter from another host organism.

Q. 3. What is host ?

The organic structure upon which parasites thrive.

Q. 4. What is definite host ?

Host harbouring the sexual form of the parasite is called definitive host.

Q. 5. What is intermediate host ?

Host harbouring the asexual or larval form or cystic stage of the parasite is called intermediate host.

Q. 6. What is infection ?

When a parasite establishes itself within a host.

Q. 7. What in infestation ?

When a parasite lives superficially on the animal host.

Q. 8. What is protozoa ? Name some protozoal diseases.

Protozoa is an unicellular organism. Protozoal diseases : Amoebiasis Kala-azar, Malaria etc.

Q. 9. Classify Protozoa. Give example.

(i) **Rhizopoda** : Protozoa with peseudopodia,-e.g. E. histolytica.

(ii) **Mastigophroa** : Protozoa with flagella e.g., T. nominis, T. Vaginalis.

(iii) **Sporozoa** : Protozoa without any organs of locomotion, e.g. Malaria parasite.

(v) **Ciliated** : Protozoa which has cilia all over body surface e.g. Balantium Coli.

Q. 10. What are different varieties of Malaria parasite ? Name them, where do they live ?

Varieties with name :

(i) Plasmodium Vivax.
(ii) Plasmodium Falciparum.
(iii) Plasmodium Malariae.
(iv) Plasmodium Ovale.

In man they live inside the R.B.C. in peripheral circulation and R.E.Cells (in liver). In mosquito they live in upper digestive tract and salivary gland.

Q. 11. What is the definite host of the Malaria parasite ?

Female Anopheline Mosquito.

12. What is incubation period or the malaria parasite ?

It varies with different species. In P. vivax, P. ovale and P. falciparum it is 10-40 days, but in P. Malariae it is 18 days to 6 weeks.

Q. 13. What is incubation period ?

It is period between the time of initial infection and the appearance of clinical manifestation.

Q. 14. What is Trophozoite ?

It is the growing stage of Malaria parasite, found inside the R.B.C.

Q. 15. What is Schizonts ?

It is the stage where parasite divides asexually.

Q. 16. What is Gametocyte ?

It is the sexual stage of the parasite.

Q. 17. What is Zygote ?

It is the fertilised female gamete.

Q. 18. What is Sporozoite ?

It is the infective form of the parasite.

Q. 19. What is the parasite of Kala azar ?

L.D. bodies.

Q. 20. Where the organism is found in blood ?

The organism is found in W.B.C.

Q. 21. What are the sources of infection of L.D. ?

Man is the sole source of infection in India. But in China and Mediterranean countries dog is the most important reservior of L.D. infection for man.

Q. 22. What are the modes of transmission of L.D.

Through female sand-fly (Phlebotomus).

Q. 23. How does the L.D. infection take place ?

Infection occurs by crushing the infected fly into the punctured skin wound caused by the bite.

Q. 24. State appearance of the skin in L.D. disease ?

The whole surface of the skin becomes dark, dry and rough with brittle lustreless scanty hair.

Q. 25. What are the parasites of blood ? Name them.

(i) Malarial parasites.
(ii) Microfilaria.
(iii) L.D. bodies.

Q. 26. (a) How will you identify parasite of blood ?

Indentify by Leishmen's Stain:
(i) Malarial parasite in R.B.C. in ring form.
(ii) L.D. bodies in W.B.C. (monocytes) and occasionally in plasma.
(iii) Microfilaria in plasma (Night Sample).

Q. 26. (b) What is Amoeba ? Name the important amoeba which causes disease ? How will you identify it ?

It is a variety of protozoa having pseudopodia e.g. Entemoeba histolytica.

It causes Amoebiasis.

It can be identify by examination of stool (usually Cystic form occasionally Vegetative form is also found.)

Q. 27. What is Helminth ?

Helminths are multicellular animal parasite.

Q. 28. Name some important intestinal Helminths ? How do they injure the host ?

Ascaris lumbricoides. Ancylostoma duodenale, Taenia salium, Taenia, saginata.

They usually injure the host by their presence in large number or size, or by their large production etc.

(a) **A. lumbricoides** : Intestinal lesion (i) obstruction of gut, appendix, common bile duct, (ii) perforation.

(b) **A. duodenale** : Chronic intestinal haemorrhage.

(c) **T. saginata** : Intestinal irritation and obstruction.

Q. 29. What is Metozoa ?

Metozoa is a multicellur organism.

Q. 30. What are Hook worms ? Name them.

The anterior end of the worm is bend like hook, so it is called Hook Wroms.

e.g. Ancylostoma duodenale, Necator americanus etc.

*** Q. 31. How does Hook worms infection occur in man ? How they produce the diseases ?**

When the filariform larvae come in contact with the skin or mucous membrane they perforate the skin or mucous membrane and enter the lymphatic or venous channel. Thus the hook worm infection occurs in man.

They produce anaemia. The causes are:

(i) Sucking the blood by worms.

(ii) Haemorrhage from the wounds by biting the wall of intestine and liberating anticoagulant.

(iii) They produce toxin which inhibit R.B.C. formation.

(iv) Interference with digestion.

Q. 32. What are the Tape worms ? Name them.

Tape like varieties of Helminths are called Tape worms.

They are: T. Solium, T. Saginata, T. Ecchinoccous, Granulosus etc.

Q. 33. How does Tape worm infection occur in man due to different varieties of Tape worms ?

(i) **T. Solium (Pork tape worm)** : In Pork eating persons. Cystasarca enter with under cooked pork.

(ii) **T. Saginata (Beef tape worm)** : In beef eating persons. Cystasarca Bovis enter with under cooked beef.

(iii) **T.E. Granulosus** : (Dog tape worm)-In dog covers enter through oral rout. Produce Hydatid cyst in body.

Q. 34. Which type of Tape worms are more dangerous ?

Taenia Echinococcus Granulosus as it forms hydadit cyst in tissue, but T. Solium are more dangerous than. T. Saginata.

****Q. 35. Defferentiate between T. Saginata and T. Solium.**

		T. Saginata	T. Solium
Length		**5 -10 metres**	**2-3 metres**
Scolex:			
	Shape	Quadrate	Globular
	Size	1-2 m.m.	Pin head
	Suker	Pigmented	Not pigmented
	Rostellum	Absent	Present
	Hooklets	None	Double
	Proglottides	1000-2000	800-900
	Segments	Disposed Singly	In chain of 5 or 6
	Testes	300-400 follicles	150-200 follicles

Ovary	Bilobed	Trilobed
Vaginal Spincter	Present	Absent

Q. 36. What is Cysticercus ?

They are the sack-like oval larvae of T. Saginata or T. Solium seen along the lingitudinal axis of muscles. They are distended with clear or opalescent fluid and the centre there is an opaque slot known as milk stot which present the site of invagination of scolex.

Q. 37. Where are the Cysticercus found ?

Brain, Eyeballs, Subcutaneous tissues, Straiated muscles i.e. anywhere in the body.

Q. 38. What is the danger of Cysticercus ?

They may be clacified and give rise to space occupy in lesions.

Q. 39. What examination would you make for identification of worms ?

Stool (and blood in case of Filaria).

Q. 40. What type of substance of worm will be found in microscope ?

Egg or Ova.

****Q. 41. What is hydatid cyst ?**

It is the cystic larvae of T. Echinoccus Granulosus.

Q. 42. Explain the structure of hydatid cyst.

There may be three layers in the hydatid cyst:

(a) **Pericyst :** It is the fibrous tissue barrier. This separates the larva from the rest of the healthy parts of the organ.

(b) **Ectocyst :** It is the outer circular layer and consists of a laminated hyaline membrane. It looks like the white portion of a boiled egg.

(c) **Endocyst :** It is the inner or germinal layer. It consists of a membrane of nuclei embedded in a protoplasmic mass. It is thin and transparent. This layer secretes the specific hydatid and forms the outer layer.

Q. 43. How hydatid disease can be detected ?

By Casoni' reaction or Allergic skin test.
By blood examination. Serological test, Aspiration of cyst etc.

****Q. 44. What is round worm ? Name it. What damage it does in man ?**

It is an unsegmented long worm with alimentary canal.
Name: Ascaris lumbricoides.
Damages: In 50% of cases no symptoms at all.
In Others :

(i) Mechanical—Irritation of stomach, perforation of stomach or intestine, obstruction of intestine, Appendix, Common bile duct etc.
(ii) Toxic — Convultion, vertigo, itching of nose and anus, dyspepsia.
(iii) Pulmonary—Loffler's syndrome.

****Q. 45. What is Loffler's Syndrome ?**

It is the Eosinophilic Pneumonia.

Q. 46. What is the mode of infection of round worm ?

By ingestion (usually by taking contaminated food or drink containing ova of worm).

Q. 47. Differences between male and female of a Lumbricodies ?

	Male	**Female**
Size	Smaller than female 15-25 cm.	Longer than male 25-40 cm.
Posterior end	Coiled	Tapering
Genital opening.	At the post. End near the anus. Spicules present corresponding to penis.	Valva at the junction. Anterior and middle third, no spicula present.

Papillae	Pre and post-anal multiple	Post anal one pair.

Q. 48. What is microfilaria ? How will you collect blood for its indetification ? What is the vector of filaria ?

It is a snake-like minute larvae of Filariae.

One drop of patient's blood is taken by pricking the finger tip at midnight when patient is asleep, and examined by drop method.

Vector — Culex mosquito.

Q. 49. What is the commonest member of Filaria parasite ?

W. bancrofti in our country.

Q. 50. What is the infective form of the parasite ?

3rd stage Larva.

Q. 51. Where do you get the adult parasite ?

(i) In lymph gland, (ii) In dilated lymph trunks and (iii) In elephantiod tissue.

Q. 52. What is elephantiasis ?

The affected skin is thickened due to hyperplasia and hypertrophy caused by the irritant action of high protein content of tissue fluid.

Q. 53. What form of parasite cause lesion ?

Adults form.

Q. 54. Differences between Male and Female W. bancrofti ?

Male	**Female**
25-30 mm long and 120 broad	80-10 mm long and 230 broad.
Two unequal, refractile Spicules present.	Two uterine tubes run along the length of body, vulva is about 12 mm from anterior extremity.

Q. 55. Name the hosts of W. bancrofti ?

Definitive host is man and intermediate host is a mosquito.

Q. 56. What is viviparous parasite ? Give example.

Viviparous parasites are those which don't lay eggs, but give birth to larva.

Example : All members of Filaria group.

Q. 57. Name the parasites causing macrocytic anaemia ?

(i) Hookworm, (ii) L.D. bodies (raely).

Q. 58. What are the parasites seen in urine ?

(i) Microfilaria, (ii) Byproducts of hydatid cyst, (iii) Eggs of S. haemotobium.

(III) GENERAL PATHOLOGY

****Q. 1. What is inflammation ?**

It is a series of changes that take place in living tissues when it is injured by various noxious agents or irritants provided the injury is not insufficient to cause immediate death of the tissues.

****Q. 2. What are signs of the inflammation ?**

(1) Rubor (redness) (2) Dolor (pain), (3) Calor (heat), (4) Tumour (swelling), (5) Functio laesa (loss of functions).

Q. 3. What are the types of inflammation ?

Types : Acute, Subacute and Chronic.

Q. 4. Name some varieties of acute inflammation ?

Varieties :

(i) Catarrhal, (ii) Membranous, (iii) Phlegmonous, (iv) Allergic, (v) Suppurative, (vi) Plastic, (vii) Serous etc.

Q. 5. What change do occur in blood in inflammation. Name some inflammatory diseases ?

Increased T.C. of W.B.C. Moreover W.B.C., R.B.C. and Plasma come out of the blood vessel and perform useful function in controlling the inflammation.

Initial vasoconstriction, vasodialation, slowing of blood flow, exudation of plasma.

Inflammatory diseases : Tonsilitis, Pneumonia etc.

Q. 6. What are the fate of inflammation ?

(i) Resolution, (ii) Fibrosis, (iii) Necrosis suppruation, Ulceration, Sinus formation, (iv) Generalisation, (v) Chronic inflammation.

****Q. 7. What is Exudated and Transudate ?**

Exudate : It is an inflammatory fluid partly divived from the blood and partly from the tissue as in cases of acute inflammation, like Tonsitis,

Appendicitis etc. Then fluid is rich in protein.

Transudate : It is a non-inflammatory fluid due to passive venous congestion as in cases of cardiac or renal failure.

****Q. 8. Mention differences between Exudate and Transudate.**

Exudate	Transudate
(i) Formed as a result of acute inflammation.	(i) Formed due to inbalance of hydrostatic pressure in intra and extra cellular components.
(ii) Sp. gr. in more than 1080	(ii) Sp. gr. in less than 1080
(iii) Rich in protein 3.4%	(iii) Protein 1%
(iv) Cell count numerous	(iv) Rarely more than 4/cu.ml.
(v) Nature of content albumin, globulin and globulin and fibrinogen.	(v) Only albumin, globulin may be present but never fibrinogen.

Q. 9. What is abscess ?

It is a suppurative inflammation in the solid tissue.

Q. 10. What is pus ?

Pus is a semifluid creamy opaque material produce in consequence of an inflammation associated with progressive polymorpho nuclear emigration and death and liquification of the polymorphs and local tissue.

Q. 11. What is pus cell ?

The dead polymorphs are known as pus cell.

Q. 12. What are the contents of pus ?

(i) Pus cell, (ii) Cell debris, (iii) Liquified necrosed tissue and cell, (v) Bacteria.

Q. 13. What is healing ?

It is a process of replacement of dead tissue by new living tissue.

Q. 14. What are stages of healing ?

(i) Stage of latent period 72 hrs., (ii) Stage of contraction and (iii) Stage of replacement by regeneration and repair.

***Q. 15. What is necrosis ?**

It is a cellular death of the living body in a localised area due to some bacteria, toxin or by chemical and mechanical injury with severe irreversible changes or death of the cells.

Q. 16. What are the various types of necrosis ?

(i) Coagulative, (ii) Colliquative, (iii) Caseous, (iv) Fibrinoid, (v) Liver necrosis, (vi) Muscle necrosis, (vii) Fat necrosis.

Q. 17. What is the fate of necrosis ?

It depends on the cause, the size and the tissue involved.

It may be (i) Absorption and Resolution, (ii) Fibrosis, (iii) Fibrous encapsulative with Central part:

Ossified, Hyalinised, or with Cystic space.

*****Q. 18. What is gangrene ?**

Gangrene is a massive death of tissue, superadded by putrefaction due to action of proteolytic enzymes liberated by saprophytic organisms.

Q. 19. What are the types of gangrene ?

It is two types : (i) Dry gangrene and (ii) Moist gangrene.

Q. 20. What is difference between dry and moist gangrene ?

Dry gangrene : The area is dried up and the colour changes from green to black.

Mosit gangrene: The area is highly offensive and the colour changes from dusky red to olive green to black.

*****Q. 21. What is thrombosis ?**

It is a pathological process by which a solid mass or a thrombus form either intracardiac or intravascular derived from elements of circulating blood during life time.

****Q. 22. What is thrombus ?**

It is an intravscular blood clot form from elements of blood i.e. W.B.C + R.B.C. + Fibrin + Plateletes.

Q. 23. What are the factors which are responsible for thrombosis?

(i) Damage to the vascular endothelium, (ii) Slowing of blood flow, (iii) Change in the constituents of blood, (iv) Inflammation of vessel wall.

Q. 24. What are the types of thrombus ?

(i) **Red thrombus** : When blood is in slow velocity i.e. in veins.
(ii) **Pale thrombus** : When blood is in high velocity i.e. in heart.
(iii) **Mixed thrombus** : When blood is in intermediate velocity i.e. in arteries.

Q. 25. What are the fate of a thrombus ?

(i) Absorption, (ii) Contraction, (iii) Calcification, (iv) Organisation, (v) Hyalinisation, (vi) Canalisation, (vii) Embolism.

****Q. 26. What is embolism ?**

It is a process by which an undisolved material is impacted in the blood vessels which is carried by the blood stream from its point of origin and ultimately lodged into the distal part of the body, causing obstruction to the lumen of blood vessels more or less completey or partially.

****Q. 27. What is embolus ?**

Solid body or air bubble transported in the circulation.

Q. 28. What are the different types of embolus ?

(i) Detached thrombus may be an embolus, (ii) Air embolus, (iii) Fat embolus, (iv) Tumour cell embolus, (v) Bacterial embolus, (vi) Gas embolus, (vii) Amniotic fluid embolus etc.

****Q. 29. What is infarction ? What is infarct ?**

Infarction : It is a process by means of which ischaemic necrosis of a tissue takes place due to the occlusion of end arteries of an organ.

Infarct : It is this ischaemic necrosis part of the tissue occurs due to infarction.

Q. 30. What are the types of infarct ?

It is two types : Pale or anaemic and Red or haemorrhagic.

Q. 31. What are the fate of an infarct ?

(i) Hayalinisation, (ii) Calcification, (iii) Ossification, (iv) Fibrosis and (v) Sepsis.

****Q. 32. What is oedema ?**

It is an abnormal accumulation of fluid in the cells or intercellular tissue spaces or serous cavities of the body due to disturbed water metabolism.

Q. 33. What are the types of oedema ?

(i) **Generalised :** Cardiac.
(ii) **Local :** (a) Pitting on pressure, e.g. inflammatory oedema, venious oedema.
(b) Nonpitting, e.g. lymphatic, angioneurotic, Myxoedema.

****Q. 34. What is degeneration ?**

It is a pathological process by which the cell component as a whole directly affected by the toxic condition or by secondary metabolic causes, accumulating abnormal material either in the cytoplasm or in intercellular ground substance.

Q. 35. What are the types of degenerations ?

(i) Cloudy swelling and hydropic degeneration, (ii) Mucoid degeneration, (iii) Hyaline degeneration, (iv) Fatty degeneration, (v) Amyloid degneration.

Q. 36. What is a tumour ?

It is an independent, uncontrolled, abnormal and autonomous new growth of cells.

Q. 37. What are the types of tumour ?

It has two types — Benign and Malignant.

Q. 38. What is fibroma ?

A Benign tumour composed of fibrous tissue.

Q. 39. What is lipoma ?

A benign tumours composed of adipose tissue.

Q. 40. What is a myoma ?

Benign tumour of muscle cells.

Q. 41. What are the types of myoma ?

It has two types :

(i) **Leimomyoma** : Smooth muscle tumour i.e. Uterus, stomach etc.

(ii) **Rhabdomyoma** : Striated muscle tumour i.e. Heart, skeletal muscle etc.

Q. 42. What is carcinoma ?

It is a malignant tumour of epithelial tissue.

Q. 43. What is sarcoma ? What are the differences between them ?

It is a malignant tumour of connective tissue.

Differences between Carcinoma and Sarcoma

Carcinoma	*Sarcoma*
(i) Origin — Epethelial tissue.	(i) Connective tissue
(ii) Stroma — Surrounds mass of cells.	(ii) Surrounds individual cells.
(iii) Spread — by Lymph.	(iii) By blood vessels.
(iv) Vessels — Contact with the cells.	(iv) Contained in stroma.

Q. 44. Give some examples of carcinoma and sarcoma.

Carcinoma : (i) Epidermoid carcinoma, (ii) Rodent ulcer, (iii) Choroeonic epithelioma.

Sarcoma : (i) Round celled sarcoma, (ii) Lympho-sarcoma, (iii) Lipo sarcoma.

Q. 45. What is cyst ?

It is a sac with membranous wall, enclosing fluid or semisolid matter.

Q. 46. What is immunity ?

Immunity means resistance or non-susceptibility to infection and diseases naturally or artificially acquired.

Q. 47. Mention classification of immunity ?

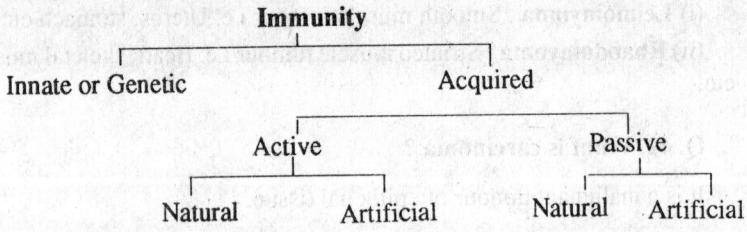

Immunity

- Innate or Genetic
- Acquired
  - Active
    - Natural
    - Artificial
  - Passive
    - Natural
    - Artificial

Q. 48. What is innate immunity ?

It means the inherited resistance power to infèction. e.g. The immunity of horse against tetanus.

Q. 49. What is acquired immunity ?

During the life time the immunity which is acquired by an individual e.g. A second attack of smallpox is rare.

Q. 50. What is active immunity ?

When any body gathers resistant power by the virtue of naturally or artificially during an infectious disease e.g. Vaccination of smallpox.

Q. 51. What is passive immunity ?

When any individual gets the maternal antibodies naturally via the placenta or in the milk or artifically by administering immune sera.

e.g. Anti—Tetanic Serum.
Anti—Diphtheric Serum.

Q. 52. What is artificial immunity ?

When the immunity power gathers artificially by an individual e.g. Vaccin, B.C.G. against tuberculosis.

Q. 53. What are the differences between active and passive immunity ?

	Active	Passive
(i) How achieved :	(i) By participation of defence force.	(i) By burrowing of defence force from outside.
(ii) Types of defence force.	(ii) Cellular and humoral.	(ii) Only humoral
(iii) Duration	(iii) Long	(iii) Short 10-14 days.
(iv) Inheritance of immunity.	(iv) No	(iv) May be from mother.
(v) Reaction on immunisation	(v) Local/Focal and General.	(v) Only general
(vi) Conterring of immunity.	(vi) Latent period present .	(vi) Immediate no latent-period.
(vii) Use	(vii) Mainly prophylactic.	(vii) Therapeutic and prophylactic
(viii) Negative phase	(viii) Presence	(viii) Absence

Q. 54. What is antigen ?

It is an agent which can produce some antibody when introduce in a living tissue.

Q. 55. What is antibody.

It is a protein like substance either in Bacteria, Rekettsia, Virus or certain cells, which when into the host produce a substance known as antibody.

Q. 56. What is B.C.G. Vaccination?

This is a bovine strain vaccine of tubercle bacilli which has been attenuated by series of subcultures. This process has found out by Calmete and Guerin. For this the vaccine in called B.C. G. Vaccine.

Q. 57. What is the use of antigen and antibody ?

It helps in the diagnosis as well as in estimating prognosis of a disease. *Examples :* (a) With known antigen — Widal test, (b) With know antibody no Bordet Durham reaction, (c) Complement fixation test Wasserman reaction etc.

[N.B. In definition of Inflammation read insufficient in place of sufficient. p. 376.]

COUNCIL OF HOMOEOPATHIC MEDICINE, WEST BENGAL

D. H. M. S. - 1987

(JUNE TERM)

Pathology

Full Marks - 100

All Questions carry equal marks.

Answer four Questions (One from each Group).

GROUP - A (Any one)

1. What is gangrene ? How does it differ from necrosis ? Describe the pathogenesis and pathology of gangrene *see P. 235

(4+4+10+7).

2. Define anaemia? Describe the morphological classification of anaemia? What are the typical haematological finding in a case of iron deficiency anaemia. *see P. 289 (4 + 12 + 9)

GROUP - B (any one)

3. Write in short, the pathogenesis of different types of ulcers in stomach. What are the complication of peptic ulcer ?

* consult Text Book of Pract. of Medicine.

(16 + 9)

4. (a) Write down the differences near, by naked eye and microscopically, in facing from faces of amoebic dysentery and bacillery dysentery.

*see P. 136

(b) Give the urinary, findings in cases of acute glomerulonephritis, nephrotic syndrome and chronic glomeralo-nephritis.

* consult Text Book of Pract, of Medicine.

GROUP - C (any one)

5. Name the Micro-organism responsible for diarrhoea and dysentery. How cholera outbreaks are diagnosed in laboratory?

*see P. 105

6. What are the different types of mycobacteria? Write the diseases produced by them. How mycobacteria tuberculosis is cultured in laboratory ? * 85 (10 + 10 + 5)

GROUP - D (any one)

7. What are the different types of malarial parasites effecting man. Give the life cycle of plasmodium vivax? How malaria fever can be diagnosed in laboratory ? (5+10+10)

* see P. 145

8. Describe the morphology of Ankylostoma. Give the life cycle. Write down the pathogonic effects caused by adult worm. (7 + 10 + 8)

* see P. 180

D. H. M. S. - 1988

Pathology, Bacteriology, Parasitology

Full Marks: 100

Answer four Questions one from each group.

All Questions carry equal marks.

GROUP - A

1. What is inflammation ? Describe the mechanism of formation of inflammatory exudate and its formation in inflamation. How an exudate differ from transudate. * See P. - 216.

2. Define Jaundice, what are the different types of Jaundices and how they can be differentiated. Describe the biochemical change in urine and blood in obstructed Jaundice. * see P. 282

(6+9+10)

3. Define Leukaemia, How leukaemia can be classified ? Describe the peripheral blood picture of chronic myeloid leukomia.

* see Text Book of Pract. of Medicine.

(4+6+15)

GROUP B

1. Classify malignant tumours of the lung. Describe the macroscopic and microscopic picture of a common variety of careinoma lung, labelled diagram. * see Special Pathology (10+ 15)

2. Describe the Aetiopathogenesis and pathology of Acute glomerulo nephritis. What changes are found in urine in different types of glomerulo-nephritis. * See Speical Pathology. (15+10)

3. Describe the actiology of gastric ulcer. How a chronic gastric ulcer can be differentiated from a malignant ulcer? How gastric juice analysis can help in diagnosis of different gastric lesions. * see Special Pathology (6+4+15)

GROUP - C

1. Enumerate the Organism responsible for a tonsilar patch. Describe the methods of laboratory procedure for their diagnosis. * see P.65 (9 + 16)

2. What are the Organisms responsible for food poisoning. Describe this laboratory diognosis of a care of food poisoning. * see P. 97+50 (7+8)

GROUP - D

1. Enumerate the species of malaria parasite which may infect man. Describe diagram of erythrocytic phase of malignant tertion malaries. Describe the clinical types of malignant.

   * see P.146 (5+10+10)

2. What are nematodes? How can they be differentiated from cestodes? Describe the life cycle of any one of the intestinal nematodes. * see P. 159 (5+10+10)

D. M. S. - 1989

Pathology

Answer any two Questions from each group.

Full Marks: 100

GROUP - 1

1. Fill in the blanks:

(a) Neutrophilic infiltration is found in ...(Acute) inflammation.

(b) Gangrene is necrosis with ... (Putrifraction)

(c) Hyperplasia mean increase in ...and size of cells. (Number of cell)

(d) Increase ...time is found in idiopathic thrombocytopenic purpura.

(e) Carcinoma is the ... tumour of ... tissue (Malignant), (Epthelial)

(f) Deficiency of vitamin ...leads to night blindness (Vit. A.)

(g) ...type of necrosis in found in brain. (Colliquative)

(h) Nutmeg liver is found in...congestive cardiae failure.

(i) Engulfment of bacteria by neutrophil is called...phagoagtosis.

(j) Oedema is the accumulation of...in extracelluler space of body. (fluid)

(k) Cloudy swelling is a type of ...(Albuminous degeneration)

(l) Megaloblastic anaemia occurs due to deficiency of vitamin ...(B12 or Folic acid).

(m) Abscess is the collection of .... in living tissue.

2. What is necrosis? How can it be differentiated from degareration? Mention the different types of necrosis. Describe the microscopic picture of a tubercle with caseation. * see P. 232 (5+5+5+10)

3. Define anaemia. How can it be classified ? Describe the laboratory diagnosis of a case of haemolytic anaemia.

* see P. 289 (5+20)

4. What is tumour? How benign tumour differs from malignant tumour? Describe the rates of metastasis of a malignant tumour.

* see P. 266 (5+10+10)

5. Describe the aetiological factor in the genesis of atherosclerosis. Mention the common sites of atherclerosis and its complication. * consult Text Book of Pract. of Medicine.

(15 + 10)

6. What is shock? How can it be classified. Describe the mechanism of formation of irreverhible shock. * consult Text Book of Pact. of Medicine. 25

GROUP - 2

7. Describe the morphological feature of C. Diphtheriae. Describe the laboratory diagnosis of a suspected care of diphtheria.
* see P. 64 (10+15)

8. What is sterilisation? Describe the different methods of sterilisation in laboratory. * consult Text Book of Pathology (5+20)

9. Mention the causative organism of typhoid fever. Describe how will you proceed for laboratory diognosis of a case of typhoid fever.
* see P. 97

10. What is streptococcus ? Give the classification of strepto coccus. Describe the toxic and enzymes of streptococcus pyogenes and lesions produced in man. * see P. 51 (5+10+10)

11. Enumerate the clostridia pathogenic to man, and the pathogenic lesions produced in man. Describe the laboratory diagnosis of a case of gangrene. * see P. 77 (5+10+10)

12. Write short notes on:
(a) Schick's test (P.-71)
(b) Bacterial capsule (P.-30)
(c) Active immunity (P.-293)
(d) Bacteriophase (P. -118)
(e) Schizont(P.-147)

(5 x 5)

University of Calcutta

B.H.M.S. (F)-Pathology

1985 Pathology

Group - A

Answer four Questions, of which question No. 1 is compulsory.

1. Pick up the correct answers (Bold is Correct) :- 20x1

(a) Keytone bodies may be present in urine in dibetes mellitus/starvation/ **both**.

(b) Low sugar in C.S.F. is usual in pyogenic tubercular/**viral maningitis**.

(c) E.S.R is low in **polycythemia**/leukaomia/both.

(d) Lymphocytosis occurs in chronic lymphatic leukaemia/whooping cough/**both**.

(e) Haematuria is best detected by **physical**/chemical/microscopical examination of urine.

(f) Langhan's type of giant cells are found in **tuberculosis**/non-specific inflammation both.

(g) Abscess contains pus cells, neocrotic tissue/**both**.

(h) Acute inflammation usually shows presence of **neutrophils**/lymphecytes/monocytes.

(i) Platelet aggregation is important in **thrombosis**/blood clot/both.

(j) Metastasis is seen in **malignant**/being neoplasm/both.

(k) Aschoff's giant cell is found in **rheumatic endocarditis**/infective endocarditis/both.

(i) Typhoid ulcer in intestine occurs in **pyer's patches**/in between pyer's patches/both.

(m) Lobar pneumonia shows massive **consolidation**/patchy consolidation/cavitation of lung.

(n) Chronic nephritis results in **small**/large/normal kidney.

(o) L.D. body is found in **Kala-azar**/malaria/filariasis.

(p) Microfilria is found in RBC/leukocytes/**extracelularly**.

Group - B

Answer any one question.

9. "Homoeopaths treat the patients not the disease"- If this is ture-Justify that knowledge of pathology is essential for a homoeopath.
See P. 5 20

10. "Hahnemannian homoeopaths must read pathology seriously" - Discuss. see P. 10 20

11. Enumerate the importance of pathological study (clinical) during the treatment of patients homoeopthically.

see P. 13

B.H.M.S. (F-1)-Pathology

1986 Pathology

Group-A

Full Marks-80

Answer four Questions, of which Question .1 is compulsory

1. Pick up th correct answers: 1x20

(a) Corynebacterium diphtheriae is demonstrated by Gram's Stain/Albert's Stain/Ziehl-Neelsenstain.

(b) Blood agar medium is enriched/indicator/both.

(c) Coagulase is produced mainly by Streptococcus.

(d) Pathogenicity of Clostridiam tetani is due to Exotoxin/Endotoxin/inflammation.

(e) Mycobacterium tuberculosis is grown in Nutrient agar/Blood agar/Lowenstain-Jensen medium.

(f) Benign tertain malaria is caused by Plasmodium vivax/Plasmodium falcimparum,/Plasmodium malarial.

(g) Microfilaria is seen within R.B.C./W.B.C./in between cells.

(h) Severe anaemia is a feature of hookworm disease/roundnorm infection/threadworm infection.

(i) Infected pork may cause infection by Taenia Solium/Taenia Saginata/ Taenia echinococcus.

(j) Stool of acute amoebic dysentery shows presence of cystic stage/ trophozoite stage/both stages of Entamoeba histolytica.

(k) Leukaemia is a neoplastic state of crythrocyte precursors/leucocyte precurors/both.

(l) Anaemia may affect haemoglobin level/total erytherocyte count/ both.

(m) Low platelet count is associated with anaemia/purpura/haemophilia.

(n) Massive albuminuria is characteristic of nephrotic syndrome/acute glomerulonephritis/chronic nephritis.

(o) Haematuria is detected by presence of RBC in Urine/Occult blood test of urine/both.

(p) Mitral stennosis is associated with normal/hypertrophied/atrophied left venrgicle.

(q) Athenoma affects the medial coast/adventilial coat/intimal coat of arteries.

(r) Adenocarcinoma is a malignent condition of glandular epithelium/ squamous epithelium/nural tissue.

(s) Caseation necrosis is found in tubercular lesion/phyogenic inflammation/psendomembranous inflammation.

(t) Typhoid ulcer is found in small intestine/large intestine/both.

2. Write short notes on any four of the following: 12

(a) M.C.H. C - 355 (b) Leucopenia-350 (c) Chyluria: (d) Microcytic anaemia (207) (e) Rothera's test (339)

3. Write short notes on any four of the following:- 5x4

(a) Bacterial capsule (30)
(b) Toxiod (79)
(c) Active Immunity (293)
(d) Koch's postulates - (28)
(e) Macconkey's Medium (37)

4. Write short notes on any four of the following: 5x4

(a) Farty liver;
(b) Hypernephroma;
(c) Lobar pneumonia; inflammation.
(d) Granular contracted Kidney;
(e) Pseudomembranous

5. Define thrombosis. Describe the stages of thrombus formation and its fates. see P. 247 5+10+5

6. Describe the steps of laboratory diagnosis of case of pulmonary tuberculosis. What is Koch's phenomenon? see P. 87 15+5

7. Name the parasites causing hookworm disease. Describe the pathology and laboratory diagnosis of hookworm disease.
see P. 190

8. What is neophlasm? How a malignant neoplasm differs from a benign one? What are the common routes of metastasis of a malignant neoplasm? see P. 266 5+10+5

Group - B

Full Marks - 20

Answer any one questions.

9. "Homoeopaths treat the patient not the disease"— Justify the place of pathology if the above statement is true. see P. 5

10. Why homoeopath should know pathology? Discuss. 20
see P.11.

11. Discuss in detail the scope of pathology and microbiology in homoeopathic medicine. see P. 13

H.M.S. (P.1) Sub-Pathology

1986 Pathology

Group - A.

Answer any four questions, of which question 10 is compulsory.

1. Pick up the correct answer (Bold is correct) answers:

(a) Granular Contracted kidney may result from chronic nephritis/prolonged benign hypertension/**both**.

(b) Fibroscacoma is a malignant neoplasm of **connective tissue**/glandular epithelium/squamous epithelium.

(c) Liver usually shows nodular appearance in falty change/neoplastic condition/**cirrhosis**.

(d) Bronchopneumonia is associated with massive **consolidation**/of lung.

(e) Aortic incompetence results in normal/hypertrophied left ventricle.

(f) Coagulation time is normal/**increased**/below normal in haemophilia.

(g) E.S.R. if normal/low/**high** in tuberculosis.

(h) Immature leucocytes are common in eosinophilia/**leukaemia**/anaemia.

(i) Ketone bodies may appear in urine in prolonged strvation/Diabetes mellitus/**both**.

(j) Turbid C.S.F. is a feature of **phypogenic meningitis**/tubercular meningitis/viral meningitis.

(k) Kala-azar is transmitted by mosquite/**sandfly**/ticks.

(i) Hydatid cyst is the **larval stage**/adult stage/host tissue reaction of Taenia echinococcus.

(m) Peripheral blood in filariasis shows adult Filaria/**microfilaria**/none of the parasite.

(n) Infective form of Entamoeba histolytica is the **cystic stage**/trophozoite stage/precystic stage.

(o) Infective from of hookworm is ova/**filariform larva**.

(p) Lowenstein-jensen medium is selective for **Mycobacterium tuberculosis**/Neisseria/Corynobacterium.

(q) Widal test helps in the diagnosis of **enteric fever**/U.T.I/ typhus fever.

(r) Pathogenic streptococcus is a haemolytic/a haemolytic/both

(s) Exotoxin is produced by **Corynebacterium diphtheriae**/vivrio cholerae/both.

(t) Clostridum tetani is **aerobe**/annerobe/microaecrophilic.

2. Write short notes on any four of the following: 5 x 4

(a) Occult blood test.
(b) Giant cells (231)
(c) Haematuria.
(d) Megaloblastic anaemia.
(e) Eosinophilia. (351)

3. Write short notes on any four of the following: 5 x 4

(a) Bacterial Flagella (30)
(b) Gram stain (37)
(c) Cell mediated immunity (293)
(d) Enriched media (35)
(e) Cloudy swelling(261)

4. Write short notes on any four of the following: 5 x 4

(a) Large white Kidney.
(b) Mitral stenosis.
(c) Caseation necrosis. (234)
(d) Hypertrophy.
(e) Fat necrosis. (235)

5. What is Oedema? Write briefly about the common causes and pathology of oedema. (p. 242) 5+7+8

6. Classify streptococcus. Enumerate the lesions produced by various species of streptococcus. Why suppurative lesions of streptococcal origin are spreading? (P. 50) 8+8+4

7. Describe the mode of infection and life cycle of Plasmodium vivax. How benign tertian malaria differs from malignant tertian malaria? What changes occur in the R.B.C in benign tertian malaria? 10+4+6